Database Annotation in
Molecular Biology

Database Annotation in Molecular Biology

EDITOR

Arthur M. Lesk

Department of Biochemistry and Molecular Biology
The Pennsylvania State University
University Park, PA 16802, USA

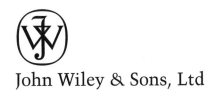

John Wiley & Sons, Ltd

Other Wiley Editorial Offices

John Wiley & Sons Inc., 111 River Street, Hoboken, NJ 07030, USA

Jossey-Bass, 989 Market Street, San Francisco, CA 94103-1741, USA

Wiley-VCH Verlag GmbH, Boschstr. 12, D-69469 Weinheim, Germany

John Wiley & Sons Australia Ltd, 33 Park Road, Milton, Queensland 4064, Australia

John Wiley & Sons (Asia) Pte Ltd, 2 Clementi Loop #02-01, Jin Xing Distripark, Singapore 129809

John Wiley & Sons Canada Ltd, 22 Worcester Road, Etobicoke, Ontario, Canada M9W 1L1

Wiley also publishes its books in a variety of electronic formats. Some content that appears in
print may not be available in electronic books.

British Library Cataloguing in Publication Data

A catalogue record for this book is available from the British Library

ISBN 0-470-85681-5

Typeset in 10.5/13pt Times by Thomson Press (India) Limited, New Delhi
Printed and bound in Great Britain by TJ International Ltd., Padstow, Cornwall
This book is printed on acid-free paper responsibly manufactured from sustainable forestry
in which at least two trees are planted for each one used for paper production.

Contents

9   Issues in the Annotation of Protein Structures   149
G. J. Swaminathan, J. Tate, R. Newman, A. Hussain, J. Ionides, K. Henrick and S. Velankar

10   Classification of Protein Function   167
A. M. Lesk, H. Parkinson and J. C. Whisstock

III   DATABASE DESIGN AND INTEGRATION

11   Information Flow and Data Integration of Databanks   187
C. H. Wu and W. C. Barker

Preface

Two factors dominate current developments in molecular biology, especially in genomics and related fields:

1. the amount of raw data is increasing, very very rapidly, and

2. successful application of the data to biomedical research requires carefully and continuously curated and accurately annotated databanks.

Annotation is currently a challenging, arguably the limiting, component of the whole enterprise. The quality of many of the experimental data – notably the nucleic acid sequences – is very satisfactory. However, much of the annotation depends on features *inferred* from the data rather than directly measured: for instance, the identification of genes in genome sequences. For people interested in analysing the protein sequences implicit in genome sequence information, errors in gene identification or functional assignment tend to vitiate the high quality of the data themselves.

A second major stream of data generation is structural and functional genomics. X-ray crystallography and NMR spectroscopy are copiously generating many new structures. However, without direct experimental evidence there is considerable difficulty in assigning function to proteins even if their amino-acid sequences and three-dimensional structures are known, and even if they are homologous to well-characterized proteins. This is because of the phenomenon of recruitment of proteins for divergent functions. Furthermore, correct classification of proteins often requires sensitivity to very delicate nuances of structure, and it requires great expertise to do this correctly. Computer programs can support and assist, but cannot do the whole job reliably. Proteomics – data on the space and time distribution of protein expression patterns, and networks of protein–protein interactions – are a third datastream.

With the recognition of the importance of accurate database annotation and the requirement for individuals with particular constellations of skills to carry it out, annotators are emerging as a specialized set of experts within the bioinformatics profession. This suggests that it would be a service to the field to collect information about annotation – its current status, what is required to improve it, and what skills must be brought to bear on database curation and hence what is the proper training for annotators.

These were the goals of a European Science Foundation training course in Functional Genomics: Curation of Databases in Molecular Biology, which took place in Paris on 11–14 October 2002, hosted by CODATA – The Committee on Data of the International Council of Scientific Unions. A. Lesk was the primary organizer, with M. Helmer-Citterich and J. Garnier. Speakers included experts in annotation from leading databases in molecular biology. The students were preparing for careers in bioinformatics, and many of them were themselves involved in database development.

The potential audience for this book is people working in the field of bioinformatics, including those carrying out research and those training students. All molecular biologists, geneticists, clinicians and drug developers now use the databanks and would find the information useful, in order to maintain appropriate reservations rather than blindly trusting the databanks on which their work depends. Some computer scientists would find it interesting to discover problems that they might be able to help solve. The book is suitable for all people at the advanced undergraduate level and higher.

I thank the European Science Foundation and CODATA for supporting the training course, K. Cass for the hospitality of the CODATA Secretariat and L. J. Kunes for expert help in preparing the manuscript.

Arthur M. Lesk

List of Contributors

Rolf Apweiler   The European Bioinformatics Institute, EMBL Cambridge Outstation, Wellcome Trust Genome Campus, Cambridge CB10 1SD, UK

Winona C. Barker   National Biomedical Research Foundation, 3900 Reservoir Road NW, Box 571414, Washington, D.C. 20057-1414, USA

Frances C. Bernstein   Bernstein + Sons, 5 Brewster Lane, Bellport, NY 11713-2803, USA

Herbert J. Bernstein   Dowling College, Kramer Science Center, Rudolph Campus, Idle Hour Blvd., Oakdale, NY 11769, USA

Philippe Bessières   INRA, Unité MIG (Mathématique, Informatique et Génome), Bat. 233, Domaine de Vilvert, 78352 Jouy en Josas Cedex, France

Harry Boutselakis   The European Bioinformatics Institute, EMBL Cambridge Outstation, Wellcome Trust Genome Campus, Cambridge CB10 1SD, UK

Hélène Chiapello   INRA, Unité MIG (Mathématique, Informatique et Génome), Bat. 233, Domaine de Vilvert, 78352 Jouy en Josas Cedex, France

Dimitri Dimitropoulos   The European Bioinformatics Institute, EMBL Cambridge Outstation, Wellcome Trust Genome Campus, Cambridge CB10 1SD, UK

Maria Garcia-Pastor   The European Bioinformatics Institute, EMBL Cambridge Outstation, Wellcome Trust Genome Campus, Cambridge CB10 1SD, UK

Jean Garnier   INRA, Unité MIG (Mathématique, Informatique et Génome), Bat. 233, Domaine de Vilvert, 78352 Jouy en Josas Cedex, France

Jean-François Gibrat   INRA, Unité MIG (Mathématique, Informatique et Génome), Bat. 233, Domaine de Vilvert, 78352 Jouy en Josas Cedex, France

Kim Henrick   EMBL Outstation, The European Bioinformatics Institute, Wellcome Trust Genome Campus, Hinxton, Cambridge CB10 1SD, UK

Mark Hoebeke   INRA, Unité MIG (Mathématique, Informatique et Génome), Bat. 233, Domaine de Vilvert, 78352 Jouy en Josas Cedex, France

Ayzaz Hussain   The European Bioinformatics Institute, EMBL Cambridge Outstation, Wellcome Trust Genome Campus, Cambridge CB10 1SD, UK

John Ionides   The European Bioinformatics Institute, EMBL Cambridge Outstation, Wellcome Trust Genome Campus, Cambridge CB10 1SD, UK

Melford John   The European Bioinformatics Institute, EMBL Cambridge Outstation, Wellcome Trust Genome Campus, Cambridge CB10 1SD, UK

Peter A. Keller   The European Bioinformatics Institute, EMBL Cambridge Outstation, Wellcome Trust Genome Campus, Cambridge CB10 1SD, UK

Graham J. L. Kemp   Department of Computing Science, Chalmers University of Technology, 41296 Göteborg, Sweden

Micah I. Krichevsky   Bionomics International, 3023 Kramer Street, Wheaton, MD 20902, USA

Arthur M. Lesk   Department of Biochemistry and Molecular Biology, The Pennsylvania State University, 512 Wartik Laboratory, University Park, PA 16802, USA

Michèle Magrane   The European Bioinformatics Institute, EMBL Cambridge Outstation, Wellcome Trust Genome Campus, Cambridge CB10 1SD, UK

Phil McNeil   The European Bioinformatics Institute, EMBL Cambridge Outstation, Wellcome Trust Genome Campus, Cambridge CB10 1SD, UK

Gertrud Mannhaupt   Department of Genome Oriented Bioinformatics, Technical University of Munich, Wissenschaftszentrum Weihenstephan, 85350 Freising–Weihenstephan, Germany

Klaus Mayer   MIPS at GSF, Research Center for Environment and Health, Ingostädter Landstr. 1, 85758 Neuherberg, Germany

Nicola Mulder   The European Bioinformatics Institute, EMBL Cambridge Outstation, Wellcome Trust Genome Campus, Cambridge CB10 1SD, UK

Richard Newman   The European Bioinformatics Institute, EMBL Cambridge Outstation, Wellcome Trust Genome Campus, Cambridge CB10 1SD, UK

Helen Parkinson   Microarray Informatics Team, The European Bioinformatics Institute, EMBL Cambridge Outstation, Wellcome Trust Genome Campus, Cambridge CB10 1SD, UK

Jorge Pineda   The European Bioinformatics Institute, EMBL Cambridge Outstation, Wellcome Trust Genome Campus, Cambridge CB10 1SD, UK

Manuela Pruess   The European Bioinformatics Institute, EMBL Cambridge Outstation, Wellcome Trust Genome Campus, Cambridge CB10 1SD, UK

Antonio Suarez-Uruena   The European Bioinformatics Institute, EMBL Cambridge Outstation, Wellcome Trust Genome Campus, Cambridge CB10 1SD, UK

Jawahar Swaminathan   The European Bioinformatics Institute, EMBL Cambridge Outstation, Wellcome Trust Genome Campus, Cambridge CB10 1SD, UK

John Tate   The European Bioinformatics Institute, EMBL Cambridge Outstation, Wellcome Trust Genome Campus, Cambridge CB10 1SD, UK

Sameer Velankar   The European Bioinformatics Institute, EMBL Cambridge Outstation, Wellcome Trust Genome Campus, Cambridge CB10 1SD, UK

James C. Whisstock   Department of Biochemistry and Molecular Biology, Victorian Bioinformatics Consortium, Monash University, Clayton Campus, Melbourne, Victoria 3168, Australia

Cathy H. Wu   Georgetown University Medical Center, 3900 Reservoir Road NW, Box 571455, Washington, D.C. 20057-1455, USA

1 Annotation and Databases: Status and Prospects

M. Hoebeke, H. Chiapello, J.-F. Gibrat, Ph. Bessières and J. Garnier

Abstract

The newly developed techniques of automated genome sequencing generate a huge amount of data that need to be securely stored, properly analysed and made easily accessible to biologists. A major challenge is the annotation of the sequences, that is, to be able to deduce from the nucleic acid sequence its biological features at all intermediate levels: molecular and cellular processes, tissues, organs, physiological processes. We first review and describe the problems related to the methods and tools in the hands of annotators to perform their task. The rest of the chapter is devoted to the computer aspect of biological databases. It first addresses the management of the biological information and the design of databases, then access by the biologist to the biological data and the problems it generates: web interfaces, automated access facilities and virtual integration of multiple databases.

Keywords

software, bioinformatics, genomics, user interfaces, web services, ontologies data management, data integration, database, annotation

1.1 Introduction

The communication of data is a requirement for the advancement of knowledge. When the data become abundant or/and worth preserving, they have to be collected, structured and recorded on a permanent device – in the past on stone, then on paper

Database Annotation in Molecular Biology   Edited by Arthur M. Lesk
© 2005 John Wiley & Sons, Ltd.   ISBN: 0-470-85681-5

and in our days as digital data on computer disks. Thanks to the astonishing development of computer technologies, biologists are seeing some hope of being able to better handle and understand the biological data, and fortunately computer scientists are giving more and more attention to their interest.

In a collection of data, each data item is labelled at least by an identifier and is usually complemented by annotations as free text or/and as codified information, including for example the names of the authors responsible for the data item, the date of deposition of the data and any information considered useful for the users. Under the general term of collection, a distinction is made between databanks, in which the data are contained in a series of flat files such as Genbank or the Protein Data Bank (PDB), and databases, in which the data are organized as relations or objects. In our prospects we shall mainly deal with databases. We shall also distinguish primary collections of data that contain a minimum of annotations given by the authors who submit the data (typically the PDB) and secondary collections of data that are derived from the primary collections by other research groups. These secondary collections contain more functionality and eventually wider biological information. Primary collections of data are also named archival databanks or databases. The International Council for Science (ICSU) has recently recommended a free access to the public of the primary collections of data (Garnier and Berendsen, 2002). The difference between primary (archival) and secondary (derived) collections of data is nevertheless not always obvious. There is also the distinction to be made between general or generic databases, for instance Genbank or Swissprot, dealing with all nucleic or amino-acid sequences, and specialized or specific databases such as the database of immunoglobin sequences. More definitions about databases will be given below.

The annotations become a challenge in biology considering the size and complexity of the biological information. There are two main sources of annotations: those given by the authors of the data themselves from their published experimental results and those that we name annotation (singular) that are obtained by an annotator or a group of annotators by a manual and computer analysis of the raw data (typically a genome sequence) with various informatics tools extracting biological information from other collections of data, or inferring these information from data of similar properties stored in other collections. Only this second source of annotation will be discussed in this chapter because of the generalization of this process in the future (see below). More recently annotation tends to include an automatic search and analysis of published experimental data (data mining, information extraction). Automatic management of annotation raises many problems that are analysed in the following sections. A more general problem concerns the inference of a biological function based on the principle of a common ancestor (homology). Annotations based on inferences need to be confirmed by experiments.

As the biological databases undergo a very rapid growth, two major consequences are emerging. First, an efficient utilization of database systems programs to provide easy management and access to these data is continuously developing, including better interfacing between servers to achieve a virtual integration of multiple databases. A second consequence is a necessary formalization of biological concepts and of the relationships among these concepts (via for example the creation of ontologies).

1.2 Annotation of Genomic Data

The ultimate goal of the annotator is to deduce from the genome of an organism all its biological features, exploring and describing all intermediate levels: molecular and cellular processes, tissues, organs, physiological processes etc. Annotation is thus a complex process that requires, besides the raw sequencing data, the integration of much additional information: the results of bioinformatic analysis tools, data extracted from generic or specific databases, biological knowledge accumulated in the literature over the years and data from genome-wide experiments such as transcriptomics or proteomics experiments (Figure 1.1).

This constitutes a huge mass of heterogeneous data that needs to be stored. Annotators must be able, readily, to retrieve and consult these data. Therefore databases and man–machine interfaces are of prime importance in genome annotations.

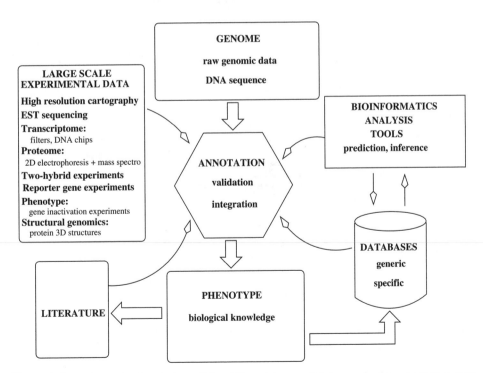

Figure 1.1   Schematic description of the different types of data required to annotate a new genome and their interactions

The efficiency and quality of the annotation of genomic data is a problem that is central to molecular biology, as one witnesses an ever widening gap between the gene products that have been studied experimentally (about a few tens of thousands) and the hundreds of thousands that come from genomic projects (as of January 2003 there are 106 prokaryotic and 17 eukaryotic genomes that have been published and 350 prokaryotic and 235 eukaryotic ongoing genome sequencing projects).[1]

Figure 1.2 presents the various stages of a genome annotation and the role played in this process by the knowledge of other genomes and data produced by genome-wide experiments.

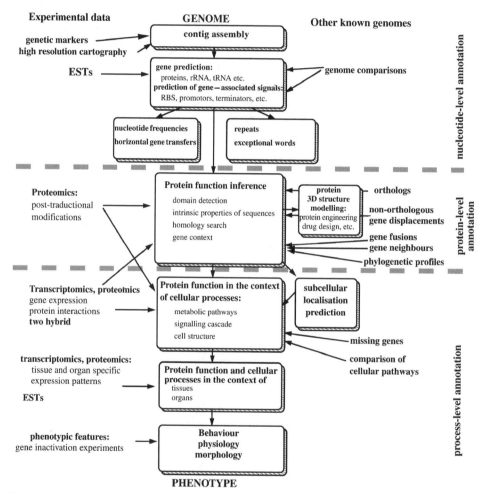

Figure 1.2   Schematic description of a typical annotation process together with the different types of additional information from genome-wide experiments on the left and the knowledge of other genomes on the right

[1]http://wit.integratedgenomics.com/GOLD

Broadly speaking the annotation process can be divided into three levels: nucleic sequence-level annotation, protein-level annotation and process-level annotation (Stein, 2001). This third level is the more challenging for actual annotation methods and requires the integration of various external data such as high-throughput experiments and data from other sequenced genomes.

Nucleic sequence annotation

After assembling the contigs to obtain the chromosomes (a task that can be facilitated by the prior knowledge of genetic markers or the availability of a physical map) the first step is to detect the genes and associated signals: ribosome binding sites (RBSs), promoters, terminators etc. Detection of genes by bioinformatics tools such as hidden Markov models (HMMs) or homology-based methods can be effectively supplemented by the knowledge of expressed sequence tags (ESTs), particularly for eukaryotes. Genome comparison can help to confirm the existence of genes or, if a close family of organisms is used, to detect regulatory regions.

Other analyses on the assembled genome can be carried out, such as overall nucleotide frequencies, identification of repeats or detection of exceptional words (that is, words that are significantly under- or over-represented in the genome and thus might have a biological role).

It is also possible to study gene transfers using either HMM methods or the identification of regions where the nucleotide frequencies differ significantly from the general use of these nucleotides made by the organism under scrutiny.

Protein sequence analysis

The second step of the genome analysis is to assign a function to the largest possible fraction of the gene products by sequence comparison to genes of known function. For coding sequences the sequence comparison is most accurately done on the amino-acid sequences from the six possible reading frames of the nucleotide sequence. Two problems must be mentioned. First, many proteins are comprised of several functional domains. Functional domains, rather than protein sequences, are the proper level at which genomes should be annotated, although the specific function of the associated domain entity has to be considered. Second, the function of a protein is usually best defined by a hierarchical approach: molecular function, cellular function, physiological function (Bork *et al.*, 1998). It is worth noticing that as one goes from the molecular to the physiological levels the function becomes more context dependent.

Three kinds of bioinformatics methods can be used to obtain information about the function of proteins. These methods are discussed in the next sections.

Methods based on intrinsic properties of the sequences

These methods are based on an analysis of sequence properties. They usually do not provide very specific information regarding the protein function. For instance, the detection of stretches of hydrophobic residues, likely to be transmembrane residues, indicates that the protein studied is a membrane protein (Krogh *et al.*, 2001). Other regions with a peculiar amino-acid composition include low complexity regions (Wootton and Federhen, 1996), for which little is known concerning their functional role, or heptad repeats of coiled-coil regions that are involved in oligomerization (Lupas, Van Dyke and Stock, 1991). From a more structural viewpoint it is useful to detect the presence of repeats in the sequence or to predict the secondary structure of the protein.

The principal use of these methods, in conjunction with domain detection methods, is to divide the protein sequence into regions that have distinct amino-acid compositions. Many regions having a biased amino-acid composition, such as low complexity regions, must be masked before applying homology search techniques.

Homology search methods

This type of method constitutes the 'work-horse' of annotation tools. They are the ones, up to now, that have provided the most detailed information about protein functions. They rely on the properties that homologous proteins show a tendency to keep similar functions. Of course this process relies on the existence of databases of carefully annotated protein sequences such as SWISSPROT (Boeckmann *et al.*, 2003) or PIR (Vinayaka *et al.*, 2002).

There are several ways of inferring a homology relationship between two proteins. The most straightforward one is to detect a significant similarity at the level of the amino-acid sequences. Methods based on this principle, such as BLAST (Altschul *et al.*, 1990), are well known and widely used by biologists. Recently, more sensitive methods based on multiple sequence alignments instead of pair sequence comparisons, such as PSI-BLAST (Altschul *et al.*, 1997) (an extension of BLAST) or methods based on HMMs have been developed. It has been shown that, on average, these methods, for the same error rate, are two to three times as sensitive as pair sequence methods (Park *et al.*, 1998).

To detect remote homologues, whose sequences have diverged beyond the point where the homology can be recognized by the simpler sequence comparison methods, new techniques, called fold recognition methods, have been developed over the past 10 years (Marin *et al.*, 2002). These are based on the fact that the core of the 3D structure of homologous proteins is extremely well conserved. Instead of aligning the sequence of the unknown protein with a database of annotated sequences, they align this sequence onto a database of known 3D *structures*. If the sequence is compatible with a family of folds it may then be possible to infer its function from the known functions of the family of folds.

Methods based on gene context

With the availability of a number of completely sequenced genomes it has become possible to obtain information about the function of proteins by studying the co-localization of genes on different genomes (Aravind, 2000).

Unlike homology search techniques that often provide information about protein molecular functions, methods based on gene context principally provide information about the interactions between proteins such that the ones occurring in various cellular processes. These techniques therefore make the transition between the protein-level annotation and the process-level annotation.

Interactions between proteins can be more or less direct. The most specific form of contextual information concerns gene fusions. If two genes that are known to exist independently in a number of organisms are fused in some others this is indicative of a tight interaction, for instance two enzymes catalysing adjacent reactions of a given biochemical pathway or two chains belonging to the same oligomeric structure. A less direct association between genes is measured by gene neighbourhood (Overbeek *et al.*, 1999). It is known that genes that are functionally co-regulated tend to be close in the genome.[2] For instance, the conservation, in several genomes, of the order of a group of genes along the genomes can be a good indication of functional interactions between these genes. The presence of an uncharacterized gene in the neighbourhood of known genes can provide some information relative to its function.

The 'weakest' form of association between genes is detected with the help of phylogenetic profiles, i.e. the pattern of orthologues in different genomes (Pellegrini *et al.*, 1999). This technique is based on the observation that orthologues involved in a particular cellular pathway are either all present if the organism exhibits this pathway or all absent if the organism does not. If an uncharacterized protein shows a pattern similar to other proteins that are known to be involved in a particular cellular pathway, this indicates that this unknown gene might be involved in the same pathway.

Process-level annotation

This is the most challenging level. After having predicted the function of as many gene products as possible, assigned their interactions and possibly analysed their expression levels, it is now necessary to put everything together in the context of cellular processes as a first step, and then in the broader context of tissues, organs etc.

To fulfil this goal, in addition to bioinformatics tools, annotators rely heavily on high-throughput experiments such as micro-array or DNA chip expression analysis, RNA interference experiments, proteomics (2D gels coupled to mass spectroscopy) to detect protein expression levels, two-hybrid studies to analyse protein interactions in genomes, transposon-mediated insertional mutagenesis to compare the mutant and

---

[2]This is epitomized by the existence of operons in bacterial genomes.

wild-type phenotypic properties, reporter genes for determining the anatomic and temporal patterns of gene expression etc.

Some important information also comes from the knowledge of other complete genomes, for instance, when comparing cellular pathways or detecting non-orthologous gene displacements.

Although this is in general true for all annotation levels, this third level will more specifically benefit from the use of a common and consistent description of living organisms amongst biologists. For the annotation of other genomes to be fully useful in the analysis of a new genome, particularly when automated methods are used, it is necessary that a structured, cross-species, vocabulary be used. Such a vocabulary has been put forward recently by the Gene Ontology Project (Gene Ontology Consortium, 2001). In this project, biomolecular functions are organized as three ontologies (hierarchies) that describe the molecular functions, the cellular processes and the cellular components (the sub-cellular localizations). It is expected that this systematic representation of biological knowledge will make the full utilization of genomic data and their integration with existing knowledge much easier than they currently are.

By now it must be clear to the reader that a genome annotation is a never ending process. Biological data and the associated knowledge increase extremely fast (one must remember that the first complete genome was published in 1995). Published genomes must therefore be continuously re-annotated to benefit from this increase in available data. Genes that a few months ago were considered 'orphans', i.e. without any homologues in the then existing databases, may very well be found to be homologous to new genes from which information is now available. Automatic annotation systems must facilitate this re-annotation process, by pointing out to the genome curators which genes need to be updated and why.

The traceability, or 'sourcing', of the information obtained from a genome analysis is very important. It is imperative to distinguish annotations that have an experimental basis from those inferred with the help of bioinformatics tools. In this latter case it is mandatory that the type of analysis software and the releases of the databases that have been used as well as some level of confidence in the inferred annotation all be included in the annotation.

Genome annotation and databases

The process of genome annotation, briefly sketched above, requires an important effort from the biological community at large to organize, standardize and rationalize biological data and concepts.

- First of all, the biological information must be defined and organized in a systematic manner in databases. In this context, computational biologists have to deal with many problems of primary databases: redundancy, low quality (errors, incorrect annotations, inconsistencies), lack of traceability, problems of nomen-clature (such as the naming of genes) etc.

- Once these data are stored in databases it is critical to be able to retrieve and consult them easily. In this respect, the development of the internet, happily coincident with the development of genomics, has had a strong impact on the accessibility of biological collections.

- As is apparent in Figure 1.1 the process of annotation relies heavily on the integration of heterogeneous biological data. Integration is thus a key concept if one wants to make full use of the biological data from various collections. Integration can be considered on a physical level: how can one interconnect various databases stored on different machines, with different operating systems and using different database management systems? Integration can also be considered on a more conceptual level. In order to be able to integrate various data it is important that the biological concepts underlying the data be agreed upon by the community.

- This leads naturally to the development of controlled vocabularies and a standardized description of the biological 'objects' and concepts manipulated by the biologists (the so-called ontologies).

1.3 Databases: Concepts and Definitions

This section provides some definitions of technical concepts used in biological data banks and databases.

Managing the biological information

Databanks: flat files

The simplest and most primitive database system consists in building a set of flat files (i.e. text files containing records with a standardized nomenclature). The typical flat file database is split up using a common delimiter such as a tab, new line or a combination of characters unlikely to be found in the data itself. Within a file record, one can organize the data using different types of field. One of the main problems with flat file databases is that they are prone to corruption because there is no inherent locking mechanism that detects when a file is being edited. A second problem is that accessing data in a flat file implementation is slow in practice due to the multiple file open operations. Addition of index files[*] (terms marked with an [*] appear in the glossary at the end of this chapter) can provide efficient access to elements of these flat files. This organization emulates some of the behaviours of a relational database and has often been used in biology in order to store or distribute banks of primary data, for example by the PDB (Bernstein et al., 1977). However, it generates many problems (inefficient access, security and administration problems, no concurrency access and no logical data model).

Databases

A database is a collection of data that is organized so that its contents can easily be accessed, managed and updated. A database can provide access only through a *logical* model of the data. The entities are no longer files (as in flat file systems) but concepts defined by the database administrator. Generally, a database management system (DBMS) is used to access information. A DBMS is a collection of programs that enables the user to enter, organize and select data in a database.

The most common type of database is the relational database, a collection of data items organized as a set of formally described tables from which data can be accessed or reassembled in many different ways. Each table (also called a relation) is defined by one or more data categories in columns (also named attributes or fields). Each row contains a unique instance of data for the categories defined by the columns. For instance, a table providing a minimal description of an EMBL entry should contain as attributes its accession number, its definition and its organism of origin. The rows of the table contain the different EMBL entries stored in the database. Relational databases provide extremely powerful procedures to build complex access to many subsets of attributes and tables. A relational database has many advantages: simplicity of creation and access, extensibility and availability of a standard user and application program interface: SQL[*] (Structured Query Language). The availability of efficient relational database management systems (RDBMSs) such as Oracle, PostgreSQL or mySQL, in mainframe as well as personal computers, explains the popularity of relational databases.

More recent object-oriented database systems (OODBMSs) are DBMSs that support the modelling and creation of data as objects. Manipulation of objects in the framework of databases provides interesting functionalities, such as manipulation of complex objects, encapsulation[*], inheritance[*] and transparently persistent data (the ability to directly manipulate data stored in the database using an object programming language). Very few biological databases use OODBMSs. The AceDB[3] (A *Caenorhabditis elegans* database) (Stein and Thierry-Mieg, 1998) uses a system in which data are stored in objects. AceDB databases store information as classes, which are a collection of information on a common topic. Typically, general classes are 'Sequence', 'Locus', 'Clone', 'Chromosome'. Objects are then entered in these defined classes. For instance, an EMBL entry would be an object of the 'Sequence' class. An advantage of AceDB is its powerful query language and browsing interface, which provide easy access and manipulation of classes and objects of the database. The problem is that there is currently no widely agreed-upon standard for OODBMS

[3]http://www.acedb.org

products. In the meantime, the idea that object-oriented database concepts can be superimposed on relational databases is more commonly encountered in products named object-relational database management systems (ORDBMSs): for instance Oracle and PosgreSQL's latest releases.

Typical design of a biological database

Usually, the creation of a biological database involves three main steps (see Figure 1.3).

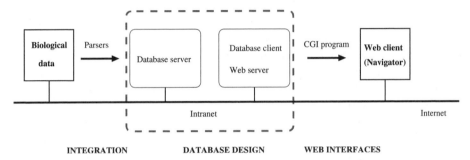

Figure 1.3 Main steps of the development of a biological database (design, integration, interfaces)

1. *The modelling and creation of the database*. For example, the definition of a relational database results in formal descriptions of tables and attributes. The DBMS (database management system) will then provide facilities to create and maintain the database. This first step is of course essential and requires a model of the data.

2. *The integration of data into the database*. This can be done either by the design of parsers or by the development of web forms. A parser is a program that is able to convert primary biological data into entities defined in the database. Typically a parser will be able to split a set of EMBL entries according to the different EMBL tags (accession, locus, features and qualifiers), to facilitate integration of entries in a database. The BioPerl toolkit (Stajich *et al.*, 2002) provides this kind of facility for the Perl language. Web forms and CGI[*] programs permit us to develop frames to submit data to a database integration procedure. Typically Perl modules such as DBI/DBD[4] provide easy procedures to embed SQL code in a Perl script. In parallel, Perl CGI[5] modules allow easy production of dynamic HTML documents.

---

[4]http://dbi.perl.org
[5]http://stein.cshl.org/WWW/software/CGI/

3. *The development of Web interfaces.* In the web area, the development of good web interfaces is essential. The problem is to produce dynamic HTML pages using data stored in a database. Many programming languages provides interfaces to retrieve data from a database (for instance the DBI/DBD Perl modules). In order to produce dynamic web pages, the older technique of CGI programming is giving way to more recent techniques such as PHP* (PHP: Hypertext Processor) or XML* (eXtensible Markup Language) provide new facilities.

CGI programs are the most common way for web servers to interact dynamically with users. Another increasingly common way to provide dynamic feedback to web users is to include scripts or programs that run on the user's machine rather than the web server, for instance Java applets or Javascript programs (see below). PHP is a widely used general-purpose scripting language that is especially suited to web development and can be embedded into HTML. The PHP commands are executed on the web server to generate dynamic HTML pages. One of the strongest and most significant features in PHP is its support for a wide range of databases. Writing a database-enabled web page is quite simple using PHP.

XML is a markup language much like HTML, but XML was designed to describe data using a hierarchical structure. An XML document uses a document type definition (DTD*) or a schema to describe the data and is designed to be self-descriptive. This point allows easy and powerful manipulation of data in XML documents. Many languages already include XML parsers. Many projects aim to define DTDs for genomic projects. Some biological databanks, including GenBank, can export data in XML format.

1.4 Access to Annotation Databases

As noted before, annotation databases have become repositories of huge amounts of heterogeneous data, and this trend is likely to increase in the foreseeable future. To extract new knowledge from these resources, access methods capable of retrieving every single entity they store, as well as synthesizing reports about specific collections of items, are of primary importance. A major issue in the deployment of access methods is the nature of the 'client' performing the requests, ranging from the casual user, personified by the laboratory biologist, to the seasoned bioinformaticist or bioanalyst mastering the arcana of a complex query language. Recently, a new category of clients is emerging, consisting of software tools designed to submit a set of queries to a database on a regular time basis, either to perform batch analyses or, more frequently, to keep local subsets of a database up to date.

Database access in the pre-web era

Digitally stored annotation information in biology was available well before the advent of the World Wide Web: the Protein Data Bank, or PDB (Bernstein *et al.*, 1977) appeared as early as 1977, GenBank (Burks *et al.*, 1985) was started in 1985, SWISS-PROT (Bairoch and Boeckman, 1994) was established in 1986 and the AceDB (Stein and Thierry-Mieg, 1998) database system has been developed since 1989. The lack of user-friendly remote access methods implied that users of these databases frequently had to obtain a copy of their entire contents. Such releases came as collections of flat files whose format was described in accompanying documentation files. Browsing these databases often meant opening files in a text editor and scrolling back and forth between relevant blocks (heavily using text search features to locate these blocks). Some of the packages came with programs capable of querying and retrieving information from the files, but these programs were highly platform dependent (for instance, at one time SWISS-PROT tools ran only on MS-DOS and Apple Macintosh computers, and AceDB software was available for Unix and Windows machines).

First generation web-based user interfaces

Subsequent to the widespread use of the World Wide Web, database access methods have been geared towards the novice-to-moderately-experienced user community. Almost every annotation database now offers a web-accessible graphical user interface (or GUI). This interface presents a series of fill-in forms allowing the user to fix the values of certain attributes, and to specify the details of the information the query should return. In its simplest form, the user is presented with a set of attributes of the database, and corresponding text fields for entering one or more values for these attributes. The resulting query then extracts all the records of the database whose attributes match these values, and displays the results as a list or a set of rows in a table. Query capabilities are frequently enhanced through the use of search patterns or Boolean expressions. Instead of entering a fixed value for a chosen attribute, search patterns may allow some ambiguity about the value to accept as a match. Such patterns can be used to search for records with attributes starting or ending with a given string, or containing potential misspellings. Boolean expressions combining attribute values using logical operators add another level of power to the query capabilities.[6]

All major publicly accessible annotation databases offer at least a minimal set of Boolean operators to combine record attributes, mostly by letting the user choose which operator to use to combine the attributes (SWISS-PROT, the PDB

---

[6]The query 'retrieve all gene names starting with the letters "rpo" and located in the first magabase of all organisms belonging to the Bacillus group' is an instance of a query mixing patterns (rpo) and logical operators (and).

and the Protein Information Resource or PIR (Wu *et al.*, 2003)). A few resources allow the user to enter a complex expression as a text string, including Entrez (Wheeler *et al.*, 2003) and SRS (Zdobnov *et al.*, 2002).

The very nature of the information stored in annotation databases is in some cases ill suited for display as text. One of the most typical operations of the initial annotation stages, the search for homologies between the DNA portion or protein to be annotated, and databases of known genes or proteins, respectively, can yield significant amounts of textual information. Although they are ranked by relevance, sifting through these results can become a time-consuming task. Displaying a graphical summary of the most salient features contained in the results (as provided by the BLAST section of Entrez, or by Prodom (Corpet *et al.*, 2000)) greatly enhances the usability of these search tools.

Graphical displays become an invaluable asset when annotations have natural mappings to graphlike structures. Hence, the Database of Interacting Proteins or DIP (Xenarios *et al.*, 2002) gives a graphical representation of the interaction network of selected proteins. In the same way, the Kyoto Encyclopedia of Genes and Genomes (Kanehisa and Goto, 2000) proposes graphical views of metabolic and regulatory pathways. Finally, as gene context becomes a source of increasing value, repositories offering graphical views of series of neighbouring genes have appeared. For instance, the Search Tool for the Retrieval of Interacting Genes/Proteins (STRING) (von Mering *et al.*, 2003) focuses on delivering displays of gene strings conserved in various genomes. The GMOD initiative (Stein *et al.*, 2002) proposes a generic genome browser, capable of displaying user-defined portions of a selection of genomes with multiple annotation tracks. The amount of detail as well as the type of annotation to be displayed can be fixed through the user interface.

Enhancing the dynamics of the interface

Most of the examples presented in the previous paragraphs describe user interfaces in which each action the user performs generates a query addressed to the server, which then returns a web page dynamically generated by an appropriate program. The benefit of this model is that it works with a minimum set of requirements on the client side: a web browser is all that is needed to access these repositories. The downside is the relative lack of reactivity of the user interface, as a round-trip to the server is needed to refresh the display.[7]

Other models of dynamic on-line content display have emerged that allow higher levels of interactivity for web-based interfaces. Undoubtedly, the most popular of these make use of the Java platform. The Java platform encompasses an object-oriented programming language and a rich set of libraries for network communications and graphical user interface design among others. Its attractiveness is related to

---

[7]Each time the user clicks on a link in a page, the browser directs a request to the server, which generates a new page and returns it to the browser.

the fact that Java programs can be transferred on demand from remote servers. A web page can contain a link to a Java program that is loaded in the web browser when viewing the page. This Java program, called an applet, then runs in the context of the web browser, either embedded in the web page or in a separate window, and is capable of communicating with the server to retrieve additional data if needed. Being run locally, Java applets offer quite the same level of reactivity as 'ordinary' local executables.

Over the last several years, web browsers have added the capability to run Java applets. Early on the entire Java runtime environment was tightly integrated in the browsers, requiring no user configuration prior to using Java programs, but as the Java platform evolved integrated runtime environments tended to lag behind in terms of functionality. This led Java developers to neglect the newest features, in order to keep the broadest possible user community. Nowadays, runtime environments are available as browser plug-ins, which keeps their installation straightforward and, at the same time, allows them to be updated more frequently than the browser itself. Examples of Java-based web interfaces are the protein interaction network visualization module provided by the DIP, or the MapView tool at the Human Genome Database (Letowsky *et al.*, 1998).

Even if Java applets have brought web interfaces a step further, they still suffer some restrictions hampering their usefulness. For security reasons, Java applets are not allowed to access data on the client machine's disks, nor are they authorized to make network connections to servers other than the one they were loaded from. This makes them impractical for user interfaces grabbing data from multiple servers or needing local persistent storage. The Java platform nevertheless offers a second category of programs, called applications, that are independent of any web browser. Java applications are also run by the Java runtime environment but as stand-alone programs.

The benefit of Java programs versus programs written in more traditional programming languages such as C/C++ is the 'write once run anywhere' paradigm. Java applications can be distributed in a compiled format independent of any hardware or operating system specifics. The mere availability of a runtime environment for a given platform guarantees that Java programs will run on that platform. Considering the diversity of workstations used in biology laboratories, Java's ubiquitous execution model came as a boon to the bioinformatics developer community.

Visualization tools

Full-blown annotation applications, able to extract entries from databases and present them to the user in a rich contextual view, have subsequently been developed. Artemis (Rutherford *et al.*, 2000), perhaps the first package in this category, offers graphical views of annotated sequences, separating each of the six reading frames both in a global overview and in a close-up view of the actual sequence with colour codes for each type of feature. Various analysis results (codon usage plots, GC content plots and others) can be drawn in these views. Not only a visualization tool, Artemis is also an annotation editor, giving users the opportunity manually to curate the loaded entries. Modifications are then made persistent by saving local copies of edited entries.

A second graphical curation tool, Apollo (Lewis *et al.*, 2002), has recently been released, emphasizing the integration of analysis results with sequence data to be annotated. Hence, graphical representations of the output of programs such as BLAST, GenScan and Genie can be superposed on the entry under scrutiny. As with Artemis, Apollo allows full editing of the annotations.

As annotation databases proliferate, the cost of developing specific graphical interfaces for each of them becomes prohibitive. Several initiatives have emerged that endeavour to standardize access to annotation repositories at different levels. At one end of the spectrum, the bioSQL group proposes a database schema capable of storing genome annotations (mainly sequence features and qualifiers with references to other databases). If this proposal catches on, developers of graphical annotation presentation and manipulation tools will have to master this single schema to build applications capable of tapping into multiple databases. However, the fact that these applications rely on SQL queries prohibits their widespread usage across large networks, partly because of potential resource problems caused by too many simultaneous complex requests, partly because the network protocol they rely on is often limited to local area networks.

Towards automated access facilities

The preceding discussion has covered access methods targeting annotation visualization by human end-users. However, automated annotation analysis tools offer some promising prospects for annotation enrichment. Such tools must be able to extract huge datasets from multiple annotation repositories in order to carry out their analysis algorithms. A first generation of tools imitated human usage patterns, to query Web annotation databases and parsed the resulting HTML pages to extract the relevant bits of information. The most blatant weakness of this approach is its tight coupling with the HTML presentation elements embedded in the results pages. A small to moderate amount of change to these elements would render the automated extraction tools almost useless until they were updated to handle the new presentation style.

Hence, the need arose for methods to access databases using protocols of a sufficiently high level to abstract the actual database structure, and adopt a format capturing the semantics of the data rather than its presentation. On the one hand, the HTTP protocol,[8] being ubiquitous, and lightweight, imposed itself as the means best suited to transfer structured information across wide networks. On the

---

[8]The hyper-text transfer protocol is the protocol used for the exchange of information between web servers and browsers.

other hand, XML has emerged as a natural format for encapsulating this structured data.

Building on these foundations, the Biodas project strives to implement a distributed annotation system, capable of pulling annotation information from a variety of annotation servers and integrating these with a reference sequence in a single view. Clients retrieve annotations from servers using a set of standardized URLs, which return the requested data formatted according to one of the DTDs issued by the DAS (Dowell *et al.*, 2001) community. Recently, the DAS specifications have evolved to adopt more general purpose web service standards. Consequently, DAS servers are now able to respond to SOAP[*]. Moreover, the services they offer can be published in the WSDL[*] web service description language, broadening their audience to any WSDL aware client.

The BioMOBY (Wilkinson and Links, 2002) project, though still in its infancy, aims to take service integration and discovery a step further. By offering a central registry for bioinformatics services, as well as a hierarchical description of the kinds of object they manipulate, BioMOBY allows its clients to propose to end users a series of operations applicable to the data at hand at each stage of the analysis. Users can build their own processing pipelines by chaining operations, whose output objects are compatible with the input objects of other services. Because BioMOBY uses mostly lightweight objects, information flow between services is streamlined as much as possible.

As these technologies mature, the shift from single annotation databases being queried by web-based scripts generating HTML pages to annotation repositories capable of exporting selected data in XML format – either to be further analysed by remote applications, or to undergo a transformation stage to be presented to the user in a web browser – will undoubtedly be one of the major evolutions of the genome annotation process. Systems leveraging these technologies will allow a community of curators located all around the world to carry out live editing of genome annotations to deliver up to date information to users world wide.

The integration challenge

Scientists today crave methods enabling them to correlate bits and pieces of information scattered among several annotation repositories. This challenge has until now been addressed in two ways.

One approach has been to perform a physical integration of all data into a single database. In practice, this amounts to building one all-encompassing data model which will be fed with data from various sources. The power of this approach is that, once this physical integration has been performed, it is possible to formulate queries involving any type of annotation the database contains. For example, considering a database containing information about microbial gene positions in their respective genomes, as well as expression data about these genes and homology relationships between them, it becomes possible to establish hypotheses about operon organization by assessing the degree of conservation across microbial genomes of neighbouring genes exposing similar expression profiles.

Unfortunately, some serious drawbacks preclude success of this approach when more than a very few data sources are to be integrated. Indeed, managing and maintaining such a database becomes highly impractical when many original databases have to be integrated: because each of these evolves at its own pace (both in their contents but also in their own data model), one must constantly amend the integrated database to keep it up to date.

The second approach tries to build an architecture in which the user has a single view of the set of data resources at hand, whatever architecture is used to tie these together. The most basic level of this so-called virtual integration is built as a federation of hyperlinks. When extracting data from one of the databases of the federation, the user also obtains links to the relevant data items in the other databases. In practice, this is the most widely used virtual integration method due to its ease of implementation. SWISS-PROT (Boeckman *et al.*, 2003), for instance, provides an extensive list of cross-references to other databases. This entry-level virtual integration nevertheless sacrifices almost all querying power as all links are hard coded.

Achieving a tighter coupling between distributed databases, and allowing queries spanning multiple sources, raises the challenge of building a more formal description of database contents. In the last decade, technical proposals have been put forward to ease the construction of such integrated resources. Undoubtedly one of the most promising has been the CORBA* initiative. CORBA has been touted as the silver bullet for distributed application development. There is even a Life Science Research Domain Task Force dedicated to the development and the adoption of standard modules for accessing and manipulating biological information (genomic maps, macromolecular structures and gene expression data among others). The fact that CORBA has not caught on as expected is tied in part to the skills required to deploy CORBA-compliant components, and in part to the fact that more often than not, information exchange between distant CORBA components is blocked by network filters (firewalls). It remains to be seen whether the emerging web services will play the role CORBA was expected to play.

These technological solutions do not solve the other obstacle to providing virtual database federations: the need for more agreed-upon semantical standards to describe biological entities. The database community must come up with clear and unambiguous definitions of at least all major biological concepts (gene, chemical reaction, cellular process) and of the relationships between them. Using such a unified controlled vocabulary, both for the annotation data types, and for the annotation data, is the key to the emergence of the much anticipated semantic web. The Gene Ontology Consortium (Gene Ontology Consortium, 2001) has undertaken the task of defining a hierarchy of terms related to genome annotation. So far, it has been used to describe the genes of several model organisms (*Saccharomyces cerevisiae, Drosophila melanogaster, Mus musculus* and others). As the consortium's proposals gain acceptance, querying multiple annotation databases starting from a single entry point may soon become the biologist's bread and butter.

Glossary

CGI: The *Common Gateway Interface* is a specification for transferring information between a World Wide Web server and a program. A CGI program is any program designed to accept and return data that conforms to the CGI specification.

CORBA: The *Common Request Broker Architecture* is a set of standards for building distributed applications. It specifies how to define interfaces for these components that are independent of any hardware platform, operating system or programming language.

DTD: A *document type definition* or DTD is used to give a formal specification of the structure of an XML document. The DTD describes the set of allowed tags and attributes, as well as the rules governing their usage, to which all XML documents using it must conform.

Encapsulation: Object-oriented programming concept promoting grouping of data and methods that manipulate them.

Index file: Index files are used in flat file databases to speed up access to data items. Thy contain pointers to the locations of these data items in the flat files, allowing one to directly retrieve data relevant to a query instead of having to search them all sequentially.

Inheritance: Object-oriented programming concept modelling the 'is a' or 'is a kind of' relationship between classes. Code and data common to a set of classes is factored out in so-called 'superclasses'. Subclasses deriving from these superclasses thus automatically 'inherit' this behaviour.

PHP: The *PHP: Hypertext Preprocessor* programming language has become quite a popular programming language for building web sites in recent years. It is an object-oriented scripting language aimed at dynamic web content generation. In contrast to the Perl/CGI paradigm, in which the output of Perl programs is sent back to web clients, PHP programs are directly embedded in HTML pages and surrounded by specific tags.

SOAP: The *simple object access protocol* defines a set of standards allowing access to computer resources across the network. Data exchange between service providers and clients is done through XML documents and often uses the HTTP protocol.

SQL: The *Structured Query Language* or SQL is the standard language used by relational database management systems. It provides constructs for the creation and modification of database tables as well as instructions for inserting, deleting and querying the data they contain.

WSDL: The *web service description language* provides a framework for describing a set of services with their names and how to invoke them (the list of parameters and parameter types they take as input and yield on return). Service descriptions are expressed in XML.

XML: The *eXtensible Markup Language* is a language for building structured documents. Information inside such documents is delimited by a set of tags denoting their very meaning. The set of allowed tags and their relationships can be specified in a DTD.

References

Altschul, S.F., Gish, W., Miller, W., Myers, E.W. and Lipman, D.J. (1990). Basic local alignment search tool. *J. Mol. Biol.* **215**, 403–410.

Altschul, S.F., Madden, T.L., Schaffer, A.A., Zhang, J., Zhang, Z., Miller, W. and Lipman, D.J. (1997). Gapped Blast and Psi-Blast: a new generation of protein database search programs. *Nucleic Acids Res.* **25**, 3389–3402.

Aravind, L. (2000). Guilt by Association: contextual information in genome analysis. *Genome Res.* **10**, 1074–1077.

Bairoch, A. and Boeckman, B. (1994). The SWISS-PROT Protein Sequence Databank: current status. *Nucleic Acids Res.* **22** (17), 3578–3580.

Bernstein, F.C., Koetzle, T.F., Williams, G.J., Meyer, E.F. Jr., Brice, M.D., Rodgers, J.R., Kennard, O., Shimanouchi, T. and Tasumi, M. (1977). The Protein Data Bank: a computer-based archival file for macromolecular structures. *J. Mol. Biol.* **112** (3), 535–542.

Boeckmann, B., Bairoch, A., Apweiler, R., Blatter, M.C., Estreicher, A., Gasteiger, E., Martin, M.J., Michoud, K., Donovan, O., Phan, I., Pilbout, S. and Schneider, M. (2003). The Swiss-Prot protein knowledgebase and its supplement trembl in 2003. *Nucleic Acids Res.* **31**, 365–370.

Bork. P., Dandekar, T., Diaz, L., Eisenhaber, F., Huynen, M. and Yuan, Y. (1998). Predicting Function: from genes to genomes and back. *J. Mol. Biol.* **283**, 707–725.

Burks, C., Fickett, J.W., Goad, W.B., Kanehisa, M., Lewitter, F.I., Rindone, W.P., Swindell, C.D., Tung, C.S. and Bilofsky, H.S. (1985). The GenBank nucleic acid sequence database. *Comput. Appl. Biosci.* **1** (4), 225–233.

Corpet, F., Servant, F., Gouzy, J. and Kahn, D. (2000). Prodom and Prodom-CG: Tools for protein domain analysis and whole genome comparisons. *Nucleic Acids Res.* **28**(1), 267–269.

Dowell, R.D., Jokerst, R.M., Day, A., Eddy, S.R. and Stein, L. (2001). The distributed annotation system. *BMC Bioinformatics* **2** (1), 7.

Garnier, J. and Berendsen, H.J.C. (2002). International unions concerned about biodata. *Nature* **419**, 777.

Gene Ontology Consortium (2001). Creating the Gene Ontology Resource: design and implementation. *Genome Res.* **11**, 1425–1433.

Kanehisa, M. and Goto, S. (2000). KEGG: Kyoto Encyclopedia of Genes and Genomes. *Nucleic Acids Res.* **28** (1), 27–30.

Krogh, A., Larsson, B., von Heijne, G. and Sonnhammer, E.L. (2001). Predicting Transmembrane Protein Topology with a Hidden Markov Model: application to complete genomes. *J. Mol. Biol.* **305**, 567–580.

Letowsky, S.I., Cottingham, R.W., Porter, C.J. and Li, P.W.D. (1998). GDB: the human genome database. *Nucleic Acids Res.* **26** (1), 94–99.

Lewis, E., Searle, S.M.J., Harris, N., Gibson, M., Lyer, V., Richter, J., Wiel, C., Bayraktaroglir, L., Birney, E., Crosby, M.A., Kaminker, J.S., Matthews, B.B., Prochnik, S.E., Smithy, C.D., Tupey, J.L., Rubin, G.M., Misra, S., Mungall, C.J. and Clamp, M.E. (2002). Apollo: a sequence annotation editor. *Genome Biol.* **3** (12), 0082.1–0082.14.

Lupas, A., Van Dyke, M. and Stock, J. (1991). Predicting coiled coils from protein sequences. *Science* **252**, 1162–1164.

Marin, A., Pothier, J., Zimmermann, K. and Gibrat, J.F. (2002). Frost: a filter based fold recognition method. *Proteins* **49**, 493–509.

Overbeek, R., Fonstein, M., Souza, D., Pusch, G.D. and Maltsev, N. (1999). The use of gene clusters to infer functional coupling. *Proc. Natl. Acad. Sci. USA* **96**, 2896–2901.

Park, J., Karplus, K., Barrett, C., Hughey, R., Haussler, D., Hubbard, T. and Chothia, C. (1998). Sequence comparisons using multiple sequences detect three times as many remote homologues as pairwise methods. *J. Mol. Biol.* **284**, 1201–1210.

Pellegrini, M., Marcotte, E.M., Thompson, M.J., Eisenberg, D. and Yeates, T.O. (1999). Assigning protein functions by comparative genome analysis: protein phylogenetic profiles. *Proc. Natl. Acad. Sci. USA* **96**, 4285–4288.

Rutherford, K., Parkhill, J., Crook, J., Horsnell, T., Rice, P., Rajandream, M.-A. and Barrell, B. (2000). Artemis: sequence visualization and annotation. *Bioinformatics* **16** (10), 944–945.

Stajich, J.E., Block, D., Boulez, K., Brenner, S.E., Chervitz, S.A., Dagdigian, C., Fuellen, G., Gilbert, J.G.R., Korf, I., Lapp, H., Lehvaslaiho, H., Matsalla, C., Mungall, C.J., Osborne, B.I., Pocock, M.R., Schattner, P., Senger, M., Stein, L.D., Stupka, E., Wilkinson, M.D. and Birney, E. (2002). The BioPerl toolkit: Perl modules for the life sciences. *Genome Res.* **12**, 1611–1618.

Stein, L. (2001). Genome Annotation: from sequence to biology. *Nat. Rev. Genet.* **2**, 493–503.

Stein, L.D., Mungall, C., Shu, S., Caudy, M., Mangone, M., Day, A., Nickerson, E., Stajich, J.E., Harris, T.W., Arva, A. and Lewis, S. (2002). The Generic Genome Browser: a building block for a model organism database. *Genome Res.* **12** (10), 1599–1610.

Stein, L.D. and Thierry-Mieg, J. (1998). Scriptable access to the *Caenorhabditis elegans* genome sequence and other AceDB databases. *Genome Res.* **8** (12), 1308–1315.

Vinayaka, L-SL Yeh, Zhang, J. and Barker, W.C. (2002). The Protein Information Resource: an integrated public resource of functional annotation of proteins. *Nucleic Acids Res.* **30** (1), 135–137.

von Mering, C., Huynen, M., Jaeggi, D., Schmidt, S., Bork, P. and Snel, B. (2003). STRING: a database of predicted functional associations between proteins. *Nucleic Acids Res.* **31** (1), 258–261.

Wheeler, D.L., Church, D.M., Federhen, S., Lash, A.E., Madden, T.L., Pontius, J.U., Schuler, G.D., Schriml, L.M., Sequeira, E., Tatusova, T.A. and Wagner, L. (2003). Database resources at the National Center for Biotechnology. *Nucleic Acids Res.* **31** (1), 28–33.

Wilkinson, M.D. and Links, M. (2002). BioMoby: an open source biological web services proposal. *Briefings Bioinformatics* **3** (4), 331–341.

Wootton, J.C. and Federhen, S. (1996). Analysis of compositionally biased regions in sequence databases. *Methods Enzymol.* **266**, 554–571.

Wu, C.H., Yeh, L.S., Huang, H., Arminski, L., Castro-Alvear, J., Chen, Y., Hu, Z.-Z., Kourtesis, P., Ledley, R.S., Suzek, B.E., Vinayaka, C.R., Zhang, J. and Barker, W.C. (2003). The protein information resource. *Nucleic Acids Res.* **31** (1), 345–347.

Xenarios, I., Salw'inski, L., Duan, X.J., Highney, P., Kim, S.-M. and Eisenberg, D. (2002). DIP, the Database of Interacting Proteins: a research tool for studying cellular networks of protein interactions. *Nucleic Acids Res.* **30** (1), 303–305.

Zdobnov, E.M., Lopez, R., Apweiler, R. and Etzold, T. (2002). The EBI SRS server – recent developments. *Bioinformatics* **18** (2), 368–373.

I
The Databanks

2 Survey of Sequence Databases: Archival Projects

M. Magrane, M. Garcia-Pastor and R. Apweiler

Abstract

A wide variety of nucleic acid and protein sequence archives exist, ranging from simple sequence repositories that store data with little or no manual intervention in the creation of the records to expertly curated universal databases that cover all species and where the original sequence data are enhanced by manual addition of further information in each sequence record. These databases play an increasingly important role as central comprehensive resources of biological information. Several of the leading nucleic acid and protein archival projects are examined in this chapter.

Keywords

bioinformatics, databases, sequence archives, protein sequences, nucleotide sequences, annotation

2.1 Introduction

What are archival databases?

Archival sequence databanks consist of nucleic acid and protein sequence collections as well as the annotation they contain. This is a very broad definition that applies to a great number of data sources available to scientists. There can, however, be many differences among these databases in relation to how the data are acquired, managed and distributed. Some sequence databases are built using voluntary contributions from researchers, who may remain owners of their data and be responsible for its

Database Annotation in Molecular Biology   Edited by Arthur M. Lesk
© 2005 John Wiley & Sons, Ltd.   ISBN: 0-470-85681-5

accuracy. In other databases, the responsibility for the accuracy and quality of the data lies with the database project. With regard to biological annotation, there is also a range of approaches, from databases that store the data as submitted with little or no extra added information to those in which the original data are enhanced by addition of further information derived from sources such as published scientific literature. In some databases, emphasis is placed on having a complete dataset, even if this results in redundancy, whereas others attempt to maximize completeness while keeping redundancy to a minimum through merging of multiple sequences that originate from the same gene. There are benefits to each approach, with the result that there are a large number of collections available and meaningful ways to extract the underlying knowledge from all types of datasets. This chapter concerns a number of the leading archival sequence databanks in both the nucleotide and protein fields, and details the structure of these databases and how they manage the vast amounts of data that they maintain.

Nucleotide database archival projects

The three primary nucleotide sequence databases are DDBJ (Tateno and Gojobori, 1996), EMBL (Stoesser *et al.*, 2003) and GenBank (Benson *et al.*, 2003). These archives include sequences provided through the voluntary cooperation of scientists from all over the world, both from individual submitters and large sequencing centres, and from patents. The databases also contain nucleotide sequences extracted from the literature, although data are no longer obtained in this way. The three databases exchange public data on a daily basis, making these resources the most complete nucleotide sequence set available to the public, at the expense of some redundancy.

There are no legal restrictions on the use of the data in these databases. In its 2002 meeting, the International Advisory Committee, made up of members of the advisory body of each database, endorsed a brief policy statement detailing the procedures followed by the three databases with regard to the availability of the data (Brunak *et al.*, 2002). The statement included a declaration on free and unrestricted access to the public data, and stated that the databases would not attach statements that restrict access or limit use of the information.

There are other databases available that contain a subset of the DDBJ/EMBL/ GenBank databases. These include species and molecule specific collections, which may expand on the original annotation, such as the Eukaryotic Promoter Database (EPD) (Praz *et al.*, 2002) or the ImMunoGeneTics database (IMGT) (Lefranc, 2003).

In this chapter, the universal primary archival databases, DDBJ/EMBL/GenBank, will be discussed in detail, as the most widely used resources to gather information on nucleotide sequence data.

Protein database archival projects

The major protein database archives include Swiss-Prot (Boeckmann *et al.*, 2003), TrEMBL (Boeckmann *et al.*, 2003), PIR (Wu *et al.*, 2003), GenPept, NCBI's Entrez

Protein and RefSeq (Pruitt, Tatusova and Maglott, 2003). Although other protein databases exist, most are specialized data collections storing information about specific families or groups of proteins. Of the above, Swiss-Prot, TrEMBL and PIR are the only annotated universal protein sequence databases, covering proteins from all species. Databases such as GenPept contain translations of coding sequences in the DDBJ/EMBL/GenBank nucleotide sequence database but lack annotation and proteins derived from amino acid sequencing. In compilations such as NCBI's Entrez Protein, which contains sequence data from the translated coding regions from DNA sequences of DDBJ/EMBL/GenBank as well as sequences from PIR, Swiss-Prot, RefSeq and the Protein Data Bank (PDB) (Westbrook *et al.*, 2003), nearly all annotated data have been curated by Swiss-Prot and PIR. NCBI's RefSeq currently contains 110 160 records, of which only approximately 10 000 have been reviewed by NCBI staff compared with the many more comprehensively annotated records in Swiss-Prot, TrEMBL and PIR. Also, while NCBI provides reference sequences for over 1000 viruses and 100 bacteria, there is still a very limited number of sequences from higher organisms. Therefore, this chapter will concentrate on the significance of the three major universal protein sequence databases, Swiss-Prot, TrEMBL and PIR, as these are the most comprehensive sources of information on proteins.

2.2 Nucleotide Sequence Databases

The EMBL Data Library was founded in 1980 as a response to the need for a repository for the increasing number of nucleotide sequences and was the first central repository of this nature in the world. Its role was to collect, organize and distribute a database of nucleotide sequences and related descriptive information extracted from publications in scientific journals. This archive was located at the main EMBL station in Heidelberg, Germany. The data library was the precursor of the EMBL Nucleotide Sequence Database. The first release by the EMBL Data Library was produced in 1982, and contained nearly 600 000 bases in approximately 600 entries.

GenBank was also founded in 1980 at Los Alamos National Laboratory (LANL), USA. The National Centre for Biotechnology Information (NCBI) took over the development and maintenance of the GenBank database in 1992. Their web site can be found at www.ncbi.nlm.nih.gov/GenBank

The collaboration between the European and American databases started soon after they were established. Initially, the databases exchanged communications, ideas and participated together in workshops, but the databases merely took each other's data and reloaded it locally, which created duplications, and incompleteness of both sets. This interaction gradually developed into a closer collaboration with sharing of data and entry identifiers.

The DNA Database of Japan (DDBJ) started collecting data in 1986 at the National Institute of Genetics (NIG). From the beginning, DDBJ joined the collaboration already in place between the other two databases. The Japanese databank adopted formats and protocols already in place that facilitated compatibility with the other databases. The DDBJ web site is at www.ddbj.nig.ac.jp

In 1994, the European repository, now known as the EMBL Nucleotide Sequence Database, was relocated to the European Bioinformatics Institute (EBI) at Hinxton, Cambridge, in the United Kingdom. This institute offers a wide range of bioinformatics services and databases to the scientific community. All resources can be accessed via the EBI home page at www.ebi.ac.uk

The international collaboration of nucleotide sequence databases

The International Nucleotide Sequence Databases (INSD) constitutes a collaboration between the three major databases: DDBJ, EMBL and GenBank.

The three databases collect and manage nucleotide sequence data, and offer their own services to the scientific community, often catering for a more or less 'local' audience. To achieve optimal synchronization, new and updated public data are exchanged on a daily basis amongst the INSD. The three databases adhere to a set of documented guidelines, The DDBJ/EMBL/GenBank Feature Table Definition Document, that regulates the content and syntax of the database entries. These guidelines ensure that the data continue to be made available in a format that can be exchanged efficiently between the databases, is compatible with current bioinformatics software and reflects the latest developments and discoveries in the fields of molecular and general biology. The Feature Table Definition Document represents the vocabulary used to describe the sequence annotations. Features, qualifiers, location descriptors etc. are listed and described and incremental versions are made available to the public from each of the databases' sites.

The comprehensive nucleotide sequence database collaborative taxonomy includes all organisms appearing in the nucleotide sequence database. This centralized database ensures that the member databases display the same organism classification at each site. Entries are not released into the public domain until the sequenced organism is classified. Organisms are identified to the species level whenever possible, as well as to subspecies level or to variety level in the case of plants. The top organisms in the database in February 2003 are shown in Figure 2.1.

The primary aim of the collaboration is to offer one central and unique repository of nucleotide sequences in the world. The collaboration has proven successful because it provides a service to users and submitters and ensures the maximum coverage of these repositories, and also because it brings ideas and resources from different institutions. This set-up has also ensured that local politics or cultural differences have not played a role in how the data are deposited and distributed back to the scientific community, so that the most complete set of sequenced nucleotide molecules is made available freely to all scientists.

Annual meetings of representatives from the databases provide a forum for technical discussions concerning detailed aspects of the work, and for discussion of

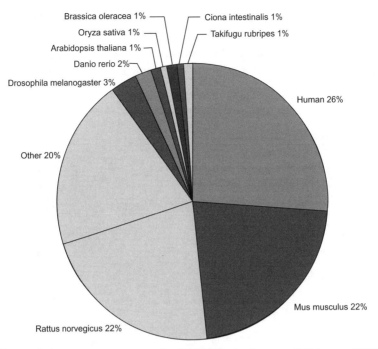

Figure 2.1 Top 10 organisms in the EMBL database on 2 February 2003

any biological developments that should find their way into the Feature Table Definition Documentation.

Data acquisition

Throughout the years, data acquisition methods have changed drastically: capturing of sequences from the literature by database staff has been replaced by direct submissions from researchers. Many journals now actively encourage scientists to submit their data to the repositories before submitting their manuscripts for publication. Each of the members of the INSD now provides stand-alone tools as well as web submission facilities for individual scientists.

Large scale sequencing centres have mechanisms to deposit their data in a much faster and automatic manner, through mail or FTP accounts. High throughput genome data (HTG) are picked up by the databases from the Genome Centres' FTP sites whenever an entry is modified. The EMBL database collects and distributes these unfinished data to make them available to users as soon as possible. Entries in the HTG division contain keywords to indicate the status of the sequencing (e.g. HTGS_PHASE1), and are grouped and distributed in a separate division. Accession numbers are assigned and maintained through subsequent updates. Once finished, the HTG entries are transferred into the relevant primary EMBL division. Quality scores from HTG data are collected, updated daily and made available on the EBI FTP server at ftp://ftp.ebi.ac.uk/pub/databases/embl EMBL Release 79 (June 2004) included over 11.7 Gb of HTG data.

Databases have therefore adapted their data submission software and protocols to the great demands of the users and the exponential growth in the influx of data (Figures 2.2 and 2.3).

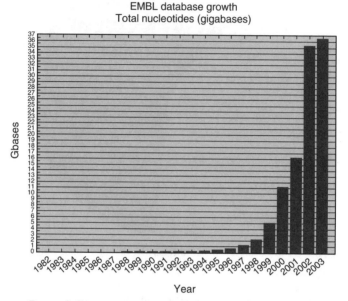

Figure 2.2 Exponential database growth by nucleotides

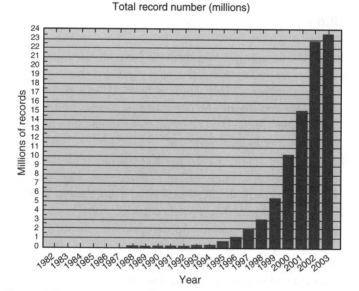

Figure 2.3 Exponential database growth by total number of entries

Biological annotation and database curation

One of the challenges of data repositories of the size and nature of the nucleotide sequence databases is to achieve accurate biological annotation while keeping up with the great influx of data. This task is complicated by the different sequence sources and different experimental efforts used to generate the data. Furthermore, the goal of completeness needs to be achieved. Hence, the large number of sequences received require different processing procedures and levels of curation of the data by the recipient database.

EMBL and its collaborative databases have teams of dedicated biologists and database specialists who manage the collection and distribution of the database. Genome project submissions are processed in large numbers using semi-automated systems. The largely computational analysis of these huge sets of data is performed at the sequencing centres, which also provide the annotation. Database biologists liaise with these genome centres to achieve the best standardization in the annotation of the biological information. Data generated by patent applications and the patent offices are also processed semi-automatically and the biological annotation of this data is generally poor.

The level of curation of sequences submitted directly by individual researchers is far greater. Such sequences have often been the subject of extensive experimental research while most genome project submissions include only preliminary gene annotations based on gene prediction programs. The databases request that submitters provide biological annotation for their sequences, with a few exceptions such as sequences that describe genomic markers, expressed sequence tag sites (ESTs) and unfinished high throughput genome sequences (HTG) (Stoesser et al., 2002). In particular, it is essential to provide locations of coding regions, even partial or preliminary, to allow inclusion of the corresponding translated protein sequences in the protein databases.

The processing of directly submitted data varies slightly between databases, but all of them perform clerical checks and history loggings that allow database staff to manage the data over time. Database curators trained in molecular biology and skilled in database production operations annotate, organize and maintain the ever-growing number of database entries. Curators ensure that all direct submissions receive a systematic quality review. Programs are used to confirm coding regions and verify amino acid translations. Using annotation and data representation guidelines, curators then create the corresponding database entry, ensuring the description lines, taxonomy classification, citation reference and biological feature annotation are correct and informative (Figure 2.4). Communication with submitters is sometimes also necessary. The databases assign accession numbers to these submitted entries and these serve as a confirmation that the sequence has been submitted and can be cited in publications. The accession number is a permanent and stable value that is used to retrieve the sequence from any of the databases that are members of the international collaboration.

```
FH    Key                Location/Qualifiers
FH
FT    source             1..1320
FT                       /db_xref="taxon:3348"
FT                       /organelle="plastid:chloroplast"
FT                       /organism="Pinus strobus"
FT                       /tissue_type="leaf"
FT    CDS                <1..>1320
FT                       /codon_start=1
FT                       /transl_table=11
FT                       /gene="rbcL"
FT                       /product="ribulose-1,5-bisphosphate carboxylase/oxygenase
FT                       large subunit"
FT                       /protein_id="AAM53143.1"
FT                       /translation="KASVGFKAGVKDYRLTYYTPEYQTKDTDILAAFRVTPQPGVPAEE
FT                       AGAAVAAESSTGTWTTUWTDGLTSLDRYKGRCYDIEPVPGEENQFIAYVAYPLDLFEEG
FT                       SVTNLFTSIVGNVFGFKALRALRLEDLRIPPAYSKTFQGPPHGIQVERDKLNKYGRPLL
FT                       GCTIKPKLGLSAKNYGRAVYECLRGGLDFTKDDENVNSQPFMRWRDRFXFCAEAINKAQ
FT                       AETGEIKGHYLNATAGTCEEMMKRAVFARELGVPIVMHDXLTGGFTANTSLAHYCRDNG
FT                       LLLHIHRAMHAVIDRQRNHGMHFRVLAKALRMSGGDHIHAGTVVGKLEGERDVTLGFVD
FT                       XLRDDFIEKDRSRGIYFTQDWVSMPGVLPVASGGIHVWHMPALTEIFGDDSVLQFGGGT
FT                       LGHPWGNAPGAVANRVALEACVQARNEGRDLAREGNEVIRE"
XX
SQ    Sequence 1320 BP; 342 A; 260 C; 334 G; 375 T; 9 other;
```

Figure 2.4 Example of the biological feature annotation in an EMBL formatted entry

Data management and representation

Data are managed internally by the collaboration member databases in different ways. For example, the EMBL nucleotide sequence database is managed in a robust relational database management system (ORACLE), using a schema that facilitates integration and interoperability with other databases. Quarterly releases and daily updates of files are generated from this system.

Database entries are distributed in flat-file format, which is supported by most sequence analysis software packages and also provides a structure that is easy to read. The format is not shared amongst the different members of the collaboration, although all of them have a similar approach to the organization of the data in an entry, which can be divided into four major blocks of data.

1. Description and identifiers.

2. Citations: citation details of the associated publications and the name and contact details of the original submitters.

3. Features: detailed source information, biological features with their associated locations with reference to the sequence contained in the entry and associated qualifiers to offer more detailed and specific information over that feature.

4. Sequence: sequence length, base composition and sequence.

The databases produce user manuals and documentation to assist users in the interpretation of the information contained in the entries.

In addition to unique and stable accession numbers, nucleotide database entries include sequence identifiers in the form of version numbers that increment with every sequence update. Protein identifiers are also assigned to every coding sequence and are later used by protein databases such as Swiss-Prot and TrEMBL.

Integration between different biomolecular databases is essential to facilitate the extraction of knowledge from the data. In EMBL Release 79, the database included links to 17 external databases, including TrEMBL, Swiss-Prot, the Gene Ontology Annotation database (GOA) and other species-specific databases such as FlyBase (FlyBase Consortium, 2003) or MaizeDB.

The database is organized into separate divisions, with each entry belonging to one. Divisions are indicated using three letter codes, e.g. PRO, Prokaryotes; HUM, human. The grouping is based mainly on taxonomy with a few exceptions, such as the already discussed HTG, or the CON division. The CON database division represents CON(structed) or CON(tig) sequences of chromosomes, genomes or other long sequences constructed from segment entries (Stoesser et al., 2003).

Third party annotated data

The sequencing centres, which produce data in massive numbers, generally provide only computational analysis and predicted features. Scientists from other groups make use of these data for further experimental analysis, which generates biological knowledge about the sequences. The nucleotide sequence databases could not include this information without prior agreement from the group that had originally submitted the sequence.

To meet the growing need for an adequate repository to store this valuable information, the international collaboration of nucleotide databases has agreed to accept re-annotations/re-assemblies of sequences already present in DDBJ/EMBL/GenBank and owned by other groups to be included in the Third Party Annotation (TPA) data collection (Stoesser et al., 2003). Consensus sequences from multiple organisms are not accepted. TPA entries are derivative but the ownership principle of the primary data archive remains: the ownership of the data lies with the submitting scientist.

To ensure the quality of the data distributed by the database, only TPA entries that are published in a peer-reviewed journal are included in the public set. TPA entries include information about the contributing sequences, including base spans, accession and version numbers of the primary entry. This information appears in specific line types in the flat file and is validated by the recipient database prior to acceptance of the sequence.

2.3 Swiss-Prot

Introduction

The Swiss-Prot protein knowledgebase is an annotated protein sequence database that was established in 1986 and is maintained collaboratively by the European

Bioinformatics Institute (EBI) (http://www.ebi.ac.uk/swissprot/) and the Swiss Institute of Bioinformatics (SIB) (http://www.expasy.org/sprot/). The database has grown
steadily since its inception, with an average of almost 6500 new entries added each
year (Figure 2.5). Swiss-Prot contains data from a wide variety of organisms: as of
August 2004, release 44.2 contained 155 596 annotated sequence entries from almost
8500 different species.

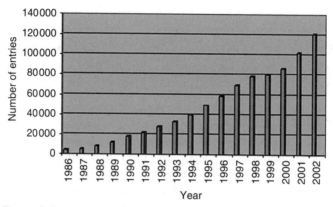

Figure 2.5   Growth of the Swiss-Prot protein sequence database

The database is non-redundant, which means that all reports for a given protein are
merged into a single entry, thus summarizing many pages of scientific literature into a
concise yet comprehensive report. Swiss-Prot also provides a high level of integration
with other databases. Cross-references are provided to other sequence databases as
well as to specialized data collections. Currently, there are cross-references to more
than 60 different databases (Gasteiger, Jung and Bairoch, 2001) and this allows users
to access a large amount of additional information related to a particular protein. The
Swiss-Prot database strives to provide a high level of annotation through a process of
literature-based manual curation and this allows the addition of as much accurate and
up-to-date information as possible about each protein. This includes descriptions of
properties such as function(s) of the protein, post-translational modifications,
domains and sites, secondary and quaternary structure, similarities to other proteins,
diseases associated with deficiencies in a protein, developmental stages in which the
protein is expressed, in which tissues the protein is found, pathways in which the
protein is involved and sequence conflicts and variants.

Entry format

The Swiss-Prot database consists of sequence entries (Figure 2.6) that are composed
of different line types, each line type having its own specified format. The large

```
ID   SPAS_MOUSE      STANDARD;      PRT;     504 AA.
AC   Q9QYY8;
DT   16-OCT-2001 (Rel. 40, Created)
DT   16-OCT-2001 (Rel. 40, Last sequence update)
DT   15-JUN-2002 (Rel. 41, Last annotation update)
DE   Spastin (Fragment).
GN   SPG4 OR SPAST.
OS   Mus musculus (Mouse).
OC   Eukaryota; Metazoa; Chordata; Craniata; Vertebrata; Euteleostomi;
OC   Mammalia; Eutheria; Rodentia; Sciurognathi; Muridae; Murinae; Mus.
OX   NCBI_TaxID=10090;
RN   [1]
RP   SEQUENCE FROM N.A.
RX   MEDLINE=20055425; PubMed=10610178;
RA   Hazan J., Fonknechten N., Mavel D., Paternotte C., Samson D.,
RA   Artiguenave F., Davoine C.S., Cruaud C., Durr A., Wincker P.,
RA   Brottier P., Cattolico L., Barbe V., Burgunder J.M., Prud'homme J.F.,
RA   Brice A., Fontaine B., Heilig R., Weissenbach J.;
RT   "Spastin, a new AAA protein, is altered in the most frequent form of
RT   autosomal dominant spastic paraplegia.";
RL   Nat. Genet. 23:296-303(1999).
CC   -!- FUNCTION: PROBABLE ATPASE INVOLVED IN THE ASSEMBLY OR FUNCTION OF
CC       NUCLEAR PROTEIN COMPLEXES.
CC   -!- SUBCELLULAR LOCATION: Nuclear.
CC   -!- TISSUE SPECIFICITY: Ubiquitous.
CC   -!- SIMILARITY: BELONGS TO THE AAA FAMILY OF ATPASES.
DR   EMBL; AJ246002; CAB60143.1; -.
DR   MGD; MGI:1858896; Spg4.
DR   InterPro; IPR003593; AAA_ATPase.
DR   InterPro; IPR003959; AAA_ATPase_centr.
DR   Pfam; PF00004; AAA; 1.
DR   SMART; SM00382; AAA; 1.
KW   ATP-binding; Nuclear protein.
FT   NON_TER       1      1
FT   NP_BIND     270    277       ATP (POTENTIAL).
SQ   SEQUENCE   504 AA;  55621 MW;  6B788BCAB4B4E47D CRC64;
     AESVRVFHKQ AFEYISIALR IDEEEKAGQK EQAVEWYKKG IEELEKGIAV IVTGQGEQYE
     RARRLQAKMM TNLVMAKDRL QLLEKLQPVL QFSKSQTDVY NESTNLTCRN GHLQSESGAV
     PKRKDPLTHA SNSLPRSKTV LKSGSAGLSG HHRAPSCSGL SMVSGARPGP GPAATTHKGT
     PKPNRTNKPS TPTTAVRKKK DLKNFRNVDS NLANLIMNEI VDNGTAVKFD DIAGQELAKQ
     ALQEIVILPS LRPELFTGLR APARGLLLFG PPGNGKTMLA KAVAAESNAT FFNISAASLT
     SKYVGEGEKL VRALFAVARE LQPSIIFIDE VDSLLCERRE GEHDASRRLK TEFLIEFDGV
     QSAGDDRVLV MGATNRPQEL DEAVLRRFIK RVYVSLPNEE TRLLLLKNLL CKQGSPLTQK
     ELAQLARMTD GYSGSDLTAL AKDAALGPIR ELKPEQVKNM SASEMRNIRL SDFTESLKKI
     KRSVSPQTLE AYIRWNKDFG DTTV
//
```

Figure 2.6   Example of a Swiss-Prot entry

numbers of different data types found in the databases are stored in a highly structured and uniform manner, which simplifies data access for users and data retrieval by computer programs. Swiss-Prot entries contain core data, which are generally provided by the submitter of the sequence. These consist of sequence data, citation information and taxonomic data that show the biological source of the protein. In addition, Swiss-Prot entries contain annotation that is added by a team of biologists during a process of literature-based curation and rigorous sequence analysis. The annotation added during this process is stored mainly in the description

(DE) and gene (GN) lines, the comment (CC) lines, the feature table (FT) lines and the keyword (KW) lines.

The description or DE line lists all the names by which a protein is known and includes standardized names assigned by official nomenclature bodies as well as Enzyme Commission numbers where applicable. An example of a Swiss-Prot description showing the main protein name, EC number and additional synonyms is shown below:

```
DE   Acid ceramidase precursor (EC 3.5.1.23) (Acylsphingosine
     deacylase)
DE   (N-acylsphingosine amidohydrolase) (AC) (Putative 32 KDA
     heart
DE   protein) (PHP32).
```

Table 2.1   Comment topics used in the Swiss-Prot database

Comment topic	Description
ALTERNATIVE PRODUCTS	Description of the existence of protein sequences produced by alternative splicing of the same gene or by the use of alternative initiation codons
BIOTECHNOLOGY	Description of the biotechnological use(s) of a protein
CATALYTIC ACTIVITY	Description of the reaction(s) catalyzed by an enzyme
CAUTION	Warns about possible errors and/or grounds for confusion
COFACTOR	Description of an enzyme cofactor
DATABASE	Description of a cross-reference to a database for a specific protein
DEVELOPMENTAL STAGE	Description of the developmental-specific expression of a protein
DISEASE	Description of disease(s) associated with a deficiency of a protein
DOMAIN	Description of the domain structure of a protein
ENZYME REGULATION	Description of an enzyme regulatory mechanism
FUNCTION	Description of the function(s) of a protein
INDUCTION	Description of compound(s) which stimulate the synthesis of a protein
MASS SPECTROMETRY	Reports the exact molecular weight of a protein or part of a protein as determined by mass spectrometric methods
MISCELLANEOUS	Any comment which does not belong to any of the other defined topics
PATHWAY	Description of the metabolic pathway(s) with which a protein is associated
PHARMACEUTICAL	Description of the use of a protein as a pharmaceutical drug
POLYMORPHISM	Description of polymorphism(s)
PTM	Description of a post-translational modification
SIMILARITY	Description of the similarity (sequence or structural) of a protein with other proteins
SUBCELLULAR LOCATION	Description of the subcellular location of the mature protein
SUBUNIT	Description of the quaternary structure of a protein
TISSUE SPECIFICITY	Description of the tissue specificity of a protein

To promote interoperability and cross-linking, Swiss-Prot carries over the unique gene identifiers assigned by genome sequencing projects. These are used in the Swiss-Prot databases to link to genome databases where possible. Where there are authoritative sources for gene names, such as the HUGO gene nomenclature committee (http://www.gene.ucl.ac.uk/nomenclature/), FlyBase or the Mouse Genome Database (MGD) (Blake *et al.*, 2003), these are used and linked.

The comment or CC lines are free text comments, which are used to convey any useful information about a protein. The information in the CC lines is contained in a number of defined topics that allow the easy retrieval of specific categories of data from the database. Although free text is permissible within the comments as this is often necessary to convey detailed and complex information about a protein, a number of comments have a standardized syntax. A list of the currently used comment topics and their definitions is shown in Table 2.1.

There are almost 553 000 comments in Swiss-Prot Release 44.2, with an average of three comments per entry. An example of the comment lines found in a single entry (Swiss-Prot Entry P14060) is shown below:

```
CC   -!- FUNCTION: 3BETA-HSD IS A BIFUNCTIONAL ENZYME, THAT
         CATALYZES THE
CC       OXIDATIVE CONVERSION OF DELTA(5)-ENE-3-BETA-HYDROXY
         STEROID, AND
CC       THE OXIDATIVE CONVERSION OF KETOSTEROIDS. THE 3BETA-
         HSD ENZYMATIC
CC       SYSTEM PLAYS A CRUCIAL ROLE IN THE BIOSYNTHESIS OF ALL
         CLASSES
CC       OF HORMONAL STEROIDS.
CC   -!- CATALYTIC ACTIVITY: 3-BETA-HYDROXY-DELTA-5-STEROID
         + NAD(+) =
CC       3-OXO-DELTA-5-STEROID + NADH (ACTS ON 3-BETA-HYDRO-
         XYANDROST-5-EN-
CC       17-ONE TO FORM ANDROST-4-ENE-3,17-DIONE AND ON 3-
         BETA-HYDROXYPREGN
CC       -5-EN-20-ONE TO FORM PROGESTERONE).
CC   -!- CATALYTIC ACTIVITY: A 3-OXO-DELTA(5)-STEROID = A 3-
         OXO-DELTA(4)-
CC       STEROID.
CC   -!- PATHWAY: STEROID BIOSYNTHESIS.
CC   -!- SUBCELLULAR LOCATION: ENDOPLASMIC RETICULUM AND
         MITOCHONDRIAL
CC       MEMBRANE-BOUND PROTEIN.
CC   -!- TISSUE SPECIFICITY: PLACENTA AND SKIN. PREDOMINANTLY
         EXPRESSED IN
CC       MAMMARY GLAND TISSUE.
CC   -!- DISEASE: CONGENITAL DEFICIENCY OF 3BETA-HSD ACTIVITY
         CAUSES A
```

```
CC       SEVERE  DEPLETION  OF  STEROID  FORMATION  FREQUENTLY
         LETHAL IN EARLY
CC       LIFE. THE CLASSICAL FORM OF THIS DISEASE INCLUDES THE
         ASSOCIATION
CC       OF SEVERE SALT-LOSING ADRENAL INSUFFICIENCY AND AMBI-
         GUITY OF
CC       EXTERNAL GENITALIA IN BOTH SEXES.
CC  -!-  SIMILARITY: BELONGS TO THE 3BETA-HSD FAMILY.
```

The feature table or FT lines provide position-specific data relating to the sequence. The lines have a fixed format and a defined set of feature keys that may be used. These feature keys describe domains and sites of interest within a sequence such as post-translationally modified residues, binding sites, enzyme active sites, secondary structure and any other regions of interest. The full list of currently defined feature keys is available in the Swiss-Prot user manual at http://www.expasy.ch/txt/ userman.txt There are 884 619 sequence features in Swiss-Prot Release 44.2 with an average of five features per entry.

The keywords are found in the keyword or KW lines of an entry. They serve as a subject reference for each sequence and assist in the retrieval of specific categories of data from the database. Swiss-Prot maintains a controlled keyword list, which currently contains approximately 840 keywords, each with a definition to clarify its biological meaning and intended usage. This list is available at http://www.expasy.org/ cgi-bin/keywlist.pl and is updated on a regular basis.

Manual annotation

Each entry in Swiss-Prot is thoroughly analysed and annotated by biologists to ensure a high standard of annotation and to maintain the quality of the database. A process of literature-based curation is used to extract experimental and validated data that will improve the content of the knowledgebase. This experimental knowledge is supplemented by manually confirmed results from various sequence analysis programs. At the time of annotation of a record, use is made of all relevant literature to ensure that the functional information included is complete and up to date. As new information arises, entries are updated so that they always reflect the current state of knowledge in the literature. A controlled list of journal names is maintained, using the journal abbreviations recommended by the National Library of Medicine (http:// www.expasy.org/cgi-bin/jourlist), and this ensures that they are added to the database in a standardized way.

The addition of a number of qualifiers in the comment and feature table lines during the annotation process allows users to distinguish between experimentally verified data, data which have been propagated from a characterized protein based on sequence similarity, and data for which no experimental evidence currently exists (Junker, Apweiler and Bairoch, 1999). The qualifiers currently in use are 'by similarity', which shows when information has been copied from a characterized entry, 'potential', which is used when there is no experimental evidence to support the data, 'probable', which is used when there is good reason to believe that a piece of information is true, or the absence of any qualifier, which shows that the information has been experimentally determined.

2.4 TrEMBL

To produce a fully curated Swiss-Prot entry is a highly labour-intensive process and is the rate-limiting step in the growth of the database. This is because, with the increased data flow from genome projects, new sequences are submitted more quickly than they can be manually annotated and integrated into the database. To address this, a supplement to Swiss-Prot was created in 1996 to fulfil the vital role of making new sequences available as quickly as possible while preventing the dilution of the high quality annotation found in Swiss-Prot. This supplement, TrEMBL (Translation of EMBL nucleotide sequence database), consists of computer-annotated entries derived from the translation of all coding sequences in the EMBL/GenBank/ DDBJ nucleotide sequence databases that are not yet included in Swiss-Prot. To ensure completeness, it also contains a number of protein sequences extracted from the literature or submitted directly by the user community.

Some data from DDBJ/EMBL/GenBank including most of the Whole Genome Shotgun (WGS) data, translations of pseudogenes, very small fragments, synthetic sequences, non-germline immunoglobulins and T-cell receptors, and most patent application sequences, are excluded from TrEMBL to prevent dilution of the database with highly unstable and low-quality data. However, these data are available in the UniProt archive (UniParc) (see below for a description of UniProt). TrEMBL has grown from 86 033 entries in release 1 of November 1996 to 1 333 917 records in release 27 of July 2004 with more than 75 000 different species represented in the database. TrEMBL follows the Swiss-Prot format and conventions described above as closely as possible.

The production of TrEMBL starts with the translation of coding sequences in the DDBJ/EMBL/GenBank nucleotide sequence database. At this stage, all annotation in a TrEMBL entry derives from the corresponding nucleotide entry. As there is a stringent requirement of minimal redundancy, which applies equally to Swiss-Prot and TrEMBL, the first post-processing step is to reduce redundancy by merging separate entries corresponding to different literature reports (O'Donovan et al., 1999). The second post-processing step is the automated enhancement of the information content in TrEMBL to bring the entries closer to Swiss-Prot standard (Apweiler, 2001). This process is based on a system of standardized transfer of annotation from well characterized proteins in Swiss-Prot to unannotated TrEMBL entries (Fleischmann et al., 1999) and its success is due to the fact that Swiss-Prot is a comprehensive, standardized database that distinguishes experimentally derived data from those which have been predicted computationally, as described above. This process brings the standard of annotation in TrEMBL closer to that found in Swiss-Prot through the addition of accurate, high quality information to TrEMBL entries, thus improving the quality of data available to the user.

2.5 PIR

Introduction

The PIR Protein Sequence Database (PIR-PSD) (Wu *et al.*, 2003) is a protein information resource initiated in 1961 by the National Biomedical Research Foundation (NBRF) and supported by the National Institutes of Health. It compiles comprehensive, non-redundant protein sequence data, organized by superfamily and family, and annotated with functional, structural, bibliographic and genetic data (Figure 2.7). In addition to the sequence data, the database contains the name and classification of the protein and the name of the organism in which it naturally occurs, references to the primary literature, function and general characteristics of the protein, sites and regions of biological interest within the sequence. The database is extensively cross-referenced with DDBJ/EMBL/GenBank nucleic acid and protein identifiers, PubMed/MedLine IDs and unique identifiers from many other source databases. In January 2003, the database contained more than 283 000 annotated and classified entries, covering the entire taxonomic range. These are organized into 36 000 superfamilies and over 100 000 families. The database is available from the PIR web site at http://pir.georgetown.edu/ and via FTP at ftp://ftp.pir.georgetown.edu/pir_databases/

Data processing

PIR-PSD data processing involves four major steps: import, merging, classification and annotation. The primary sources of PSD data are naturally occurring wild-type sequences from DDBJ/EMBL/GenBank translations, published literature and direct submission to PIR-International. Once imported, unique protein sequence reports are assigned an accession number and enter PIR-PSD for further merging, annotation and classification. The PIR-PSD has comprehensive coverage across the entire taxonomic range. To provide a truly non-redundant database, both identity and non-identity merges are performed to generate reliable reference sequences (the same protein from the same species) for annotation. The original sequences can be regenerated from residue lines in accession blocks nested within reference blocks.

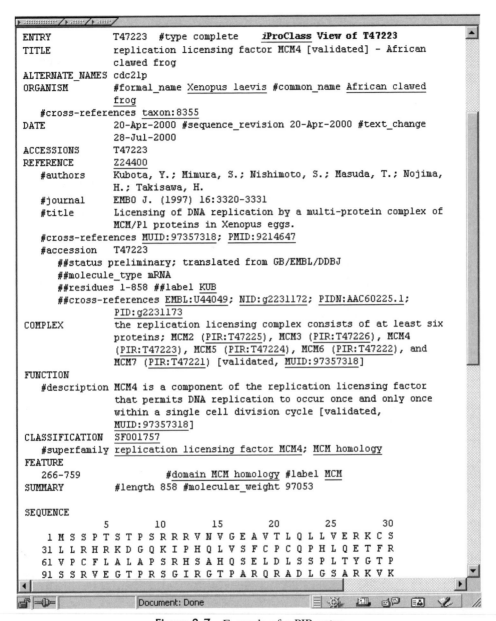

```
  ┌▶::::::::::::/ ▶:::::/ ▶:::::/
  ENTRY             T47223  #type complete      iProClass View of T47223       ▲
  TITLE             replication licensing factor MCM4 [validated] - African
                    clawed frog
  ALTERNATE_NAMES   cdc21p
  ORGANISM          #formal_name Xenopus laevis #common_name African clawed
                    frog
     #cross-references taxon:8355
  DATE              20-Apr-2000 #sequence_revision 20-Apr-2000 #text_change
                    28-Jul-2000
  ACCESSIONS        T47223
  REFERENCE         Z24400
     #authors       Kubota, Y.; Mimura, S.; Nishimoto, S.; Masuda, T.; Nojima,
                    H.; Takisawa, H.
     #journal       EMBO J. (1997) 16:3320-3331
     #title         Licensing of DNA replication by a multi-protein complex of
                    MCM/P1 proteins in Xenopus eggs.
     #cross-references MUID:97357318; PMID:9214647
     #accession     T47223
        ##status preliminary; translated from GB/EMBL/DDBJ
        ##molecule_type mRNA
        ##residues 1-858 ##label KUB
        ##cross-references EMBL:U44049; NID:g2231172; PIDN:AAC60225.1;
                    PID:g2231173
  COMPLEX           the replication licensing complex consists of at least six
                    proteins; MCM2 (PIR:T47225), MCM3 (PIR:T47226), MCM4
                    (PIR:T47223), MCM5 (PIR:T47224), MCM6 (PIR:T47222), and
                    MCM7 (PIR:T47221) [validated, MUID:97357318]
  FUNCTION
     #description MCM4 is a component of the replication licensing factor
                    that permits DNA replication to occur once and only once
                    within a single cell division cycle [validated,
                    MUID:97357318]
  CLASSIFICATION    SF001757
     #superfamily replication licensing factor MCM4; MCM homology
  FEATURE
     266-759                    #domain MCM homology #label MCM
  SUMMARY           #length 858 #molecular_weight 97053

  SEQUENCE
                    5         10        15        20        25        30
        1 M S S P T S T P S R R R V N V G E A V T L Q L L V E R K C S
       31 L L R H R K D G Q K I P H Q L V S F C P C Q P H L Q E T F R
       61 V P C F L A L A P S R H S A H Q S E L D L S S P L T Y G T P
       91 S S R V E G T P R S G I R G T P A R Q R A D L G S A R K V K  ▼
  ◀                                                                     ▶
  ┌─┐═◑═┐            Document: Done             ☰ ⚙ ▦ ◙ ▣ ✎
```

Figure 2.7   Example of a PIR entry

Annotation

PIR-PSD employs controlled vocabularies for most annotations and adopts standard nomenclature whenever applicable. The use of status tags such as 'validated' or 'similarity' in entry titles and function and complex annotations, as well as tags such as 'experimental', 'predicted', 'absent', or 'atypical' in feature annotations helps in distinguishing experimental from predicted data. Rule-based and classification-driven procedures are used to propagate annotations among similar sequences and to perform integrity checks based on PIR controlled vocabulary and thesaurus of synonyms or alternative names.

Family classification

Protein family classification is central to the organization and annotation of PIR-PSD. A unique characteristic of the PIR-PSD is its non-overlapping classification of full length protein sequences based on the superfamily concept developed by Margaret O. Dayhoff (1976). Automated procedures have allowed the placement of more than 99 per cent of sequences into families and more than 70 per cent into superfamilies. Sequences in PIR-PSD are also classified with homology domains and sequence motifs. Homology domains, which are shared by more than one superfamily, may constitute evolutionary building blocks, while sequence motifs represent functional sites or conserved regions. The classification approach improves the sensitivity of protein identification, helps to detect and correct genome annotation errors systematically and allows a more complete understanding of sequence-function–structure relationships.

2.6 UniProt

With the recent accumulation of genome sequences for many organisms, most notably the draft human sequence, attention is now turning to the identification and function of proteins encoded by these genomes. This means that complete and up-to-date protein databases are vital for the increasingly information-dependent biological and biotechnological research. With the increasing volume and variety of protein sequences and functional information, a central database of protein sequence and function is essential for a wide range of scientists active in modern biological research, particularly in the field of proteomics. Swiss-Prot, TrEMBL and PIR currently provide different coverages of protein sequences with varying types of information annotated in each database. However, a single central resource would ensure that scientists receive rich and non-redundant information at one location. To achieve this goal, the Swiss-Prot, TrEMBL and PIR databases have recently joined forces to form the United Protein Databases (UniProt). This project will be funded by the US National Human Genome Research Institute, in cooperation with five other institutes and centres at the National Institutes of Health. The UniProt website can be accessed at www.uniprot.org

The broad, long term objective of UniProt is to create, maintain and provide a stable, comprehensive, fully classified, richly and accurately annotated protein sequence knowledgebase, with extensive cross-references and querying interfaces, which will build upon the foundations laid down by the three UniProt consortium members. This will involve the development and maintainance of a central database of curated protein sequences with annotations of sequence and functional information, facilitating use of the database by providing user-friendly interfaces and tools for queries and for retrieval of large datasets and the flexibility and adaptability needed to be responsive to the changing needs of the scientific community. The UniProt website can be accessed at www.uniprot.org

References

Apweiler, R. (2001). Functional Information in Swiss-Prot: the basis for large-scale characterisation of protein sequences. *Briefings Bioinformat.* **2**, 9–18.

Benson, D.A., Karsch-Mizrachi, I., Lipman, D.J., Ostell, J. and Wheeler, D.L. (2003). GenBank. *Nucleic Acids Res.* **31**, 23–27.

Blake, J.A., Richardson, J.E., Bult, C.J., Kadin, J.A. and Eppig J.T. (2003). MGD: the mouse genome database. *Nucleic Acids Res.* **31**, 193–195.

Boeckmann, B., Bairoch, A., Apweiler, R., Blatter, M., Estreicher, A., Gasteiger, E., Martin, M. J., Michoud, K., O'Donovan, C., Phan, I., Pilbout, S. and Schneider, M. (2003). The Swiss-Prot protein knowledgebase and its supplement TrEMBL in 2003. *Nucleic Acids Res.* **31**, 365–370.

Brunak, S., Danchin, A., Hattori, M., Nakamura, H., Shinozaki, K., Matise, T. and Preuss D. (2002). Nucleotide sequence database policies. *Science* **298**, 1333.

Dayhoff, M.O. (1976). The origin and evolution of protein superfamilies. *Fed. Proc.* **35**, 2132–2138.

Fleischmann, W., Moeller, S., Gateau, A. and Apweiler, R. (1999). A novel method for automatic and reliable functional annotation. *Bioinformatics* **15**, 228–233.

FlyBase Consortium. (2003). The FlyBase database of the *Drosophila* genome projects and community literature. *Nucleic Acids Res.* **31**, 172–175.

Gasteiger, E., Jung, E. and Bairoch, A. (2001). SWISS-PROT: connecting biomolecular knowledge via a protein database. *Curr. Issues Mol. Biol.* **3**, 47–55.

Junker, V., Apweiler, R. and Bairoch, A. (1999). Representation of functional information in the Swiss-Prot data bank. *Bioinformatics* **15**, 1066–1067.

Kersey, P., Hermjakob, H. and Apweiler, R. (2000). VARSPLIC: alternatively-spliced protein sequences derived from Swiss-Prot and TrEMBL. *Bioinformatics* **16**, 1048–1049.

Lefranc, M.P. (2003). IMGT, the international ImMunoGeneTics database. *Nucleic Acids Res.* **31**, 307–310.

O'Donovan, C., Martin, M.J., Glemet, E., Codani, J. and Apweiler, R. (1999). Removing redundancy in Swiss-Prot and TrEMBL. *Bioinformatics* **15**, 258–259.

Praz, V., Périer, R.C., Bonnard, C. and Bucher P. (2002). The eukaryotic promoter database, EPD: new entry types and links to gene expression data. *Nucleic Acids Res.* **30**, 322–324.

Pruitt, K.D., Tatusova, T. and Maglott, D.R. (2003). NCBI Reference Sequence Project: update and current status. *Nucleic Acids Res.* **31**, 4–37.

Stoesser, G., Baker, W., van den Broek, A., Camon, E., Garcia-Pastor, M., Kanz, C., Kulikova, T., Leinonen, R., Lin, Q., Lombard, V., Lopez, R., Redaschi, N., Stoehr, P., Tuli, MA., Tzouvara, K. and Vaughan, R. (2002). The EMBL Nucleotide Sequence Database. *Nucleic Acids Res.* **30**, 21–26.

Stoesser, G., Baker, W., van den Broek, A., Garcia-Pastor, M., Kanz, C., Kulikova, T., Leinonen, R., Lin, Q., Lombard, V., Lopez, R., Mancuso, R., Nardone, F., Stoehr, P., Tuli, M.A., Tzouvara, K. and Vaughan, R. (2003). The EMBL Nucleotide Sequence Database: major new developments. *Nucleic Acids Res.* **31**, 17–22.

Tateno, Y. and Gojobori, T. (1996). DNA data bank of Japan in the age of information biology. *Nucleic Acids Res.* **25**, 14–17.

Westbrook, J., Feng, Z., Chen, L., Yang, H. and Berman, H.M. (2003). The protein data bank and structural genomics. *Nucleic Acids. Res.* **31**, 489–491.

Wu, C.H., Yeh, L.S., Huang, H., Arminski, L., Castro-Alvear, J., Chen, Y., Hu, Z., Kourtesis, P., Ledley, R.S., Suzek, B.E., Vinayaka, C.R., Zhang, J. and Barker, W.C. (2003). The protein information resource. *Nucleic Acids Res.* **31**, 345–347.

3 Survey of Sequence Databases: Derived Databases

M. Pruess, N. Mulder and **R. Apweiler**

Abstract

Data derived from primary nucleotide and protein sequence databases can be used to develop new resources, in which information from different databases is combined. In most of these resources, additional software and/or annotation are added to the data, much to the benefit of the users. Protein and gene family databases describe in detail subsets of sequences, with specific value-added information, while clustering databases cluster sequences to identify relations between them. Protein signature databases help to assign certain properties to sequences by detecting specific domains, and integrated derived databases integrate results from these different resources, thus combining their individual strengths. The general purposes of derived databases are to assist in elucidation of protein function and to provide the means for organized storage and display of known biological information. They also make valuable contributions to the annotation of newly sequenced genomes and large-scale protein function prediction.

Keywords

bioinformatics, database, protein signature, protein domains, protein family, protein function, annotation, proteome analysis, proteomics

3.1 Introduction

Sequence databases are comprehensive sources of information on nucleotide and protein sequences. The most important sequence databases are the DDBJ/EMBL/ GenBank Nucleotide Sequence Database (Stoesser *et al.*, 2003), the Swiss-Prot/

Database Annotation in Molecular Biology   Edited by Arthur M. Lesk
© 2005 John Wiley & Sons, Ltd.   ISBN: 0-470-85681-5

TrEMBL Protein Knowledgebase (Boeckmann *et al.*, 2003) and the PIR International Protein Sequence Database (Barker *et al.*, 2000). These databases are described in detail in the previous chapter, 'Survey of Sequence Databases: Archival Projects'. But it is not only the information in these resources that is of use for the scientific community. Parts of the data in the sequence databases can be used to build up new resources by combining information from different databases and adding additional value by applying certain programs and/or additional annotation. These new resources can either describe in detail a subset of sequences, with added specific information, as databases about certain protein and gene families do, or they can cluster sequences to find relations between them, or help to assign certain properties to sequences by detecting specific domains or motifs. Information about the family a protein may belong to, or about its functional domains, is especially useful for the identification and characterization of newly sequenced proteins, and of sequences derived from the large scale sequencing projects where no function is known.

Model organism databases (MODs) also belong to the group of derived databases, since they gather data from different classes of databases – not limited to primary data such as genomic sequences – and are very comprehensive. FlyBase (a database of

Table 3.1   List of all databases described in this chapter, and their URLs

Resource	Database (short name)	URL
Protein and gene family databases	MEROPS	http://www.merops.ac.uk
	CAZy	http://afmb.cnrs-mrs.fr/~cazy/CAZY/
	TC-DB	http://tcdb.ucsd.edu/tcdb/
	TRANSFAC	http://www.gene-regulation.com/pub/databases. html#transfac
	EPD	http://www.epd.isb-sib.ch/
Clustering databases	CluSTr	http://www.ebi.ac.uk/clustr
	COG	http://www.ncbi.nlm.nih.gov/COG/
	ProDom	http://prodes.toulouse.inra.fr/prodom/2002.1/html/ home.php
	SYSTERS	http://systers.molgen.mpg.de/
	ProtoMap	http://protomap.cornell.edu/
Protein signature databases	PROSITE	http://ca.expasy.org/prosite/
	PRINTS	http://www.bioinf.man.ac.uk/dbbrowser/PRINTS/
	Pfam	http://www.sanger.ac.uk/Software/Pfam/
	SMART	http://smart.embl-heidelberg.de/
	TIGRFAMs	http://www.tigr.org/TIGRFAMs/
	BLOCKS	http://blocks.fhcrc.org
Integrated derived databases	MetaFam	http://metafam.ahc.umn.edu/
	iProClass	http://pir.georgetown.edu/iproclass/
	CDD	http://www.ncbi.nlm.nih.gov/Structure/cdd/cdd.shtml
	InterPro	http://www.ebi.ac.uk/interpro/

genetic and molecular data for *Drosophila*) and the Mouse Genome Informatics (MGI) database, for example, not only present the nucleotide sequences, but also contain lists of genomic clones and information about natural and engineered transposons and other molecular constructs.

Therefore there are archival biological databases available, databases derived from these and even databases that use specific data from derived databases to provide different views and new possibilities of data analyses. In this chapter, some examples of different types of derived database are presented. All databases described in this chapter and their URLs are shown in Table 3.1.

3.2 Protein and Gene Family Databases

The major sequence databases aim at providing the known nucleotide or amino acid sequences of all species. To present detailed data about certain protein or gene families, subject- and function-specific compendia derived from the major sequence databases are available. They organize specific information and online tools concerning families, which are of particular importance in medicine or biotechnology. Usually these databases provide the protein or gene sequences and additional information about them, such as their role in metabolism. Classification is often an important focus.

Three examples for protein family databases are MEROPS (Rawlings, O'Brien and Barrett, 2002), CAZy (Coutinho and Henrissat, 1999) and TC-DB (Saier, 2000); TRANSFAC (Matys *et al.*, 2003) provides information about both genes and proteins involved in the process of transcription, and EPD (Praz *et al.*, 2002) is a database about a certain class of nucleotide sequences.

MEROPS

MEROPS (Rawlings, O'Brien and Barrett, 2002) is a protease database that provides a catalogue and a structure-based classification of proteases – called 'peptidases' within the database – which account for about two per cent of all proteins. The information in the database is structured into 'cards'. PepCards are a set of files, each of which provides information on classification and nomenclature for a single protease. Also provided is an interface to the relevant entries in databases for human genetics, amino acid and nucleotide sequences and tertiary structures.

The proteases are classified into families on the basis of statistically significant similarities between the protein sequences in the part termed the 'peptidase unit' that is most directly responsible for activity. Families that are thought to have common evolutionary origins because they have similar tertiary folds are grouped into 'clans'. The MEROPS database provides sets of pages called FamCards and ClanCards describing the individual families and clans. Each FamCard page provides links to other databases of sequence motifs and secondary and tertiary structures, and shows the distribution of the family across the major kingdoms of living creatures, a sequence alignment and a cladogram.

MEROPS allows a variety of searches and contains representations of three-dimensional structures of protease molecules. It additionally includes alignments and data tables for ESTs for human, mouse and rat peptidases. MEROPS is linked at the protease level amongst others to Swiss-Prot, TrEMBL and PIR, and at the family level to CATH, Pfam, PROSITE and SCOP, which will be described later on in this chapter.

CAZy

The CAZy database of carbohydrate-active enzymes (Coutinho and Henrissat, 1999) describes the families of structurally related catalytic and carbohydrate-binding modules (or functional domains) of enzymes that degrade, modify or create glycosidic bonds. Data are structured according to enzyme functional family and organism. CAZy is linked to GenBank, Swiss-Prot and PDB, the Protein Data Bank (Westbrook et al., 2003).

TC-DB

TC-DB, the Transport Protein Database (Saier, 2000), provides a functional–phylogenetic classification system for membrane transport proteins known as the Transport Commission (TC) system. The TC system is analogous to the Enzyme Commission (EC) system for the classification of enzymes, except that it incorporates both functional and phylogenetic information. Transport systems serve the cell in numerous capacities, for example in metabolism, regulation of metabolite concentrations, mediating the active extrusion of drugs and other toxic substances from either the cytoplasm or the plasma membrane, mediating uptake and efflux of ionic species that must be maintained at certain concentrations, secretion of macromolecules, which play a variety of biologically important roles, secreting toxins and the uptake and release of signalling molecules.

The TC-DB classification system is based on transporter class and subclass (mode of transport and energy coupling mechanism), protein phylogenetic family and subfamily and substrate specificity. Descriptions, TC numbers and examples of families of transport proteins are provided. Data sources of TC-DB are Swiss-Prot, TrEMBL and Pfam.

TRANSFAC

TRANSFAC (Matys et al., 2003) is a database on eukaryotic transcriptional regulation. This process is regulated in a complex way, through an intricate system of mutual interactions of transcription factors, whose effects – activation or repression of transcription – are mediated via DNA-binding sites on their target genes. TRANSFAC comprises protein sequences and other data on transcription factors, on their target genes and on experimentally proven regulatory binding sites, which are usually relatively short DNA elements of about 5–25 bp. Transcription factors are grouped into classes according to their DNA-binding domain, and a hierarchical factor classification system has been developed.

The database aims at the modelling of factor–site interactions, for a better understanding of how genes are regulated. A further intention is to explain the tissue specific expression of genes with the help of specific expression patterns of the regulating transcription factors. Search tools help to find potential binding sites for transcription factors in DNA sequences, using single site sequences or a library of weight matrices, derived from these sites, respectively. TRANSFAC is linked to the EMBL nucleotide sequence database and Swiss-Prot for the sequences, and to PROSITE for factor classes.

EPD

The Eukaryotic Promoter Database (EPD) (Praz *et al.*, 2002) is another resource that deals with eukaryotic transcription regulation, but it is even more specialized than TRANSFAC, and is restricted to a certain type of nucleotide sequence. EPD is a collection of promoters recognized by the RNA Pol II system of higher eukaryotes (multicellular plants and animals), gene regions immediately upstream of a transcription initiation site; for all promoters in the database the transcription start site has been determined experimentally. The main purpose of the database is to keep track of experimental data that define transcription initiation sites of eukaryotic genes. This type of functional information is linked to promoter sequences, to which access is provided by pointers to positions in nucleotide sequence entries.

EPD is linked to the EMBL nucleotide sequence database, Swiss-Prot, TRANS-FAC and other databases. In the near future, EPD plans to process data directly submitted from genome and cDNA sequence centres, including promoter sets contributed by the *Drosophila* genome annotation team and by collaborators from the Mammalian Gene Collection (MGC) (Strausberg *et al.*, 1999) and NEDO full-length cDNA sequencing projects (Suzuki *et al.*, 2001).

Clustering databases

With sequencing projects producing large amounts of data lacking functional characterization, there is an increasing need for automated sequence analysis procedures to predict molecular functions and biological roles for the predicted gene products. One approach is to pre-process a protein database into sets of homologous proteins (i.e. proteins that have evolved from the same ancestor) and use derived information for further analysis.

Most approaches for the tentative assignment of functions to predicted proteins are based on pair-wise sequence similarity searches against known proteins using sequence comparison programs such as FASTA (Pearson and Lipman, 1988) and BLAST (Altschul *et al.*, 1990). Sequence-cluster databases are derived automatically from sequence databases using different clustering algorithms. Since they do not depend on manual crafting or validation of family discriminators, these databases are relatively comprehensive although the biological relevance of clusters can be ambiguous and can sometimes be an artefact of particular thresholds (Kriventseva, Biswas and Apweiler, 2001).

CluSTr

The CluSTr (Clusters of Swiss-Prot and TrEMBL proteins) database (Kriventseva, Servant and Apweiler, 2003) offers an automatic classification of Swiss-Prot and TrEMBL proteins into groups of related proteins. The clustering is based on analysis of all pair-wise sequence comparisons between proteins using the Smith–Waterman algorithm (Smith and Waterman, 1981). A Monte Carlo simulation, resulting in a Z-score (Comet *et al.*, 1999), is used to estimate the statistical significance of raw Smith–Waterman scores between potentially related proteins. Clustering is carried out at different levels of protein similarity, yielding a hierarchical organization of the protein groups. The database provides links to InterPro (see below), HSSP, the Homology-Derived Secondary Structure of Proteins database (Holm and Sander, 1999) and the PDB.

COG

The database of Clusters of Orthologous Groups of proteins (COGs) (Tatusov *et al.*, 2001) provides a phylogenetic classification of proteins encoded in complete genomes. Each COG includes proteins that are thought to be orthologous, i.e. connected through vertical evolutionary descent. Orthology may involve not only one-to-one, but also, in cases of lineage-specific gene duplications, one-to-many and many-to-many relationships (hence orthologous groups of proteins). The purpose of the COG database is to serve as a platform for functional annotation of newly sequenced genomes and for studies on genome evolution. In order to facilitate functional studies, the COGs have been classified into four broad functional categories, information storage and processing, cellular processes, metabolism and poorly characterized. Each of these categories contains a number of sub-categories.

ProDom

ProDom (Servant *et al.*, 2002) provides automated analysis of protein domains. It assumes that the shortest full length sequence in the Swiss-Prot and TrEMBL database is single domain proteins and uses PSI-BLAST (Altschul *et al.*, 1997) to find the homologous domains that are then clustered in the same ProDom entry. The sequences that hit form a new ProDom domain family and are removed from the protein database. The remaining sequences are once again sorted by size, and the smallest sequence is used as a query sequence. This process is repeated until there are no more sequences in the protein database. In this way ProDom groups all the non-fragment sequences in Swiss-Prot and TrEMBL into more than 150 000 families. The consistency of a family is measured using the diameter (maximal distance between two domains in a family) and radius of gyration (root mean square of distance between domain and family consensus), both counted in PAM (percent accepted mutations – number per 100 aa). The lower these values, the more homogeneous the family. An interactive graphical interface allows for the navigation between schematic domain arrangements, multiple alignments, phylogenetic trees, Swiss-Prot entries, PROSITE patterns, Pfam-A families (Bateman *et al.*, 2002) and 3D structures in the PDB. Alignments and trees can be reduced or developed to facilitate the analysis of sequence relationships within large domain families.

SYSTERS

SYSTERS (SYSTEmatic Re-Searching, Krause, Stoye and Vingron, 2000) classifies the whole of Swiss-Prot and PIR into disjoint protein family clusters, which are then related hierarchically as family and superfamily clusters. The database applies iterative gapped BLAST searches to cluster the proteins. For each seed protein, all BLAST hits higher than a pre-set threshold are retained and the lowest scoring sequence is used for the next query. The process repeats until no new sequences above the cut-off value are found. The clusters are available for searching using the SSMAL search tool, BLAST or FASTA. A multiple sequence alignment for each cluster is generated and, where possible, may be annotated using Pfam domains (Pfam is described below). Additional search facilities allow querying of the database by cluster number, organism, protein accession number, keywords etc. It is therefore possible to use SYSTERS to classify a query protein sequence on the family and superfamily levels, and retrieve additional functional information from the databases from which the clusters are derived.

ProtoMap

ProtoMap is an automatic hierarchical classification of all Swiss-Prot and TrEMBL proteins that works with complete protein sequences. The classification is based on analysis of all pairwise similarities among protein sequences, combining Smith–Waterman, FASTA, and BLAST searches with two different scoring matrices (blosum 50 and blosum 62) to create an exhaustive list of neighbouring sequences. The analysis makes essential use of transitivity to identify homologies among proteins.

Within each group of the classification, every two members are either directly or transitively related. A statistical algorithm is used to identify groups of possibly related clusters. Within these groups clusters are interactively merged when the similarity between the closest clusters is higher than the threshold. The classification is done at different levels of confidence, and results in a hierarchical organization of all the proteins. The ProtoMap database aims at serving as a complementary tool for sequence analysis, and at helping to elucidate new relationships that might not be discovered by other methods (Yona, Linial and Linial, 2000).

Protein signature databases

There are currently (July 2004) over 1 520 000 protein sequences in the Swiss-Prot and TrEMBL Protein Knowledgebases alone, and this number is increasing exponentially as more genome sequencing projects emerge and develop. More than 150 000 of these are in Swiss-Prot and therefore have been manually curated, although many of these are annotated as 'hypothetical protein'. Needless to say there is an overabundance of proteins in the knowledgebase that are as yet uncharacterized, and this number is increasing. Some methods and derived databases that attempt to group related proteins, ultimately to help with function elucidation, have already been described above. While sequence clustering methods and FASTA or BLAST searches are useful for grouping or identifying related proteins, these methods have their limitations. Sequence clustering methods are automated and thus provide little or no additional biological information about a query protein. These and sequence similarity searches are not optimal for identifying distantly related proteins, and may incur problems with multi-domain proteins.

These drawbacks were tackled by protein signature databases, which use different methods to create signatures diagnostic for protein families, domains or functional sites. All of these databases are themselves derived from the protein sequence databases. Protein sequences belonging to a family are used in multiple sequence alignments, which form the base from which a signature is derived. From one sequence it is difficult to identify important sites in the protein; however, from a number of related sequences in an alignment it is possible to create a consensus for protein families, or identify conserved domains or highly conserved residues that may be important for function, e.g. an active site. These conserved areas of a protein family, domain or functional site can be used to recreate identifiable features using several different methods. There are many protein signature databases in the public domain, some of which use similar methods for signature creation, but are driven by different ultimate goals. The methods primarily used are hidden Markov models (HMMs), profiles and regular expressions, and the major databases using these methods, PROSITE (Falquet et al., 2002), PRINTS (Attwood et al., 2003), Pfam (Bateman et al., 2002), SMART (Letunic et al., 2002), TIGRFAMs (Haft, Selengut and White, 2003) and Blocks (Henikoff et al., 2000) are described in more detail below.

PROSITE

PROSITE (Falquet *et al.*, 2002) is a database of patterns and profiles. PROSITE patterns are built from sequence alignments of related sequences taken from a variety of sources, e.g. from a well characterized protein family or derived from the literature. The alignments are checked for conserved regions, which may have been experimentally shown to be involved in the catalytic activity or to bind a substrate. A core pattern is created in the form of a regular expression, which specifies which amino acid may occur at each position. In this regular expression, where a position is conserved throughout the alignment, only one amino acid is specified; however, it may be that one of two amino acids may occur at a position, and this is described symbolically by [AC], which suggests that this position may be occupied by either alanine (A) or cysteine (C). An x is used to indicate that any amino acid may occur for this or more than one position (x(3)), and curly brackets { } are used to indicate which amino acids may not occur at a given position. As an example, the pattern [AC]–x–V–x(4)–{ED} describes a region of sequence where position 1 is occupied by A or C, position 2 may be any amino acid, position 3 is a valine (V), positions 4 to 7 may be occupied by any amino acid, and position 8 may be any amino acid except glutamic acid (E) or aspartic acid (D). Once a core pattern has been identified, this is tested against the sequences in Swiss-Prot. If the correct set of proteins match this pattern then it is kept; if it fails to pick up some family members or picks up too many unrelated proteins, the pattern is refined and retested until it is optimized.

Patterns have many advantages, but they also have their limitations across whole sequences, which is why PROSITE also creates profiles for their database to complement the patterns. A profile is built starting with multiple sequence alignments, and using a symbol comparison table to convert residue frequency distributions into weights, resulting in a table of position specific amino acid weights and gap costs (Gribskov, Luthy and Eisenberg, 1990). In other words, profiles are matrices describing the probability of finding an amino acid at a given position in the sequence. The numbers in the table (scores) are used to calculate similarity scores between a profile and a sequence for a given alignment. For each set of sequences a threshold score is calculated so that only sequences scoring above this threshold are true matches (considered to be related to the original set of sequences in the alignment). The profile is tested against sequences in Swiss-Prot, and the profile is refined until only the intended set of protein sequences scores above the threshold score for the profile. Profiles produced by the PROSITE database begin as preliminary profiles, and once they have been tested and approved they become integrated as new members of the database.

PRINTS

The PRINTS database (Attwood *et al.*, 2003) uses fingerprints as diagnostic signatures, a variation on the profile method described above. A fingerprint is a group of conserved motifs, which characterizes a protein family. Instead of focusing on a single conserved area, the occurrence of multiple small conserved areas across the sequence alignment is taken into account. The starting point in the fingerprinting process is a curated multiple sequence alignment. Conserved regions within this alignment are excised as motifs, which are used to scan a protein sequence database. The scanning algorithm interprets the motifs essentially as a series of frequency matrices: identity searches are made, with no mutation or other similarity data to weight the results. Diagnostic performance is enhanced by iterative database scanning. The motifs therefore grow in size and become more mature with each database pass as more sequences are matched and assimilated into the process. Sequences, which match all motifs in order, are considered to be true fingerprint matches. Additional potency is gained from the mutual context provided by motif neighbours, which allows sequence identification even when parts of the signature are absent. Many fingerprints have been created to identify proteins at the superfamily as well as the family and subfamily levels. Consequently, many of the fingerprints are related to each other in an ordered, hierarchical structure, although each motif set is unique for the superfamily, family or subfamily that it represents.

Pfam

There are a number of protein signature databases that use HMMs instead of patterns or profiles. HMMs are like profiles but with a more complex probabilistic scoring mechanism. Pfam (Bateman *et al.*, 2002) is a collection of multiple protein sequence alignments and HMMs, and provides a good resource of models for identifying protein families, domains and repeats. There are two parts to the Pfam database, PfamA, which is a set of manually curated and annotated models, and PfamB, which has higher coverage, but is fully automated with no manual curation. PfamB is created from automatic clustering of the protein sequences in Swiss-Prot and TrEMBL by ProDom. The Pfams are coverage driven and strive to include the largest families they do not already have. Where possible their domains are based on 3D structure knowledge of the proteins. Pfam provides additional information on its website, including information on the taxonomic range of each domain, and links to other databases.

SMART

The SMART database (a Simple Modular Architecture Research Tool) (Letunic *et al.*, 2002) produces HMMs that facilitate the identification and annotation of genetically mobile domains and the analysis of domain architectures. The database is highly populated with models for domains found in signalling, extracellular and chromatin-associated proteins. The models rely on hand-curated multiple sequence alignments of representative family members based on tertiary structures where possible, otherwise those found by PSI-BLAST (Altschul *et al.*, 1997). Once the models are created they are used to search the database for additional members to be included in the sequence alignment. This iterative process is repeated until no further homologues are detected. Like Pfam, SMART also provides information on the taxonomic range of each domain.

TIGRFAMs

TIGRFAMs (Haft *et al.*, 2003) creates HMMs, which group homologous proteins that are conserved with respect to function. The models are produced in a similar way to those in Pfam and SMART, but should only hit equivalogues, i.e. proteins that have been shown to have the same function. The TIGRFAMs project currently consists of over 1000 HMMs, of which a large proportion are of type 'equivalog' (conserved function) and make strong predictions of known conserved protein function. TIGR-FAMs have a strong focus on microbial genomes driven by the projects at TIGR to annotate newly sequenced microbial genomes. The database has specific strengths in enzyme and transport protein families.

Blocks

Blocks (Henikoff *et al.*, 2000) is a collection of multiply aligned ungapped segments corresponding to the most highly conserved regions of proteins. These alignments are represented in profiles, built up using a tool called PROTOMAT (Henikoff and Henikoff, 1991). The profiles are calibrated against the Swiss-Prot database, and the LAMA software tool (Pietrokovski, 1996) is used to search new blocks against existing blocks.

Integrated derived databases

Many of the derived databases described above have interactions and exchange of data between them. PfamB, for example, uses ProDom families as a starting point for its automatically built HMMs. Blocks previously used alignments from PROSITE, Prints, PfamA and ProDom as a starting point for the creation of the Blocks database, and now uses InterPro, an integration of these databases (described below). Each method has its own advantages; for example, patterns are relatively simple to build, and are very useful for small regions of conserved amino acids such as active sites or binding sites, but fail to provide information about the rest of the sequence, and due to the constraints on which amino acids may be found in a given area of the sequence, patterns fail to pick up related sequences with a small divergence in that particular area. Profiles and HMMs compensate for these shortcomings in that they generally cover larger areas of the sequence, and since all amino acids have a chance of occurring at a given position, albeit with a lower probability or score, more divergent family members may still be included in the match list.

The big question is which database to use, and how to integrate results from the different databases which all have their own formats and outputs. A solution has been provided by several groups, which have made an effort to integrate these derived databases into a single coherent protein signature resource. The integrated database resources include MetaFam (Silverstein *et al.*, 2001), iProClass (Wu *et al.*, 2001), CDD (Wheeler *et al.*, 2001) and InterPro (Mulder *et al.*, 2003).

MetaFam

MetaFam (Silverstein *et al.*, 2001) is a protein family classification system that automatically creates supersets of overlapping families from Blocks+, DOMO, Pfam, PIR-ALN, Prints, PROSITE, ProDom and SBASE using set theory to compare these databases. In the first step MetaFam produces a non-redundant protein sequence set, which is then used to determine protein sets for each family from the member databases. A pairwise correspondence for each pair of families between two databases is measured. When the intersection of two families from different databases is more significant than any other family pairings then these two families form a match. These 'matches', or two-way correspondences, are then clustered into super-sets grouping related family pairs. Some families may not cover the whole protein sequence, while others do, therefore some families may occur in multiple supersets. The domain members of the superset are the unions of all members of the constituent families. A set of reference domains, calculated using similar algorithms and covering the total area, is provided for use in certain applications. In this way MetaFam provides a method for functional classification of proteins, and has high coverage due to the extensive list of databases included, but has limitations in the fact that the procedure is automated and not manually curated by biologists.

iProClass

iProClass (Wu *et al.*, 2001) links ProClass, PIR-ALN, PROSITE, Pfam and Blocks into a single database providing family relationships and structural features of protein sequences. ProClass is a protein family database that integrates PIR superfamilies and PROSITE. iProClass is derived from protein sequences in PIR and Swiss-Prot, and is organized into different components: the ClassSeQuence (CSQ), which describes the protein sequence entries; the ClassSuperFamily (CSF), ClassDoMain (CDM) and ClassMoTif (CMT), which define family relationships at the superfamily, domain and motif levels, and the ClassFuNction (CFN) and ClassSTructure (CST), which describe protein function and structure. iProClass provides an automatic means for classifying proteins at all these different levels of information.

CDD

CDD (Wheeler *et al.*, 2001) is a database of domains derived from SMART, Pfam and contributions from NCBI LOAD (Library Of Ancient Domains). CDD uses a reverse-position BLAST algorithm to identify conserved domains in protein sequences. Query sequences are compared with the resulting position-specific score matrix. Each CDD entry provides a description of the protein family or domain and a consensus reference sequence, with additional protein examples. Where possible 3D structure information is provided, as well as options for launching applications for creating alignments and sequence similarity searches. The Domain Architecture Retrieval Tool (DART) provided within CDD facilitates identification of sequences with the same domain architecture.

InterPro

InterPro (Mulder *et al.*, 2003) integrates diagnostic protein signatures from PRO-SITE, PRINTS, Pfam, ProDom, SMART and TIGRFAMs. Signatures from the different databases that describe the same protein family, domain, repeat or post-translational modification (PTM) are integrated into a single InterPro entry with a unique InterPro accession number. The guidelines for integration are that the signatures must overlap, at least in part, in position on the protein sequence; they should have at least 75 per cent overlap in the protein match lists and they must all describe the same biological entity, whether it be a family, domain etc. New signatures from member databases are manually integrated by biologists using a list of protein matches for the new signatures and a list of overlaps between new and existing signatures. New signatures are either integrated into existing InterPro entries or assigned unique InterPro accession numbers, following the guidelines described above. Each InterPro entry (see Figure 3.1) is described by one or more signatures, corresponding to a biologically meaningful family, domain, repeat or PTM. Two types of relationship can exist between InterPro entries: the parent/child and contains/found in relationships. Parent/child relationships are used to describe a common ancestry between entries whereas the contains/found in relationship generally refers to the presence of genetically mobile domains. The hits of all protein signatures in InterPro against all Swiss-Prot and TrEMBL protein sequences are precomputed and the matches are available for viewing in each InterPro entry in different formats, including a match table, a detailed graphical view and a condensed graphical view.

The integrated resources all appear to have similar functions, but InterPro has the advantage of being manually curated. A new project has been initiated to integrate PIR superfamilies into InterPro, which will enhance its effectiveness as a powerful protein classification system. Additional plans of InterPro include extending into the field of protein structure by the incorporation of data from SCOP (Structural Classification of Proteins, Lo Conte *et al.*, 2002), CATH (Class, Architecture, Topology, Homology, Pearl *et al.*, 2002) and the PDB (Berman *et al.*, 2000). These

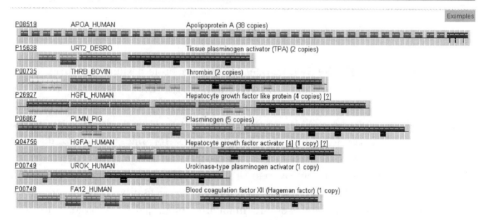

InterPro	Kringle	
IPR000001 Kringle	Matches: 147 proteins View matches: [Overview][Detailed view][Table view][Common domain architecture explorer]	
Name [help]	Kringle	
Signatures [help]	PD000395;Kringle (138 proteins) PF00051;kringle (140 proteins) PR00018;KRINGLE (127 proteins) PS00021;KRINGLE_1 (172 proteins) PS50070;KRINGLE_2 (138 proteins) SM00130;KR (135 proteins)	
Type [help]	Domain	
Dates [help]	1999-10-08 17:07:25.0 (created) 2001-01-15 11:37:21.0 (modified)	
Process [help]	mitochondrion inheritance (GO:0000001) vision (GO:0007601) phototransduction (GO:0007602)	
Function [help]	adenine deaminase (GO:0000034)	
Abstract [help]	Kringles are autonomous structural domains, found throughout the blood clotting and fibrinolytic proteins. Kringle domains are believed to play a role in binding mediators (e.g., membranes, other proteins or phospholipids), and in the regulation of proteolytic activity [17, 2, 3]. Kringle domains [18, 5, 6] are characterised by a triple loop, 3-disulphide bridge structure, whose conformation is defined by a number of hydrogen bonds and small pieces of anti-parallel beta-sheet. They are found in a varying number of copies, in some serine proteases and plasma proteins.	

Examples

P08519 APOA_HUMAN   Apolipoprotein A (38 copies)

P15638 URT2_DESRO   Tissue plasminogen activator (TPA) (2 copies)

P00735 THRB_BOVIN   Thrombin (2 copies)

P26927 HGFL_HUMAN   Hepatocyte growth factor like protein (4 copies) [?]

P06867 PLMN_PIG   Plasminogen (5 copies)

Q04756 HGFA_HUMAN   Hepatocyte growth factor activator [4] (1 copy) [?]

P00749 UROK_HUMAN   Urokinase-type plasminogen activator (1 copy)

P00748 FA12_HUMAN   Blood coagulation factor XII (Hageman factor) (1 copy)

Figure 3.1 Example of an InterPro entry. The entry describes the kringle domain, which is represented by signatures from ProDom, Pfam, Prints, Prosite and SMART

databases are derived from known protein structures, but can, through residue mapping, be linked to protein sequences in Swiss-Prot and TrEMBL. Structure information sheds more light on protein function and evolutionary relationships.

3.3 Discussion

Just as the protein sequence databases are primarily derived from nucleotide sequence databases, so too a large number of protein and gene family databases, clustering databases and protein signature databases are derived from the protein sequence databases. Both the derived protein signature databases and the resources that unite them rely on the quality of the protein sequence databases from which they are derived. These derived databases are created for the purposes of aiding in elucidation of protein function or for organized storage and display of known biological information, and each has made valuable contributions to the annotation of newly sequenced genomes and large scale protein function prediction.

There is much inter-cooperation between the different resources either directly by using the data, or indirectly by linking to other resources where appropriate. The integrated resources such as InterPro, CDD, MetaFam and iProClass go even further in cooperation by incorporating several derived databases into one, providing a 'one-stop shop' for protein sequence, family and domain information. In so doing, a feedback loop is formed to improve the quality of all the individual parts. Sequences from Swiss-Prot and TrEMBL form the basis for the protein signature databases, which, in turn, form the basis for InterPro. InterPro classifies Swiss-Prot and TrEMBL proteins into protein families and domains, and in turn is used for the automatic annotation of TrEMBL. Increased availability of annotation in the protein sequence databases then provides more scope for protein family identification for signature databases. The integration of protein signatures from different member databases into InterPro entries also provides a method for quality assessment of each method, and highlights where methods have drawbacks or lack representation.

Proteome Analysis @EBI

InterPro top 200 entries for *H. sapiens* [help]			
InterPro	Proteins matched (Proteome coverage)	Rank *	Name
IPR007087	946(3.3%)	1	Zn-finger, C2H2 type
IPR003006	883(3.1%)	2	Immunoglobulin/major histocompatibility complex
IPR000276	826(2.9%)	3	Rhodopsin-like GPCR superfamily
IPR007110	804(2.8%)	4	Immunoglobulin-like
IPR000719	687(2.4%)	5	Protein kinase
IPR000725	477(1.7%)	6	Olfactory receptor
IPR002290	472(1.7%)	7	Serine/Threonine protein kinase
IPR001680	386(1.4%)	8	G-protein beta WD-40 repeat
IPR001841	367(1.3%)	9	Zn-finger, RING
IPR006209	357(1.3%)	10	EGF-like domain
IPR000504	342(1.2%)	11	RNA-binding region RNP-1 (RNA recognition motif)
IPR001849	331(1.2%)	12	Pleckstrin-like
IPR003599	327(1.1%)	13	Immunoglobulin subtype
IPR002965	324(1.1%)	14	Proline-rich extensin
IPR001245	314(1.1%)	15	Tyrosine protein kinase
IPR001909	314(1.1%)	15	KRAB box
IPR002048	298(1.0%)	17	Calcium-binding EF-hand
IPR007086	286(1.0%)	18	Zn-finger, C2H2 subtype
IPR001452	280(1.0%)	19	SH3 domain
IPR002110	259(0.9%)	20	Ankyrin
IPR003598	259(0.9%)	20	Immunoglobulin C-2 type
IPR001356	254(0.9%)	22	Homeobox
IPR003961	232(0.8%)	23	Fibronectin, type III
IPR003596	223(0.8%)	24	Immunoglobulin V-type

Figure 3.2 Example of a proteome analysis entry. The entry shows some of the top 200 InterPro hits for the human proteome

An example for an integrated resource that makes further use of data both from sequence databases and from derived databases is the Proteome Analysis database (Pruess *et al.*, 2003). This resource provides comprehensive statistical analyses of the predicted proteomes of fully sequenced organisms, thus aiming at overcoming the lack of *in vivo* gathered knowledge about the functions of predicted proteins (Figure 3.2 shows an example for the statistical analysis of *Homo sapiens*).

Complete proteome sets as well as functional annotation are derived directly from Swiss-Prot and TrEMBL, whereas InterPro is used for the classification of proteins and protein families in these proteomes, and the CluSTr database for the clustering of proteins (see Figure 3.3). The InterPro analysis on complete proteomes in the Proteome Analysis database also highlights the protein space that InterPro signatures do not cover. Therefore, not only do derived databases provide the user with biological information at different levels; they can also contribute to adding value to the original data.

Proteome Analysis @EBI

Protein set for InterPro entry IPR001818

Protein_ac	Protein_id	Description	InterPro hits			
O60882	MM20_HUMAN	Matrix metalloproteinase-20 precursor (EC 3.4.24.-) (MMP-20) (Enamel metalloproteinase) (Enamelysin).	8		CluSTr	STRING
P03956	MM01_HUMAN	Interstitial collagenase precursor (EC 3.4.24.7) (Matrix metalloproteinase-1) (MMP-1) (Fibroblast collagenase).	8		CluSTr	STRING
P08253	MM02_HUMAN	72 kDa type IV collagenase precursor (EC 3.4.24.24) (72 kDa gelatinase) (Matrix metalloproteinase-2) (MMP-2) (Gelatinase A) (TBE-1).	8		CluSTr	STRING
P09237	MM07_HUMAN	Matrilysin precursor (EC 3.4.24.23) (Pump-1 protease) (Uterine metalloproteinase) (Matrix metalloproteinase-7) (MMP-7) (Matrin).	8		CluSTr	STRING
P22894	MM08_HUMAN	Neutrophil collagenase precursor (EC 3.4.24.34) (Matrix metalloproteinase-8) (MMP-8) (PMNL collagenase) (PMNL-CL).	8		CluSTr	STRING
P45452	MM13_HUMAN	Collagenase 3 precursor (EC 3.4.24.-) (Matrix metalloproteinase-13) (MMP-13).	8		CluSTr	STRING
P51511	MM15_HUMAN	Matrix metalloproteinase-15 precursor (EC 3.4.24.-) (MMP-15) (Membrane-type matrix metalloproteinase 2) (MT-MMP 2) (MTMMP2) (Membrane-type-2 matrix metalloproteinase) (MT2-MMP) (MT2MMP) (SMCP- 2).	8		CluSTr	STRING
P39900	MM12_HUMAN	Macrophage metalloelastase precursor (EC 3.4.24.65) (HME) (Matrix metalloproteinase-12) (MMP-12) (Macrophage elastase) (ME).	8		CluSTr	STRING

Figure 3.3 A proteome analysis entry that shows the human protein set for the protein family Matrixin (InterPro entry IPR001818) and links to InterPro, CluSTr and the STRING, a database of predicted functional associations among genes/proteins

References

Altschul, S.F., Gish, W., Miller, W., Myers, E.W. and Lipman, D.J. (1990). Basic local alignment search tool. *J. Mol. Biol.* **215**, 403–410.

Altschul, S.F., Madden, T.L., Schaffer, A.A., Zhang, J., Zhang, Z., Miller, W. and Lipman, D.J. (1997). Gapped BLAST and PSI-BLAST: a new generation of protein database search programs. *Nucleic Acid Res.* **25**, 3389–3402.

Attwood, T.K., Bradley, P., Flower, D.R., Gaulton, A., Maudling, N., Mitchell, A.L., Moulton, G., Nordle, A., Paine, K., Taylor, P., Uddin, A. and Zygouri, C. (2003). PRINTS and its automatic supplement, prePRINTS. *Nucleic Acids Res.* **31**, 400–402.

Barker, W.C., Garavelli, J.S., Huang, H., McGarvey, P.B., Orcutt, B., Srinivasarao, G.Y., Xiao, C., Yeh, L.S., Ledley, R.S., Janda, J.F., Pfeiffer, F., Mewes, H.W., Tsugita, A. and Wu, C. (2000). The protein information resource (PIR). *Nucleic Acids Res.* **28**, 41–44.

Bateman, A., Birney, E., Cerruti, L., Durbin, R., Etwiller, L., Eddy, S.R., Griffiths-Jones, S., Howe, K.L., Marshall, M., Sonnhammer, E.L.L. (2002). The Pfam protein families database. *Nucleic Acids Res.* **30**, 276–280.

Berman, H.M., Westbrook, J., Feng, Z., Gilliland, G., Bhatm T.N., Weissig, H., Shindyalov, I.N. and Bourne, P.E. (2000). The protein data bank. *Nucleic Acids Res.* **28**, 235–242.

Boeckmann, B., Bairoch, A., Apweiler, R., Blatter, M., Estreicher, A., Gasteiger, E., Martin, M.J., Michoud, K., O'Donovan, C., Phan, I., Pilbout, S. and Schneider, M. (2003). The Swiss-Prot protein knowledgebase and its supplement TrEMBL in 2003. *Nucleic Acids Res.* **31**, 365–370.

Comet, J.P., Aude, J.C., Glemet, E., Risler, J.L., Henaut, A., Slonimski, P.P. and Codani, J.J. (1999). Significance of Z-value statistics of Smith–Waterman scores for protein alignments. *Comput. Chem.* **23**, 317–331.

Coutinho, P.M., Henrissat, B. (1999). Carbohydrate-active Enzymes: an integrated database approach. In Gilbert, H.J., Davies, G., Henrissat, B. and Svensson, B., eds., *Recent Advances in Carbohydrate Bioengineering*, Royal Society of Chemistry, Cambridge, pp. 3–12.

Falquet, L. Pagni, M., Bucher, P., Hulo, N., Sigrist, C.J.A., Hofmann, K. and Bairoch, A. (2002). The PROSITE database, its status in 2002. *Nucleic Acids Res.* **30**, 235–238.

Gribskov, M., Luthy, R. and Eisenberg, D. (1990). Profile analysis. *Methods Enzymol.* **183**, 146–159.

Haft, D.H., Selengut, J.D. and White, O. (2003). The TIGRFAMs database of protein families. *Nucleic Acids Res.* **31**, 371–373.

Henikoff, J.G., Greene, E.A., Pietrokovski, S. and Henikoff, S. (2000). Increased coverage of protein families with the Blocks database servers. *Nucleic Acids Res.* **28**, 228–230.

Henikoff, S. and Henikoff, J.G. (1991). Automated assembly of protein blocks for database searching. *Nucleic Acids Res.* **19**, 6565–6572.

Holm, L., Sander, C. (1999). Protein folds and families: sequence and structure alignments. *Nucleic Acids Res.* **27**, 244–247.

Krause, A., Stoye, J., Vingron, M. (2000). The SYSTERS protein sequence cluster set. *Nucleic Acids Res.* **28**, 270–272.

Kriventseva, E.V., Biswas, M. and Apweiler, R. (2001). Clustering and analysis of protein families (Review). *Curr. Opin. Struct. Biol.* **11**, 334–339.

Kriventseva, E.V., Servant, F. and Apweiler, R. (2003). Improvements to CluSTr: the database of Swiss-Prot+TrEMBL protein clusters. *Nucleic Acids Res.* **31**, 388–389.

Letunic, I., Goodstadt, L., Dickens, N.J., Doerks, T., Schultz, J., Mott, R., Ciccarelli, F., Copley, R.R., Ponting, C.P. and Bork, P. (2002). Recent improvements to the SMART domain-based sequence annotation resource. *Nucleic Acids Res.* **30**, 242–244.

Lo Conte, L., Brenner, S.E., Hubbard, T.J., Chothia, C., Murzin, A.G. (2002). SCOP Database in 2002: refinements accommodate structural genomics. *Nucleic Acids Res.* **30**, 264–267.

Matys, V., Fricke, E., Geffers, R., Gößling, E., Haubrock, M., Hehl, R., Hornischer, K., Karas, D., Kel, A.E., Kel-Margoulis, O.V., Kloos, D.-U., Land, S., Lewicki-Potapov, B., Michael, H., Münch, R., Reuter, I., Rotert, S., Saxel, H., Scheer, M., Thiele, S. and Wingender, E. (2003). TRANSFAC®: transcriptional regulation, from patterns to profiles. *Nucleic Acids Res.* **31**, 374–378.

Mulder, N.J., Apweiler, R., Attwood, T.K., Bairoch, A., Barrell, D., Bateman, A., Binns, D., Biswas, M., Bradley, P., Bork, P., Bucher, P., Copley, R.R., Courcelle, E., Das, U., Durbin, R., Falquet, L., Fleischmann, W., Griffiths-Jones, S., Haft, D., Harte, N., Hulo, N., Kahn, D., Kanapin, A.,

Krestyaninova, M., Lopez, R., Letunic, I., Lonsdale, D., Silventoinen, V., Orchard, S.E., Pagni, M., Peyruc, D., Ponting, C.P., Selengut, J.D., Servant, F., Sigrist, C.J.A., Vaughan R. and Zdobnov, E.M. (2003). The InterPro Database, 2003 brings increased coverage and new features. *Nucleic Acids Res.* **31**, 315–318.

Pearl, F.M, Lee, D., Bray, J.E., Buchan, D.W., Shepherd, A.J. and Orengo, C.A. (2002). The CATH Extended Protein-Family Database: providing structural annotations for genome sequences. *Protein Sci.* **11**, 233–244.

Pearson, W.R. and Lipman, D.J. (1988). Improved tools for biological sequence comparison. *Proc. Natl. Acad. Sci. USA* **85**, 2444–2448.

Pietrokovski, S. (1996). Searching databases of conserved sequence regions by aligning protein multiple-alignments. *Nucleic Acids Res.* **24**, 3836–3845.

Praz, V., Périer, R.C., Bonnard, C. and Bucher, P. (2002). The Eukaryotic Promoter Database, EPD: new entry types and links to gene expression data. *Nucleic Acids Res.* **30**, 322–324.

Pruess, M., Fleischmann, W., Kanapin, A., Karavidopoulou, Y., Kersey, P., Kriventseva, E., Mittard, V., Mulder, N., Phan, I., Servant, F. and Apweiler, R. (2003). The Proteome Analysis Database: a tool for the in silico analysis of whole proteomes. *Nucleic Acids Res.* **31**, 414–417.

Rawlings, N.D., O'Brien E. and Barrett, A.J. (2002). MEROPS: the protease database. *Nucleic Acids Res.* **30**, 343–346.

Saier, M.H. Jr. (2000). A functional–phylogenetic classification system for transmembrane solute transporters. *Microbiol. Mol. Biol. Rev.* **64**, 354–411.

Servant, F., Bru, C., Carrere, S., Courcelle, E., Gouzy, J., Peyruc, D. and Kahn, D. (2002). ProDom: automated clustering of homologous domains. *Brief. Bioinform.* **3**, 246–251.

Silverstein, K.A., Shoop, E., Johnson, J.E. and Retzel, E.F. (2001). MetaFam: a unified classification of protein families. I. Overview and statistics. *Bioinformatics* **17**, 249–261.

Smith, T.F., Waterman, M.S. (1981). Identification of common molecular subsequences. *J. Mol. Biol.* **147**, 195–197.

Stoesser, G., Baker, W., van den Broek, A., Garcia-Pastor, M., Kanz, C., Kulikova, T., Leinonen, R., Lin, Q., Lombard, V., Lopez, R., Mancuso, R., Nardone, F., Stoehr, P., Tuli, M., Tzouvara, K. and Vaughan, R. (2003). The EMBL Nucleotide Sequence Database: major new developments. *Nucleic Acids Res.* **31**, 17–22.

Strausberg, R.L., Feingold, E.A., Klausner, R.D. and Collins, F.S. (1999). The Mammalian Gene Collection. *Science* 286, 455–457.

Suzuki, Y., Tsunoda, T., Sese, J., Taira, H., Mizushima-Sugano, J., Hata, H., Ota, T., Isogai, T., Tanaka, T. and Nakamura, Y. (2001). Identification and characterization of the potential promoter regions of 1031 kinds of human genes. *Genome Res.* **11**, 677–684.

Tatusov, R.L., Natale, D.A., Garkavtsev, I.V., Tatusova, T.A., Shankavaram, U.T., Rao, B.S., Kiryutin, B., Galperin, M.Y., Fedorova, N.D. and Koonin, E.V. (2001). The COG Database: new developments in phylogenetic classification of proteins from complete genomes. *Nucleic Acids Res.* **29**, 22–28.

Westbrook, J., Feng, Z., Chen, L., Yang, H. and Berman, H.M. (2003). The protein data bank and structural genomics. *Nucleic Acids Res.* **31**, 489–491.

Wheeler, D.L., Church, D.M., Lash, A.E., Leipe, D.D., Madden, T.L., Pontius, J.U., Schuler, G.D., Schriml, L.M., Tatusova, T.A., Wagner, L. and Rapp, B.A. (2001). Database resources of the national center for biotechnology information. *Nucleic Acids Res.* **29**, 11–16.

Wu, C.H., Xiao, C., Hou, Z., Huang, H. and Barker, W.C. (2001). iProClass: an integrated, comprehensive and annotated protein classification database. *Nucleic Acids Res.* **29**, 52–54.

Yona, G., Linial, N. and Linial, M. (2000). A Brief Description of the Methodology, and an Overview of the Database and the Website: ProtoMap: automatic classification of protein sequences and hierarchy of protein families. *Nucleic Acids Res.* **28**, 49–55.

4 Databanks of Macromolecular Structure

H. J. Bernstein and F. C. Bernstein

Abstract

Structural databases are highly accessible, well indexed repositories of information about the three-dimensional structures of biologically interesting molecules that play a central role in the biological sciences. These databases make a large volume of experimental data visible for observation with different viewing paradigms. They allow users to pose questions and make an immediate start on verification of their hypotheses. We review the history of structural databases, beginning with the Cambridge Crystallographic Data Centre Structural Data File (CSD) and the Brookhaven National Laboratory Protein Data Bank (PDB) and the many internet-driven secondary databases they have spawned. Easy access to structural databases is a recent development. Changes in database technology in the 1970s and 1980s made creation of such databases more practical and the rise of the internet in the 1990s lowered the cost of making such databases accessible. Questions of data uniformity, data validation, data annotation, funding models, national and regional politics and changes in data distribution technology have had a strong influence on how one is able to do science.

Keywords

structural biology, structural databases, crystallography, NMR, Protein Data Bank, PDB, Cambridge Structural Data File, CSD, data validation, archives

4.1 Introduction

In this chapter we review the history of structural databases, beginning with the Cambridge Crystallographic Data Centre Structural Data File (CSD) (Allen *et al.*,

1973) and the Brookhaven National Laboratory Protein Data Bank (PDB) (Bernstein *et al.*, 1977) and the many internet-driven secondary databases they have spawned. Questions of data uniformity, data validation, data annotation, funding models, national and regional politics and changes in data distribution technology have had a strong influence on how one is able to do science.

4.2 Background

Establishment of the CSD and the PDB

For many decades, crystallography was the only experimental technique able to provide reliable information on the three-dimensional atomic structure of complex molecules. Making the data from these experiments generally available was a problem, especially as the number of solved structures grew at an ever increasing rate. When the number of solved structures was small, it was practical for individual scientists to extract published lists of atomic coordinates from journal articles or to request paper tapes, punch cards or magnetic tapes from authors with interesting structures, but by the 1960s it was clear that something better was needed. 'The Cambridge Crystallographic Data Centre [(CCDC)] was established in 1965... to undertake the compilation of a computerised database containing comprehensive data for organic and metal-organic compounds studied by X-ray and neutron diffraction' (CCDC history on Edubiotech web page). The CCDC began by transcribing published lists of coordinates from publications. Typically the molecules handled by the CCDC had at most a few tens of atoms.

For protein structures this is a far from optimal approach. Protein structures are large, typically ranging in size from hundreds to many thousands of atoms. Transcription from publications was likely to introduce many errors and introduce delays in processing. It was better to request the data from the original authors in machine-readable form. In addition, in those days, each protein structure might require many months or years of attention from the authors, even after coordinates had been generated. The Protein Data Bank was established at Brookhaven National Laboratory in 1971 as an archive of macromolecular structural information. The PDB dealt directly with the authors of the structures, often prior to publication of the relevant journal articles.

Approaches to software for data access, data formats and funding

The CSD and the PDB differed in many other ways. The CSD was an integrated software system centred around a database. Both the software and the database were distributed on magnetic tape for people to use on their local computers. The developers of the software had to be concerned with portability of the software across the multiple computer systems used by crystallographers, but they retained control of the design of the retrieval software and a core suite of applications. On the other hand, the PDB was an archive, rather than a database. Some software and the data were distributed on magnetic tape, but the application development model was what would now be called 'open', with users and software developers taking the data plus the PDB format specification and creating software that would do useful things with PDB entries.

The CSD had a large volume of data useful to a significant number of researchers throughout the world, and it was feasible to recover all costs through usage fees (especially national subscriptions). The PDB had a small number of large data sets of critical value to a small number of researchers, and it was primarily funded through US government grants. A small portion of the PDB funding was obtained from user fees and from arrangements with centres in other countries.

The CSD had agreed internal formats (CSD, 1978). However, as noted by Hall and McMahon (2004), there were many different formats in use for small molecule crystallography and related fields. Each author could work with his or her data in any appropriate internal format, and, for example, extract atomic coordinates for presentation in a paper. The coordinates in that paper would then be extracted from the paper for use in the CSD. (This inefficient heterogeneity of formats for small molecule crystallography started to change in the 1990s with the adoption of CIF by the International Union of Crystallography; see below.)

The PDB went through an early format change and then achieved a stable format for more than two decades. The PDB depended on user deposition of data prior to publication. The better a depositor conformed to PDB data format conventions, the more efficiently the data could move from deposition to release.

The initial standard PDB format (PDB, 1974) was derived from the format used in a popular refinement program of the day (Diamond, 1971) and had 132 character records identified by the character strings in the first six columns. Starting in 1976 the PDB spent more than a year (PDB, 1976a, 1976b, 1977) converting to an 80-column format, which is still in use to this day, although with extensions to carry additional information. (The choice of 80 or 132 columns was strongly influenced by the media and hardware available at the time: 80-column punch card equipment and 132-column printers using fan-fold paper.) Many independent programs were developed using this 80-column format, and it has become the major standard for macromolecular software applications. Disciplines other than macromolecular crystallography shared the small molecule penchant for multiple formats, even when using macromolecular structures.

In the early days of both CSD and PDB, the difference in funding models did not lead to a significant difference in access to the data they held. The CCDC would negotiate access fees with commercial firms and representatives of various countries. The end users tended not to see much of this cost. In the United States, for example, an end user would simply pay a modest fee for the tapes of each data release. The PDB had direct government funding that covered the costs of processing the data, but faced significant unfunded costs for the distribution of data on magnetic tape, and therefore also had to charge end users a modest fee for the tapes of each data release. In recent years, however, the difference in funding models allowed a rapid transition to on-line database access to the PDB data, while the move towards on-line access of the CSD data has not gone as smoothly.

Data validation and annotation

From their inception, both the CSD and the PDB put in considerable effort trying to establish a uniform representation for the data they handled, as well as a uniform format. This did not meet with universal approval. The two major objections to such modification to structural data is that it distorts the original presentation by the author and delays access to the data. However, one must now applaud the wisdom of the creators of the CSD and the PDB in resisting the pressure to lower their standards and produce the data more quickly. The design of software, especially of database software, is much simpler when the data to be processed are consistent, always representing the same information in the same way. This is particularly important with structural data that admit many different views of the same information. For example, if one has an amino acid residue to which some atoms have been added, should one present the residue as the original amino acid along with a supplemental covalently bound ligand or should one define a new, modified residue to use in place of the original amino acid? If each data set does not use the same presentation of the same data, then comparisons and data mining become very difficult.

There are many challenges in annotation of data to achieve uniformity of representation. Automated systems have much to contribute, but human guidance and intervention is also essential. In normal crystallographic studies, multiple alternative molecular conformations are averaged, resulting in what appears to be a blurred image of the molecule with partially occupied 'disordered' atomic positions. Consider the case of a structure with a disordered pair of atoms of the same atomic type assuming three alternative overlapping conformations. For ease in refinement, a depositor might fit the density with three atom sites, each with its own name, each two-thirds occupied. An annotator, trying to achieve a uniform chemical view of all the structures in a database, might argue for the more complex, but more 'physical', representation with three pairs of atom sites, six sites in all, but using only two atom names, each pair one-third occupied. As unusual situations are encountered, auto-mated programs can and should be modified to deal with them, but it is most important to preserve and record such annotation metadata to help both annotators and software developers to make informed judgments about what to do when the next unusual case arises.

The transition to database standards

Most of the early formats for sharing structural data were fixed-field, fixed-order formats. The result was that adapting an application to a data format was simple if the processing flow of the application conformed to the fixed order of the data. When it did not conform, programs became complicated using temporary files or large amounts of memory. As files became larger with more complex and interdependent data, it became clear that the cleanest solution was to base an application on an internal database and to populate the database as the data were processed. When data were to be written by an application, those data could be extracted from the database in whatever order was required.

In the 1970s commercial database application support packages became commonly available, and, more importantly, general agreement was reached to use the 'relational database' concepts of E.F. Codd (1970). Relational databases work with named tables with self-identifying named columns of data and content-identified rows, allowing software developers to free themselves from the fixed-field, fixed-order conventions of common procedural programming languages, and to search through complex data quickly and efficiently. By the late 1980s, database software was an inexpensive 'commodity' item, and anyone with access to PDB data and an interesting idea for a view of those data could create a database at reasonable cost.

The rise of the world wide web

Through the 1970s and the 1980s the costs of distributing data declined slowly. The costs of computing fell and capacities rose. The ARPANET-based internet became ubiquitous. Gradually the need to transfer data on magnetic tape was replaced by ftp and gopher-hole access. By the late 1980s anyone who needed a PDB data set could have access to it for whatever it cost them to access the internet. What was missing was an easy way to decide which data sets it would be interesting to access. Database queries could be triggered by email or gopher queries, but such mechanisms were clumsy and unsatisfactory.

Tim Berners-Lee provided the missing link by designing the world wide web built on top of the internet (Berners-Lee, 1989). Now a user can generate a database query on-line by filling out a form on the web and obtain a list of appropriate data sets to examine in seconds.

Distributed access to data

In the 1970s most structural data were distributed on magnetic tape. Because international mails were slow, from very early on the PDB arranged for secondary data distribution from the CCDC in Cambridge, UK, and from the University of Tokyo in Japan (PDB, 1976b). In 1977, the PDB added CSIRO in Melbourne, Australia, as a secondary data distribution centre. In 1979, the Japanese secondary data distribution centre moved from the University of Tokyo to Osaka University. During the late 1970s and early 1980s, due to the massive increase in air traffic, mail between the United States and Europe improved. In 1986 secondary distribution of the PDB on tape by CSD ended (PDB, 1986).

In addition to tape distribution, the PDB was available 'on line' to a limited community of people with remote access to BNL computers from the early 1970s (Bernstein *et al.*, 1974) and efforts were made to incorporate on-line access to both the CSD and the PDB into the NIH/EPA Chemical Information System in the late 1970s (Heller, Milne and Feldmann, 1977; Andrews and Bernstein, 1979). In general, distribution by both the PDB and the CSD was via magnetic tape in the early 1980s. Users then gained access to the data by connections to their local computers.

By the late 1980s remote network access was commonly available, albeit slow by modern standards. Connections between countries were particularly slow and over-loaded. If on-line access was to be practical, it was necessary to create additional on-line access points throughout the world, so called 'mirror sites'.[‡] A peak of 22 secondary distribution sites for the PDB was reached in mid-1994 (PDB, 1994), at which time the improved performance of the internet was starting to reduce the need for mirror sites. The PDB started to run a web site, a much more convenient mode of operation and much less prone to congestion than ftp sites. This was the beginning of the end of the need for large numbers of formal mirror sites. Formal and informal mirror sites still exist, but they now provide convenient alternative access, rather than being a necessity. At the same time the increasing bandwidth of the internet and the ease of use of new unix-based system software allowed many informal PDB mirror sites to be created around the world, and for those mirror sites to spawn value-added PDB-based databases.

4.3 Archival Structural Databases Now

The two original archival structural databases, CSD and PDB, have been joined by the Nucleic Acid Database (NDB) (Berman *et al.*, 1992). The CSD remains at CCDC in Cambridge, UK, but in 1998 the PDB moved from Brookhaven National Laboratory to the Research Collaboratory for Structural Bioinformatics (RCSB). For all three databases, both data ingestion and data distribution have become more efficient.

During the 1990s small molecule crystallography became a routine analytical tool, creating an ever-increasing flow of solved structures. A highly automated publication and deposition process based on a well defined ontology and the Crystallographic Information File (CIF) format (Hall, Allen and Brown, 1991) was established. Small-molecule structures moved quickly and efficiently through this system. The success of the various genome sequencing projects created a popular expectation of a similarly rapid growth in the rate of solution, deposition and publication of macromolecular structures as a consequence of high throughput structure solution in the so-called 'structural genomics' project (Burley and Bonanno, 2004).

[‡]Please note that the concept of a miror site predates the existence of the world wide web, and can be applied to ftp sites, gopher holes, databases, web sites and many other on-line data compendia.

It is now clear that the pioneers in high throughput structure determination underestimated the difficulty of the task they faced. Early efforts focused on so-called 'low hanging fruit', structures that could be solved quickly, but consistently high yields have not yet been achieved. One must recall that, in any flow through a system, the capacity of the system is determined by the capacity of the narrowest bottleneck (Elias, Feinstein and Shannon, 1956; Ford and Fulkerson, 1956). As of this writing, the only stages of high throughput structure determination not faced with serious bottlenecks are the computational aspects of crystallography, showing the results of many decades of concerted effort.

The perception in the mid-1990s of an approaching flood of macromolecular structural data led to intense discussions about the need for highly automated structure deposition and a reduction on human involvement in deposition and processing.

In the early 1990s, the PDB had offered an email list server, general on-line access to its data from an anonymous ftp server and uploads of data via ftp as an alternative to submission of data on magnetic tape (PDB, 1991). Many of the PDB's communications with depositors had already been done via email, but electronic submission of the data removed a significant bottleneck from the processing flow. It also raised expectations as to how quickly data would be made available to the community. Experiments were made with so-called 'pre-release' of partially processed data, but for structural genomics and drug design the real need was for rapid release of fully processed entries. CSD was buffered from similar pressure by working mainly after the fact of publication, but the 1990s was a time of rising expectations for the PDB, and the perception of a failure to meet those expectations. There was an expectation of immediate access to all data fully integrated into on-line accessible databases. The PDB went through a series of management changes in the 1990s, including two hotly contested funding competitions, the second of which the BNL group lost to RCSB.

The BNL PDB produced a deposition system called AutoDep (Lin *et al.*, 2000) (descendants of which are still available), which was replaced at RCSB by a more robust CIF-based system called ADIT (Berman *et al.*, 2000). The current rate of deposition is several thousand structures per year (not the predicted tens of thousands of structures per year) and this fortunate turn of events has allowed powerful automated deposition and validation software to be coupled with detailed human examination of the data, helping to maintain reasonable standards of quality.

Issues of division of labour, timely local support and regional pride have led to the creation of a distributed data deposition system. European and Japanese depositors have had the option of using deposition sites in their time zones for several years. Depositors of nucleic acid structures have had the option of sending their data to the NDB. This adds another dimension of stratification of annotation styles to the natural stratification imposed by the simple passage of time. Therefore, the central archive has to be concerned with a continuing effort at achieving data uniformity by reviewing and, if necessary, revising and updating the data it provides (RCSB PDB uniformity web page).

Cambridge structural database (CSD)

The CSD is the primary world depository for the three-dimensional structures of small molecules. These structures are distributed along with database and visualization software in forms suitable for loading onto local host machines. In some areas, local versions are made available to large network communities, but the subscription-based funding model of the CSD has not admitted general free web-based access to the full structural data.

In recent years, however, CCDC has provided increasing numbers of data on the internet. Since 2002, it has been possible to make an internet request for any specific data deposition for which the user has a literature citation and CCDC deposition number (CCDC request web page). In addition, the Relibase database (see below) allows on-line searching of protein-ligand complexes.

The CSD plays a definitive role in supplying the biological research community with structures of small molecules, both as independent entities and as templates for ligands and for polymeric residues. The deposition of structural data for small molecules is increasingly handled on-line, and primarily uses CIF.

World wide protein data bank (wwPDB)

The PDB is the primary world depository for the three-dimensional structures of macromolecules. Most deposition is done on the web, primarily to the RCSB deposition site at Rutgers. Some depositions are done to sites in the UK (MSD/ePDB) and Japan (PDBj). A single archive of annotated data is managed at RCSB. Mirror sites are available worldwide. The major international collaborations between RCSB, MSD/ePDB and PDBj have been formalized in the wwPDB Charter Agreement (wwPDB charter web page).

The RCSB is a consortium of the Department of Chemistry and Chemical Biology at Rutgers, the State University of New Jersey, the San Diego Supercomputer Center (SDSC) at the University of California, San Diego (UCSD) and the Center for Advanced Research in Biotechnology (CARB) at the National Institute of Standards and Technology (NIST) (Berman et al., 2000). The Department of Biochemistry at the University of Wisconsin has joined the RCSB. The RCSB group at Rutgers manages the PDB, the NDB and TargetDB, a database of target sequences used to help coordinate the structural genomics efforts. The RCSB group at SDSC maintains a database of obsolete structures that is used in historical reviews of entries, a structural homology database and a protein kinase resource. The RCSB group at CARB-NIST maintains a Biological Macromolecule Crystallization Database (BMCD). The RCSB group at the University of Wisconsin maintains the BioMag-ResBank, an archive of NMR experimental data.

Collectively, the RCSB provides the central PDB data repository. Other groups contribute to the deposition and annotation effort, but the RCSB has sole 'write-access' for the publicly distributed archive, in order to help reduce the chances of creation of divergent versions of the archive. Within the RCSB, the primary focus of the annotation effort is at Rutgers.

'The European Bioinformatics Institute [(EBI)] is a non-profit academic organisation that forms part of the European Molecular Biology Laboratory (EMBL).... The roots of the EBI lie in the EMBL Nucleotide Sequence Data Library, which was established in 1980 at the EMBL laboratories in Heidelberg, Germany and was the world's first nucleotide sequence database. The original goal was to establish a central computer database of DNA sequences, rather than have scientists submit sequences to journals. What began as a modest task of abstracting information from literature, soon became a major database activity with direct electronic submissions of data and the need for highly skilled informatics staff. The task grew in scale with the start of the genome projects,... There was also a need for research and development to provide services, to collaborate with global partners to support the project, and to provide assistance to industry. To this end, in 1992, the EMBL Council voted to establish the European Bioinformatics Institute and to locate it at the Wellcome Trust Genome Campus in the United Kingdom [at Hinxton, south of Cambridge] where it would be in close proximity to the major sequencing efforts at the Sanger Institute and RFCGR. From 1992 through to 1995, a gradual transition of the activities in Heidelberg took place, till in September 1995 the EBI occupied its current location on the Wellcome Trust Genome Campus' (EBI about web page).

EBI uses an updated version of BNL's AUTODEP software to accept deposition of data and forwards processed entries to RCSB for inclusion in the archive.

The Protein Data Bank Japan (PDBj) is part of the Japanese National Project on Protein Structural and Functional Analyses to 'study both structures and functions of proteins in a selected target of biological systems' (PDBj NPPSFA web page).

The PDBj 'maintains the database for protein structures with financial assistance from the Institute for Bioinformatics research and Development of Japan Science and Technology Corporation (BIRD-JST)' collaborating with RCSB and EBI.

The PDBj accepts depositions from depositors in Asia and Oceania using the RCSB ADIT software and forwards the processed entries to RCSB for inclusion in the PDB archive.

Nucleic acid database (NDB)

The Nucleic Acid Database (NDB) was first made publicly available in late 1989 as a 'database of bibliographic references and crystallographic coordinates of oligonucleotides with two or more bases... [with an] interactive query program NDB... set up to run on [local] computers...' (PDB, 1989).

The Nucleic Acid Database (NDB) was established as a distinct facility in late 1991 and began releasing data in early 1992 (NDB, 1991). Until the NDB was established, deposition of DNAs and RNAs was divided between the CSD and the PDB on the basis of size or the desires of the depositors. At its inception, the NDB took data from the PDB and from the literature and organized it into a database. Later, the NDB assumed responsibility for annotation of data as it came from depositors and sent their processed data to the PDB.

The creation of the NDB was intended to improve the uniformity of representation of the data in its own domain. The NDB also was a leader in efforts to improve the match between the PDB archival format and the demands of modern relational databases. In particular, the NDB was an early leader in the effort to create a macromolecular version of the Crystallographic Information File (mmCIF) and is still the home of the mmCIF effort.

The NDB proposed and implemented a much finer grained description of information about the experimental context of crystallographic experiments than was then the case for the PDB format. The PDB formalized changes to the 'REMARK' records of the PDB format to carry similar information in an extended version of the PDB format, and added supplemental record types. Efforts are underway at the PDB to obtain this detailed information for the older PDB entries, starting by making the 'remediated mmCIF files' available.

CIF and mmCIF

Internally the PDB maintains the detailed information about structures in mmCIF (Bourne *et al.*, 1997), the macromolecular version of the Crystallographic Information File, and uses extensions to mmCIF to maintain metadata about the processing of entries. The mmCIF data sets differ from the fixed field PDB data sets in format and, in some ways, in content. mmCIF provides a more detailed, database-oriented view of the information in a data set. The same information may be presented in different orders and with different spacing in equivalent mmCIF files. Rather than identifying data in major blocks, as is the practice in the fixed field PDB format, data are identified item by item.

One may appreciate the differences in style between the fixed field PDB format and mmCIF format by comparing the crystallographic cell information for the entry 3CRO (Hendrickson and Teeter, 1981; Teeter, 1984). The fixed field PDB format presents the cell information as a single 'CRYST1' record:

```
CRYST1  40.960  18.650  22.520  90.00  90.77  90.00 P 21      2
```

In mmCIF format, the same information is given field by field, with an identifying tag for each field:

```
_cell.entry_id              1CRN
_cell.length_a              40.960
_cell.length_b              18.650
_cell.length_c              22.520
_cell.angle_alpha           90.00
_cell.angle_beta            90.77
_cell.angle_gamma           90.00
_cell.Z_PDB                 2
_symmetry.space_group_name_H-M       'P 1 21 1'
```

PDB entries have been released in both the fixed field PDB format and in mmCIF format since 1996 (Bernstein, Bernstein and Bourne, 1998). The original mmCIF releases were based on the PDB format entries. Recently the PDB has made truly native CIF entries based on their internal extension dictionary available (RCSB PDB (2003q3) new features). These entries include detailed information not yet made available in the fixed field PDB format data sets.

4.4 Contextual Databases

Much of the value of structural data comes when it is placed in the context of related experimental, chemical, biological and bibliographic information. The CSD is effectively a contextual database for ligand and residue chemical information needed for the PDB. The PDB archives experimental structure factor information for PDB entries resulting from crystallographic experiments. The BioMagResBank archives the experimental data for PDB entries resulting from NMR experiments. For any given structural data set there may be entries in many other databases that should be cited for context.

Contextual coverage of deposited structures is not uniform. While there is now wide acceptance of the importance of deposition of structural coordinates, experimental data have not always been made available. As of the summer of 2003, structure factors were available for only half the crystallographically determined coordinate files in the PDB (RCSB PDB (2003q2) structure factor data). As of December 2003, the situation had not improved significantly (Uppsala Electron Density Server update).

When full experimental data are available one can attempt to reproduce the original structure solution to gain confidence in its accuracy and, as better solution and refinement methods become available, perhaps even to obtain more accurate structure solutions from the original data. The authors of this chapter join in the call for the deposition of experimental data.

Sequence databases

The first major effort at the creation of a sequence database was the work of Margaret Dayhoff and her coworkers (Dayhoff et al., 1965, 1978) at Georgetown University Medical Center. With the rise of the internet many other sequence databases were created.

The major sequence databases are discussed in their own right in Chapter 2. PDB data sets may have links to Blocks (Henikoff et al., 2000), the EMBL nucleotide sequence database (EMBL-bank) (Baker et al., 2003), GenBank (Benson et al., 2003), the Genome Database (GDB) (Talbot and Cuticchia, 1999), the Protein Identification Resource (PIR) (Wu et al., 2003), Swiss-Prot and TrEMBL (Bairoch and Apweiler, 2000). Swiss-Prot with the translations from EMBL-bank is the most common sequence reference.

PDB entries may also have links to ProSite (Sigrist *et al.*, 2002) for relevant motifs. Prosite uses similarities in sequences to group proteins into families. Prosite identifies 'biologically significant sites, patterns and profiles'.

Users of the PDB should be aware that the structures given do not necessarily agree precisely with the cited sequences. Any differences known at the time of annotation of the entry are documented in the entries. Older entries may not have current information. A crystallographic experiment may result in identification of residues different from those assumed in the reference sequences, portions of chains may not be observed, mutations may have been made, or changes may have been made in the sequence to achieve observable density.

BioMagResBank (BMRB)

The BioMagResBank (BMRB) 'database contains NMR chemical shifts derived from proteins and peptides, reference data, amino acid sequence information, and data describing the source of the protein and the conditions used to study the protein. In constructing the database, proteins and larger peptides have been given priority. Shift assignments for hemes, cofactors, and substrates of a protein are also included, when they are reported as part of a complex' (Seavey *et al.*, 1991).

The BMRB serves as the repository for experimental data for the NMR coordinate entries in the PDB (BMRB web page).

Biological macromolecule crystallization database (BMCD)

The Biological Macromolecule Crystallization Database (BMCD) 'contains crystal data and the crystallization conditions, which have been compiled from literature' (Gilliland *et al.*, 1994). It also holds data from NASA on crystallization in microgravity conditions. The data on crystallization conditions are contextual data of critical importance for high throughput structural determination.

4.5 Derived Structural Data Databases

With the improvements in performance of the internet and in computing speed, communications and computational resources are no longer barriers to creating databases derived from the PDB and other archival databases. There are many production systems and many experimental systems, and many more can be expected in the future. The RCSB (RCSB database list), EBI (EBI services web page), and NCBI (NCBI cross-database search page) provide extensive lists of searchable databases, and web searches (see e.g. the Google web page) will yield other resources. The following are examples.

Protein fold classification

Some of the derived databases focus on organizing proteins into groups according to similarities in their secondary structures.

The Distance Matrix Alignment (Dali) Fold Classification Database (Holm and Sander, 1994, 1996) provides a mapping of similarity of folding patterns from the PDB, organizing the known proteins into a tree of fold families. The Dali search engine keeps the database updated and is available to use to compare a probe structure to the PDB (Dali web page).

The Structure Classification of Proteins (SCOP) Database (Murzin *et al.*, 1995; Conte *et al.*, 2002) uses the PDB structural data to classify fold families of proteins and tries to illuminate evolutionary relationships. 'Nearly all proteins have structural similarities with other proteins and, in some of these cases, share a common evolutionary origin. The SCOP database, created by manual inspection and abetted by a battery of automated methods, aims to provide a detailed and comprehensive description of the structural and evolutionary relationships between all proteins whose structure is known. As such, it provides a broad survey of all known protein folds, detailed information about the close relatives of any particular protein, and a framework for future research and classification' (SCOP web page).

The Class, Architecture, Topology and Homologous superfamily (CATH) Database (Orengo *et al.*, 1997; Pearl *et al.*, 2000) classifies protein structures by a combination of automatic and manual techniques. 'Class, derived from secondary structure content, is assigned for more than 90% of protein structures automatically. Architecture, which describes the gross orientation of secondary structures, independent of connectivities, is currently assigned manually. The topology level clusters structures according to their toplogical connections and numbers of secondary structures. The homologous superfamilies cluster proteins with highly similar structures and functions. The assignments of structures to toplogy families and homologous superfamilies are made by sequence and structure comparisons' (CATH web page).

Other derived structural data

Other derived data databases extract significant interaction information or look for other levels of classification and similarity.

Relibase (Hendlich *et al.*, 2003) is a database of protein–ligand interactions. It can be probed by 2D substructure and 3D protein–ligand structure (Relibase web page). Relibase is free and web accessible. An enhanced version, Relibase+, is not free.

The National Center for Biotechnology Information (NCBI) of the U.S. National Library of Medicine maintains access to 19 bioinformatics databases and other tools in the Entrez system (NCBI Entrez web page). Among these databases are the Vector Alignment Search Tool (VAST), Conserved Domain Database (CDD) and Molecular Model Database (MMDB). The MMDB (Ohkawa, Ostell and Bryant, 1995) provides a searchable view of the experimentally determined structures in the PDB. 'Protein sequences from MMDB are extracted and available in the Entrez protein sequence database. They are linked to the 3D structures; therefore, it is possible to determine whether a protein sequence in Entrez has homologs among known structures by examining its "Related Sequences" or "Protein Neighbors" and checking whether this set has any "Structure Links'" (NCBI MMDB web page).

The asymmetric unit seen in crystallographic structural studies may or may not be the biologically active form of a molecule. The Protein Quaternary Structure Database (PQS) (Henrick, 1998) generates the biologically active multimers from PDB entries. The algorithm is based on the PDB entries, plus processing, plus human analysis.

For PDB entries prior to 1999, the depositors may not have provided information on the biologically active form and PQS can be very helpful in determining the biologically active form of an entry. For later entries, information on the biologically active form has been requested from the depositors. In some cases, the biologically active form of a molecule cannot be provided, either by the author, or by the PDB or by the PQS, because the biologically active form and perhaps even the function of the molecule is not known.

4.6 Summary and View of the Future

Molecular biology is an empirical science. 'Empirical science characteristically begins with some observation, which prompts the observer to ask a question. The new question is then subjected to some kind of verification. . .' (Valiela, 2001). Structural databases are highly accessible, well indexed repositories of information about the three-dimensional structures of biologically interesting molecules that play a central role in this process. These databases make a large volume of experimental data visible for observation with different viewing paradigms. They allow users to pose questions and make an immediate start on verification of their hypotheses. Easy access to structural databases is a recent development. Changes in database technology in the 1970s and 1980s made creation of such databases more practical and the rise of the internet in the 1990s lowered the cost of making such databases accessible.

The study of biological processes at the molecular level continues to grow and will produce increasing volumes of important data. The increasing ease and decreasing cost of creation and dissemination of data on the internet will encourage the establishment and maintenance of multiple databases providing differing views of this data enhanced in new ways. Some of these databases will be very specialized; some will be very general. The challenge one will face is to provide effective links among these databases, dealing with the highly dynamic nature of some of the data in a way that avoids stale links, and coping with the transient nature of web pages.

The value of these derived databases will depend on the continued production of high quality data by the structural databases. Long term, stable funding must be assured for the structural databases using a model which encourages widespread on-line dissemination of data of very high quality and consistency.

References

BMRB web page: http://www.bmrb.wisc.edu

CATH web page: http://www.biochem.ucl.ac.uk/bsm/cath/

CCDC history on Edubiotech web page: cited text formerly in http://www.ccdc.cam.ac.uk/about/history.html, now in http://www.edubiotech.com/study.htm

CCDC request web page: http://www.ccdc.cam.ac.uk/products/csd/request/

Dali web page: http://www.ebi.ac.uk/dali/

EBI about web page: http://www.ebi.ac.uk/Information/About_EBI/about_ebi.html#ab_1_his

EBI services web page: See http://www.ebi.ac.uk/services/index.html

Google web page: http://www.google.com

NCBI cross-database search page: http://www.ncbi.nlm.nih.gov:80/gquery/gquery.fcgi

NCBI Entrez web page: See http://www.ncbi.nlm.nih.gov/Entrez

NCBI MMDB web page: http://www.ncbi.nlm.nih.gov:80/Structure/MMDB/mmdb.shtml

PDBj NPPSFA web page: http://pdbj.protein.osaka-u.ac.jp/NPPSFA/index.html

RCSB database list: http://www.rcsb.org/pdb/links.html#Databases

RCSB PDB (2003q2) structure factor data: http://www.rcsb.org/pdb/newsletter/2003q2/sf_data.html

RCSB PDB (2003q3) new features: http://www.rcsb.org/pdb/newsletter/2003q3/new_features.html

RCSB PDB uniformity web page: http://www.rcsb.org/pdb/uniformity/

Relibase web page: http://relibase.ccdc.cam.ac.uk

SCOP web page: http://scop.mrc-lmb.cam.ac.uk/scop/

Uppsala Electron Density Server update: http://fsrv1.bmc.uu.se/eds/eds_update.html

wwPDB charter web page: http://www.wwpdb.org/wwpdb_charter.html

Allen, F.H., Kennard, O., Motherwell, W.D.S., Town, W.G. and Watson, D.G. (1973). Cambridge crystallographic data centre. II. Structural data file, *J. Chem. Doc.* **13**, 119–123.

Andrews, L.C. and Bernstein, H.J. (1979). 'The NIH-EPA chemical information system', *ONLINE* 35–49.

Bairoch, A. and Apweiler, R. (2000). 'The Swiss-Prot protein sequence data bank and its supplement TrEMBL in 2000', *Nucleic Acids Res.* **28**, 45–48.

Baker, W., van den Broek, A., Garcia-Pastor, M., Kanz, C., Kulikova, T., Leinonen, R., Lin, Q., Lombard, V., Lopez, R., Mancuso, R., Nardone, F., Stoehr, P., Tuli, M.A., Tzouvara, K., and Vaughan, R. (2003). 'The EMBL Nucleotide Sequence Database: major new developments', *Nucleic Acids Res.* **31** (1), 17–22.

Benson, D.A., Karsch-Mizrachi, I., Lipman, D.J., Ostell, J. and Wheeler, D.L. (2003). 'GenBank', *Nucleic Acids Res.* **31**, 23–27.

Berman, H.M., Olson, W.K., Beveridge, D.L., Westbrook, J., Gelbin, A., Demeny, T., Hsieh, S.-H., Srinivasan, A.R. and Schneider, B. (1992). 'The Nucleic Acid Database: A comprehensive relational database of three-dimensional structures of nucleic acids', *Biophys. J.* **63**, 751–759.

Berman, H.M., Westbrook, J., Feng, Z., Gilliland, G., Bhat, T.N., Weissig, H., Shindyalov, I.N. and Bourne, P.E. (2000). 'The protein data bank', *Nucleic Acids Res.* **28**, 235–242.

Berners-Lee, T. (1989). *Information Management: a Proposal*, proposal, CERN. http://www.w3.org/History/1989/proposal.html

Bernstein, F.C., Koetzle, T.F., Williams, G.J.B., Meyer, Jr., E.F., Brice, M.D., Rodgers, J.R., Kennard, O., Shimanouchi, T. and Tasumi, M. (1977). 'The Protein Data Bank: a computer based archival file for macromolecular structures', *J. Mol. Biol.* **112**, 535–542.

Bernstein, H.J., Andrews, L.C., Berman, H.M., Bernstein, F.C., Campbell, G.H., Carrell, H.L., Chiang, H.B., Hamilton,W. C., Jones, D.D., Klunk, D., Koetzle, T.F., Meyer, E.F. Jr., Morimoto, C.N., Sevian, S., Stodola, R.K., Strongson, M.M. and Willoughby, T.V. (1974). *Second Annual AEC Scientific Computer Information Exchange Meeting, Proceedings of the Technical Program*, chapter CRYSNET – A Network of Intelligent Remote Graphics Terminals, pp. 149–161. Brookhaven National Laboratory Report #18803.

Bernstein, H.J., Bernstein, F.C. and Bourne, P.E. (1998). 'CIF applications. VIII. PDB2CIF: Translating PDB entries into mmCIF format', *J. Appl. Crystallogr.* **31**, 282–295. Software available at http://www.bernsteinplussons.com/software/pdb2cif

Bourne, P.E., Berman, H.M., McMahon, B., Watenpaugh, K.D., Westbrook, J. and Fitzgerald, P.M. D. (1997). 'The macromolecular Crystallographic Information File (mmCIF)', *Methods Enzymol.* **277**, 571–590.

Burley, S.K. and Bonanno, J.B. (2004). Structural genomics. In Bourne, P.E. and Weissig, H., eds, *Structural Bioinformatics*, Wiley-Liss, Hoboken, NJ, chapter 29, pp. 591–612.

Codd, E.F. (1970). 'A relational model of data for large shared data banks', *Commun. ACM* **13** (6), 377–387.

Conte, L.L., Brenner, S.E., Hubbard, T.J.P., Chothia, C. and Murzin, A. (2002). 'SCOP Database in 2002: refinements accommodate structural genomics', *Nucleic Acids Res.* **30** (1), 264–267.

CSD. (1978). *Cambridge Crystallographic Database User Manual*, Crystallographic Data Centre, Cambridge.

Dayhoff, M.O., Eck, R.V., Chang, M.A., and Sochard, M.R. (1965). *Atlas of Protein Sequence and Structure*, vol. 1.

Dayhoff M.O. (editor), Hunt, L.T., Barker, W.C., Schwartz, R.M., Orcutt, B.C. and Young, C.L. (1978). *Atlas of Protein Sequence and Structure*, Vol. 5, National Biomedical Research Foundation, Silver Spiring, MD.

Diamond, R. (1971). 'A real-space refinement procedure for proteins', *Acta Crystallogr.* **A27**, 436–452.

Elias, P., Feinstein, A. and Shannon, C.E. (1956). 'A note on the maximum flow through a network', *IRE Trans. Information Theory* **IT2**, 117–199.

Ford, L.R. and Fulkerson, D.R. (1956). 'Maximal flow through a network', *Can. J. Math.* **8**, 399–404.

Gilliland, G.L., Tung, M., Blakeslee, D.M., and Ladner, J. (1994). 'The Biological Macromolecule Crystallization Database, Version 3.0: new features, data, and the NASA archive for protein crystal growth data', *Acta Crystallogr.* **D50**, 408–413.

Hall, S.R., Allen, F.H. and Brown, I.D. (1991). 'The Crystallographic Information File (CIF): a new standard archive file for crystallography', *Acta Crystallogr.* **A47**, 655–685.

Hall, S.R. and McMahon, B. (2004). Genesis of the crystallographic information file. In *Volume G: Definition and Exchange of Crystallographic Data, International Tables For Crystallography*, Kluwer, Dordrecht, Chapter 1.1.

Heller, S.R., Milne, G.W.A. and Feldmann, R.J. (1977). 'A computer-based chemical information system', *Science* **195**, 253–259.

Hendlich, M., Bergner, A., Gunther, J. and Klebe, G. (2003). 'Relibase – design and development of a database for comprehensive analysis of protein–ligand interactions', *J. Mol. Biol.* **326**, 607–620.

Hendrickson, W.A. and Teeter, M.M. (1981). PDB Entry 1CRN, 30 April 1981.

Henikoff, J.G., Greene, E.A., Pietrokovski, S. and Henikoff, S. (2000). 'Increased coverage of protein families with the Blocks database servers', *Nucleic Acids Res.* **28** (1), 228–230.

Henrick, K. (1998). 'PQS: a protein quaternary structure file server', *Trends Biochem. Sci.* **23** (9), 358–361.

Holm, L. and Sander, C. (1994). 'The FSSP database of structurally aligned protein fold families', *Nucleic Acids Res.* **22**, 3600–3609.

Holm, L. and Sander, C. (1996). 'The FSSP Database: fold classification based on structure alignment of proteins', *Nucleic Acids Res.* **24**, 206–210.

Lin, D., Manning, N.O., Jiang, J., Abola, E.E., Stampf, D., Prilusky, J. and Sussman, J.L. (2000). 'AutoDep: a web based system for deposition and validation of macromolecular structural information', *Acta Crystallogr.* **D56**, 828–841.

Murzin, A.G., Brenner, S.E., Hubbard, T. and Chothia, C. (1995). 'SCOP: a structural classification of proteins database for the investigation of sequences and structures', *J. Mol. Biol.* **247**, 536–540.

NDB. (1991). *Nucleic Acid DataBase Newsletter*, Rutgers, State University of New Jersey.

Ohkawa, H., Ostell, J. and Bryant, S. (1995). 'MMDB: an ASN.1 specification for macromolecular structure', *ISMB* **3**, 259–267.

Orengo, C.A., Michie, A.D., Jones, S., Jones, D.T., Swindells, M.B. and Thornton, J.M. (1997). 'CATH – a hierarchic classification of protein domain structures', *Structure* **5**(8), 1093–1108.

PDB. (1974). *PDB Newsletter*, Brookhaven National Laboratory.

PDB. (1976a) *PDB Newsletter*, Brookhaven National Laboratory.

PDB. (1976b) *PDB Newsletter*, Brookhaven National Laboratory.

PDB. (1977). *PDB Newsletter*, Brookhaven National Laboratory.

PDB. (1986). *PDB Newsletter*, Brookhaven National Laboratory.

PDB. (1989). *PDB Newsletter*, Brookhaven National Laboratory.

PDB. (1991). *PDB Newsletter*, Brookhaven National Laboratory.

PDB. (1994). *PDB Newsletter*, Brookhaven National Laboratory.

Pearl, F.M.G., Lee, D., Bray, J.E., Sillitoe, I., Todd, A.E., Harrison, A.P., Thornton, J.M. and Orengo, C.A. (2000). 'Assigning genomic sequences to CATH', *Nucleic Acids Res.* **28** (1), 277–282.

Seavey, B., Farr, E., Westler, W. and Markley, J. (1991). 'A relational database for sequence-specific protein NMR data', *J. Biomol. NMR* **1**, 217–236.

Sigrist, C.J., Cerutti, L., Hulo, N., Gattiker, A., Falquet, L., Pagni, M., Bairoch, A. and Bucher, P. (2002). 'PROSITE: a documented database using patterns and profiles as motif descriptors', *Brief Bioinform.* **3**, 265–274.

Talbot, C.C. Jr. and Cuticchia, A.J. (1999). Human mapping databases. In *Current Protocols in Human Genetics*, Wiley, New York, Chapter 1.13, pp. 1.13.1–1.13.12.

Teeter, M.M. (1984). 'Water structure of a hydrophobic protein at atomic resolution. pentagon rings of water molecules in crystals of crambin', *Proc. Natl. Acad. Sci. USA* **81**, 6014–6018.

Valiela, I. (2001). *Doing Science: Design, Analysis and Communication of Scientific Research*, Oxford University Press, Oxford.

Wu, C.H., Yeh, L.-S. L., Huang, H., Arminski, L., Castro-Alvear, J., Chen, Y., Hu, Z.-Z., Ledley, R.S., Kourtesis, P., Suzek, B.E., Vinayaka, C.R., Zhang, J. and Barker, W.C. (2003). 'The protein information resource', *Nucleic Acids Res.* **31**, 345–347.

5 Gene Expression Databases

H. Parkinson

Abstract

The study of gene expression is now an achievable goal for biologists.

However, the complexity and diversity of the experimental processes used present significant challenges for scientists. In addition to the purely technical problems, in order to make data comparable within and between communities bench biologists must also manage their data, describe it adequately and, in order to publish, may need to comply with community standards such as MIAME.

Here we discuss standardization for microarray experiments, meta-data description, data management and quality assurance. These issues are discussed with examples from the microarray gene expression and other communities.

Keywords

microarray, standards, database, ArrayExpress, MIAME, functional genomics, ontology

5.1 Introduction

Advances in technology and the completion of several eukaryotic genomes have presented biologists with a new range of experimental possibilities in addition to traditional gene-by-gene and one post-doc–one gene approaches. With these opportunities come the practical problems of complex experimental design, large scale data analysis and data storage: proteomics and transcriptomics data are not interpretable without detailed protocols and sample information. Biological databases now face the

Database Annotation in Molecular Biology   Edited by Arthur M. Lesk
© 2005 John Wiley & Sons, Ltd.   ISBN: 0-470-85681-5

challenges of storing these new data types and integrating huge new datasets with existing resources.

The long established model organism databases provide vital information on genes and sequences, serve species and domain specific data and provide literature curation services. They are an invaluable resource for the bench biologist, but do not provide a local solution to data management and annotation problems for individual biologists. The scale of functional genomics experiments means that the gene model used by species specific databases may not be the most appropriate for storing large scale transcript level data. It should also be recognized that the use of transcriptomics by clinicians and toxicologists for organisms of biological interest, where these are not the subject of model-organism database, creates a data storage problem for communities that may not have any experience in dealing even with sequence data. Transcriptomic, and specifically microarray data present analysis problems for some scientists who have little training in statistical analysis and who often have no local bioinformatic resources.

Microarray technology is now financially within reach of even very small groups, but commercial database solutions are expensive and the problem of data comparison has not been helped by the existence of multiple data formats. Public data are often dispersed among journal and laboratory websites, and are often lacking in basic sample information. This information is essential for interpretation, but requires some effort to find it, and import it into local databases. Analysis is complicated by the fact that even in relatively well understood systems like yeast we still do not have a complete 'parts list' – that is a complete list of genes, gene products and functions. Therefore, preservation of data for reanalysis when the parts lists are complete, or at least extended, seems prudent.

There are three hurdles for the biologist to jump when interpreting public-domain microarray data. To what genes do the spots correspond? What samples were used and how were they treated? What statistical analysis was performed on the data files to produce biological conclusions? It is also desirable that data from high-throughput experiments should be integrated with the existing databases to provide a common discovery platform for scientists. This is a huge challenge for bioinformaticians, and we are still some way from fully integrated queries running across multiple databases.

This is partly because this is an active area of research in bioinformatics, and partly because a unified solution may not meet all the needs of prospective users. Journals, local analysis systems and databases (LIMS) and public repositories have overlapping needs and interests. Cooperation between these groups is necessary to produce useful solutions for all. This will also result in a resource saving. Journals should not need to archive on a website all material relating to a publication; rather it should be in a repository in a common format. The solutions of data storage and annotation problems are likely to be expensive and users will require training to use them. The rewards for the researcher come once they have a common discovery platform and clean data for analysis.

5.2 What Do We Mean by Microarray Gene Expression Data?

Microarray gene expression experiments allow biologists to make a snapshot of the transcriptional state in a given tissue culture or even a single cell. The various methodologies for this technology provide us with information about amounts of transcript by measuring hybridization to sequences on an array. However, how the data are reported depends upon the technology used to generate them.

There are two main technologies used in microarray experiments: (1) 'two colour' or 'two channel' experiments in which two nucleic acid (usually RNA) samples are extracted from samples of interest, differentially labelled, typically with fluorescent dyes Cy3 and Cy5; (2) alternatively, single channel platforms report gene expression data in a single sample. In both case samples are hybridized to an array, usually on a glass slide, on which the sequences of interest are spotted. These 'probes' may be generated by PCR from cDNA clones; oligonucleotide arrays use synthetic 'long' oligonucleotides, and photolithographic arrays such as those generated by Affymetrix synthesize 'short' 25-mer oligonucleotides *in situ*.

In the case of two colour arrays the differentially labelled samples are hybridized to the same array and the array is then scanned at the two wavelengths at which the labels fluoresce. The data are typically reported as 'heat maps' using a red/green colour scheme. If both samples contain a given sequence in equal amounts the colour is represented as yellow; if one or the other labels is in excess the dye in excess is represented either as red or green. Typically the ratio of the signal in the two channels is measured and the data are reported as a matrix.

The Affymetrix system is slightly different as a single sample is extracted, biotinylated and hybridized to a single array. Each gene on an Affymetrix array is represented by a set of probes. Each probe consists of a pair of oligonuclotides, a perfect match (PM) and a mismatch (MM) oligonucleotide and the intensities of each oligonucleotide are measured and the intenstity of the MM oligo is subtracted from the intensity of the PM oligo to provide an 'average difference value'. Details of the Affymetrix system can be found at their website, http://www.affymetrix.com/support/technical/whitepapers.affx

5.3 Data Complexity

Gene expression experiments are necessarily complex, and generate both numeric data – in the form of gene expression values – and meta-data, which describe how that value was obtained. (Meta-data simply means data about data.)

In order to support the types of query that biologists want to ask of their data (whether stored locally or externally in a database), the meta-data relating to gene expression values themselves need to be recorded. For example, the query 'show me the top 10 up-regulated genes in organism x, treated with compound y' requires that all the data on genes, organism and compound treatments are stored. For such a query to run efficiently in a database that contains millions of rows, the text values need to be constrained. The likely follow-up query, 'show me information on sequence and annotation of my gene list', requires either that links are made to external databases, or that these data are held locally within the gene expression database or file which is being analysed. As sequence and gene annotation data are typically in flux, considerable efforts are required to update the data to obtain accurate analysis. This is a non-trivial task as the arrays can contain sequences representing $\sim$30 000 genes, and this number is rising all the time as technology develops.

Different types of data need to be stored about both the samples used and the sequences (genes) on the array. Many meta-data are in free text format and are context or domain dependent, e.g. relating to a sequence present on the array, some treatment or characteristic of the biological sample that was used in the experiment, the technology type or the mathematical transformation that produced the data. While humans are well equipped for free text processing, there are huge computational costs in searching free text. If free text is constructed independently by a large number of humans, the results are likely to have many errors and inconsistencies. Typographical errors, synonyms and abbreviations all confound computational queries but are processed effectively by humans.

The natural language processing community is now expending a great deal of effort to process resources such as Medline abstracts to extract information, e.g. about protein interaction. However, natural language processing never performs as well as an expert human, and is limited by the format, volume and content of data. Medline abstracts may just not contain information about protein interaction, even if it is expressed elsewhere in the paper (Blaschke, Hirschman and Valencia, 2002). In addition to the problems of meta data as free text, the data files for gene expression experiments can be huge – megabytes or gigabytes – as there may be multiple measurements corresponding to each sequence on the array, and the data are transformed many times as duplicate sequences are resolved, averaging is performed across biological replicates and normalization and clustering are performed.

The extent of the problems with microarray data has been widely recognized. The result was the establishment of the Microarray Gene Expression Database (MGED) Society in 1999 (www.mged.org). MGED provides a forum for those interested in the problems of microarray data storage, exchange, analysis and annotation. Four working groups were set up to address the development of a standard for data description, creation of a common terminology for data annotation, methods for data processing, and development of a database model for data storage and a format for data exchange. Many founder members of MGED represent groups that generate or analyse large numbers of data and therefore had a pressing problem and the most to gain by working cooperatively. The first achievement of MGED was the development of a standard for microarray data.

5.4 Minimum Information About a Microarray Experiment (MIAME)

MIAME addresses all parts of a microarray gene expression experiment and the goal of the developers '... *is to establish a standard for recording and reporting microarray gene expression data which will in turn facilitate the establishment of databases and public repositories and enable the development of analysis tools'*. The draft standard was published in 2001 (Brazma *et al.*, 2001) and has been widely adopted by data producers and array and software manufacturers. It should be noted that while MIAME addresses what should be reported about a microarray experiment it makes no recommendations about what format data should be stored or exchanged in.

MIAME divides a microarray experiment into six component parts: *experiment, sample, hybridization, array, data* and *normalization*. This is represented schematically in Figure 5.1. MIAME makes recommendations about what information should be provided, if data are made public. Some relevant information is contained in existing resources, such as those relating to the sequences of reporters (probes) on the array, publication details and certain sample data; for some of these it is considered sufficient to reference existing resources. These are shown in Figure 5.1.

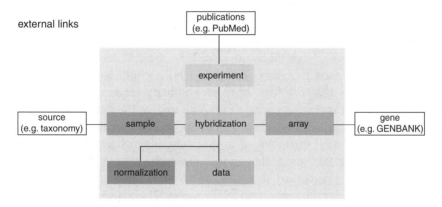

Figure 5.1 Schematic representation of MIAME concepts. Reproduced with permission from *Nature*

Some of the important MIAME terms have specific meanings that may differ from those commonly used in the laboratory. (A full glossary for MIAME and MAGE-OM can be found at http://www.mged.org/Workgroups/MIAME/miame_glossary.html).

Experiment

An experiment is considered to be a group of biologically related hybridizations. An experiment is therefore the 'container' for samples, hybridizations, arrays, normalization and data. Experiments should be uniquely identified, described simply in a single sentence. A free text full description of the experiment may also be provided. Separating all the things that happen during an experiment from the experimental design and key parameters is needed when querying data. For example, a series of hybridizations within a time course experiment are related by sampling interval, for instance, 1 h, 2 h etc.

The author or submitter of the experiment should be named along with appropriate contact details. Lastly, details of the quality control measures that were taken are required. For example, if biological or technical replicate hybridizations were performed, this should be recorded. The practical outcome of recording this data is that the reader can easily identify the rationale for and design of the experiment, identify critical variables and the constituent parts of the experiment, without having to know a great deal of detail about the experiment itself. Often such information is dispersed throughout publications, or omitted entirely. Needless to say, this makes interpretation of the results difficult.

Array design

The array design component describes the number of arrays used, their respective layout and the technology or platform used. Detailed information is also required on genes represented on the array. As already discussed, gene lists can be incomplete and in flux; therefore, it is critical that gene level information and details of each reporter (probe) located on the array should be provided. It is essential to ensure that in case of instability in gene lists, there is enough information to remap each sequence on the array. This information could be in the form of the sequence itself or at the very least links to a primary sequence database such as DDBJ/EMBL/Genbank. In cases where cDNA clones are used as templates for PCR reactions primer sequences and clone identifiers should also be supplied to allow others to reproduce the experiment or to make meaningful comparisons. This is a critical part of MIAME given the known problems with cDNA clones. Some researchers consider it necessary to re-sequence and consequently to re-annotate all clones used in the generation of cDNA arrays. Clone providers now provide mechanisms for reporting problems with clones and many laboratories are moving to long (typically $\sim$70-mer) oligonucleotide arrays to avoid problems inherent to cDNA arrays.

Samples

The sample is the material from which nucleic acid is obtained. Descriptors of the source material include those intrinsic to the material before the experiment. For example, if a breast cancer sample is used, appropriate descriptors could include species, tissue, disease state etc. Experimental treatments are also described; for example, if the breast cancer sample were subsequently cultured *in vitro* and treated with a compound, then these treatments should be described. Finally all steps of the microarray experiment are described: nucleic acid extraction, labelling and hybridization etc. These steps are often invariant within a single experiment or laboratory and are consequently easy to describe. It is harder to annotate properties of the sample and sample treatments, which are far more variable. The MGED ontology (Stoeckert and Parkinson, 2002) was initially developed to describe this part of the experiment in a controlled way. It is outside the scope of MIAME itself and will be addressed separately. Details of what should be described for different types of microarray experiment are also beyond the scope of MIAME. However, some communities are extending MIAME for specific domains and organisms.

Hybridizations

MIAME requires that the technical details of the hybridization conditions be described and that certain parameters, for example hybridization time, temperature and solution should be described.

Measurements

Measurements refer to the numeric data, often stored as a matrix in which samples are the columns and genes are the rows. Many published experiments contain only a gene list obtained by some clustering method. Format is also a problem. Affymetrix has its own format and many journals supply only a pdf file.

In order to address this lack of disclosure of the measurement data MIAME requires that all stages of the data generation be provided. This includes the processing of image data, to 'raw data' and finally details of the data processing that produced what is often referred to as the *final gene expression data matrix* and is often the basis of a publication. In addition to the data derived from the image itself, details of the scanner and image acquisition software used must also be supplied, as must details of quantitation type – mean, median etc. for each column of data. MIAME requires this level of detail, as reanalysis of data matrices is only possible if quantitation types are supplied. This is particularly true in cases when non-standard image analysis systems are being used. For example, if user-generated software is used MIAME does not dictate the format, requiring only that adequate description should be provided. It is desirable that quality indicators are provided for each data point and many commercial systems now support this.

It should be noted that although the MIAME publication refers to deposition of images in any of the current image formats (tiff, gif etc.) corresponding to each array, the public repositories do not necessarily require image submission before assigning an accession number. The main reason for this deviation is the storage costs of image data and the computational resources required to serve images in real time. It is stated that the requirement for image deposition may be 'revisited'. In practice individual experimenters store their own image files and commonly these are not made publicly available.

Normalization

The final matrix of genes and values is likely to be generated through a series of data processing and data transformation steps. The data processing steps preceding clustering or other analysis are commonly referred to as normalization. Normalization is required to adjust for variation within a single array, such as that introduced by printing the array. There is also variation that derives from actually performing the experiment, such as the differences in labelling efficiencies in two colour systems, or differences between replicate hybridizations. MIAME makes no recommendations on what normalization method is used for a given data set, but the chosen method should be reported in sufficient detail to be comprehensible. Details of spikes, so-called housekeeping gene sets and whether all genes were used to normalize the data are also required in this section.

Conclusion

Taken in small sections MIAME appears to be an exacting standard for the average bench biologist. However, it is important to remember that the experimenter already has all this information. Now that fewer experimenters are generating their own arrays, much of the information required by MIAME is supplied by the microarray facility, the array manufacturer, the scanner manufacturer and suppliers of kits used, e.g. for nucleic acid extraction. Many of the standard protocols and academic array designs are already present in the public repositories and can simply be cited, leaving the biologist to provide details of the experiment design and the samples. An inherent advantage in storing array designs centrally is that they can be comprehensibly reannotated, as annotation in the underlying sequence databases changes.

5.5 Journals and MIAME

An increasing number of journals now require MIAME-compliant data as a condition for publication. (A list can be found at www.mged.org.) Several of the high impact factor journals, such as *Cell* and *Nature*, require not only that the data are MIAME compliant, but that the data also be publicly available in one of the public repositories (see 5.11). Standards do not exist in isolation and the take-up of MIAME by the journals, funding bodies and manufacturers has been critical for its success. Indeed, other communities are now adapting the MIAME standards for microarray experiments where specific domains are addressed. These include the MIAME-Env and MIAME-Tox projects, which are developing standards for the toxicogenomics and environmental genomics communities respectively. Other standards efforts include the HUPO effort on standardization for proteomics, in which standards are being developed for mass spectrometry, protein–protein interaction etc. (Orchard, Hermjakob and Apweiler, 2003).

The proteomics and transcriptomics standards efforts described above are accompanied by open source (freely available) tools, interfaces and databases. Here we will explore some of the solutions available for microarray data.

The members of MGED have developed and also use the MAGE object model and related data exchange for microarray data (Spellman *et al.*, 2002). This is an important advance, as a common format and tools for generating and reading this format mean that individual groups need not develop their own. An object model was required because microarray data are too complex for a flat file format, such as that used by Genbank for sequence data. It is important to note that a community standard is of little use if there are no tools which make the standard easy to use.

5.6 Storage and Exchange Formats: MAGE-OM and MAGE-ML

MIAME represented a significant advance in standardization in the microarray field. However, without a data exchange format recommendations about what should be stored are of limited use. Several groups responded to the Object Management Group (OMG) call for proposals for a gene expression data exchange standard. Separate efforts, termed MAML and GEML, coalesced into the MAGE (or microarray gene expression) object model and associated data exchange format MAGE-ML, a flavour of XML. The full MAGE-OM specification is publicly available (Spellman *et al.*, 2002) and parts of it are described here.

Like the MIAME specification, MAGE is also composed of parts, called packages. Each package describes a part of the microarray experiment. MAGE is more complex and detailed than MIAME and is extremely flexible. Because of this, MAGE is suitable for any hybridization-centric experiment, such as CGH or protein arrays. Flexibility also incurs a cost as in some parts of the model information can be stored in more than one way. In practice this problem is addressed by having *de facto* rules for coding data in MAGE. These 'rules' have been developed consensually by the MAGE community and have been driven by those groups working directly with a relational database implementation of the MAGE model, and those who export data as MAGE-ML to such a database.

The key parts of MAGE map to the MIAME concepts, though this mapping is not one to one. For example, BioAssayData stores actual measurements. BioMaterial holds information on samples and treatments, BioSequence holds annotation on the

Table 5.1   Mapping of MIAME to MAGE package(s)

MIAME	MAGE package
Experiment	Experiment
Sample	BioMaterial, Protocol
Array	ArrayDesign, BioSequence, DesignElement, Array
Hybridization	BioAssay, Protocol
Data	BioAssayData, HigherLevelAnalysis, QuantitationType
Normalization	Protocol, BioAssayData

Table 5.2   Non-'MIAME' mapped MAGE packages

MAGE package	Data stored in package
Audit and Security	Contact data, creation and editing details for document
BibliographicReference	Publication details
Protocol	All protocols, hardware and software relating to sample, array and data treatments
Description	Details of references to external databases, database entries and ontology entries
Measurement	Measurements corresponding to arrays, samples, data

sequences represented on the array. Additional utility packages hold information on publication, people, contact details etc. A mapping of the MAGE packages to the six parts of MIAME and extra packages is shown in Tables 5.1 and 5.2.

Although MAGE is more complex than MIAME, the core structure is essentially preserved. Consider the example of Array in MIAME, which is split into four distinct parts in MAGE. Information that MIAME requires about an array is the following: What biological sequences are represented on the array? What is their annotation? How are they laid out and related? Which arrays were used in a given experiment? These are split in MAGE: biological sequences are contained in the BioSequence package; annotation is also stored here, excepting database information, which is stored in the Description package. The layout of the array in zones, number of spots and their physical distance apart is stored in the ArrayDesign package. As arrays can be spotted in duplicate or the same transcript represented by different sequences – say several exons of the same gene – we need to know how spots relate to each other. This is stored in the DesignElement package. Finally, the information on which particular arrays were used in a given experiment (serial numbers etc.) and what the design is called is stored in the Array package. MAGE also has a new package – Protocol – which is used to store details of all protocols, and in this example it would be used to store array manufacture protocols.

As the various MAGE packages interact, information stored in one package can be referenced by another. So there is a relationship between the annotation in the BioSequence package and which spots correspond to it. This cross-referencing is achieved by using unique identifiers for each MAGE object. BioSequence in this case links to Reporter(s) from the DesignElement package, which in turn links to a Feature (spot) in the ArrayDesign package. Relationships in MAGE have different cardinalities, meaning that there are rules in the model about how many links there can be between certain objects and these links are also directional.

MAGE-OM is described in detail elsewhere and there are MAGE tutorials for those who want to use it practically. Many projects using MAGE are accessible from the MAGE project site at source forge http://sourceforge.net/projects/mged/.

Community advice on MAGE can be accessed via a mailing list also described on the website. As MAGE is a community project, it represents a general solution for data storage and a standard format for data exchange. Although the MAGE-OM can be implemented as a relational database, many microarray databases predate MAGE and MIAME and such databases are unlikely to implement a new model, especially as they have legacy data. However, as MAGE is both an object model and a data exchange format, complete re-implementation is not necessary. Mapping an existing database to MAGE is relatively simple, and once the mapping has been achieved there is open source software (MAGEstk) that can be used to export data, to external databases such as ArrayExpress (Brazma *et al.*, 2003), and also to applications such as Bioconductor (Dudoit *et al.*, 2003), for data analysis. Several institutions have performed this mapping and can now successfully export MAGE-ML. These include the Stanford Microarray Database, RZPD and TIGR.

5.7 ArrayExpress

ArrayExpress is the public European repository for microarray data (Brazma *et al.*, 2003) maintained at the European Bioinformatics Institute in the United Kingdom (Brooksbank *et al.*, 2003). ArrayExpress offers an archiving service for data that are linked to publications and links submitted datasets to other bioinformatic resources at the EBI, such as those developed by Ensembl (Clamp *et al.*, 2003). It is also developing a data warehouse to store microarray data that can be queried in a gene-centric way. ArrayExpress is the first implementation of the MAGE model and is implemented in Oracle; queries are achieved using a java-based web application (www.ebi.ac.uk/arrayexpress).

Supported queries in the current query interface include query by accession number (experiments or arrays designs), author, laboratory, experimental design, experimental factor and protocol type. Once an experiment, array or protocol is returned the user sees a short text description with clickable links to specific parts of the experiment. These can be explored, and data or array details downloaded as tab-delimited or Excel files. Array information is presented in a format called the Array Definition Format (ADF), which is also used to submit array information to the database. Data are available for both raw and processed data (where these have been provided by the submitter) and can be either exported as a tab-delimited file for use in commercial analysis tools, or exported directly to Expression Profiler, the

EBI's own analysis tool. The database also has a browse function, whereby users can see all the experiments, arrays or protocols in the database organized by various criteria.

5.8 Annotation Tools

Data submission to ArrayExpress is either by MAGE-ML pipeline from an external database or via the MIAMExpress submission tool. MIAMExpress is the preferred submission method for biologists. It is a completely generic tool, which is not species or domain specific and requires only a web browser to use. It is designed for users with little experience of bioinformatics and requires no knowledge of MAGE or MIAME. Data are entered by a series of web forms. Array designs and protocols may be used in the submission of different experiments. This means that they need only be submitted once, thereby making multiple submissions faster. Users of commercial arrays need not submit their array designs as the ArrayExpress curation team works with vendors to make these available.

Users submit their data in the order Array Design, Protocols, Experiments and are taken through a series of forms to do this. If at any point they are unsure what to do simply clicking on the help icon will provide help of two types: help on what to do, upload a file, check a box etc., and help in the form of an example or description of what is expected in a given field, such as species, or example format of data files. Many of the fields in MIAMExpress contain drop-down lists from which users are invited to select terms. These terms are drawn from the MGED ontology. Users may also provide their own terms; these are curated and if appropriate added to both MIAMExpress and the ontology. MIAMExpress users are supported by the ArrayExpress curation team throughout the submission process, after which data are exported from the database as MAGE-ML, assigned an accession number and loaded into the database. Submitters are asked to provide a hold date on which their data will be released. They are provided with an account for the ArraysExpress database so they can see their own data once a submission has been completed. The parts of the submission and curation process are shown schematically in Figure 5.2.

5.9 Curation

Curation of the data is performed by a specialist team of data curators using a local java tool MAGEvalidator and perl scripts. Although submission routes may vary, coming via pipelines and MIAMExpress, the curation process is similar as the final file format is common. MAGEvalidator processes the MAGE-ML file and checks that the file is well formed, checks content for MIAME compliance and reports

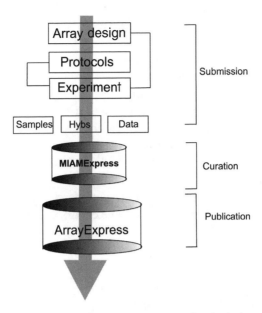

Figure 5.2 Schematic diagram showing the process of submission to ArrayExpress via MIAMExpress

novel terms to the curator, who will make any necessary changes. These are of two main types: when data are under-annotated and when information is missing altogether. In cases where terms supplied are not in the MGED ontology these will be considered for inclusion. If an incorrect term has been applied these will be corrected by the data curator and the submitter informed. Finally data are loaded either publicly or to the restricted part of the databases and the submitter is notified of the accession number. ArrayExpress accession numbers have the format A-XXXX-1, E-XXXX-1 and P-XXXX-1, for array designs, experiments and protocols respectively. The four alphabetic characters indicate the software that generated the file, so MIAMExpress has the code A-MEXP-1 and The Institute for Genomic Research (TIGR) has the code A-TIGR-1.

5.10 Standardization and Semantics

One of the outcomes of standardization is that large scale data mining becomes possible. Knowledge about the experiment is not only gained by humans reading papers but is stored with the data and can be used computationally. To do this effectively one must have access to data, a place to store and access it from, a common format and some knowledge about how the data and meta-data are described. Data descriptions need to be machine-readable to do this. Therefore, although a human may know that drugs have both generic and trade names (synonyms) a query tool would need to 'know' all possible drug names for a given compound and to look for all known variations. A simpler solution is to use ontology to represent the domain of interest which is used by multiple applications. The Gene Ontology is a good example of this system. This ontology, developed to describe gene products, is now used in many applications and development of the vocabularies continues. In some cases there is a requirement for an ontology for use in an existing application. This is the case in the MAGE model. The developers identified areas which should be described by an ontology and the ontology was largely developed after the model was complete.

The MAGE model requires Ontology Entries to describe some Objects where the developers considered that there should be some control over how certain information should be expressed. The MGED ontology specifically addresses the requirements of MAGE, but is usually useful in other contexts.

5.11 Public Microarray Databases

There are several public microarray databases, ArrayExpress at the EBI, GEO at NCBI, SMD at Stanford and plans for another in Japan at NIG and countless smaller institute specific databases who make their data public once a local researcher publishes a paper. However, here we will focus on ArrayExpress, as it is a public MIAME-compliant database whose schema, source code and data are freely available.

5.12 ArrayExpress, an Example of a Public Repository

ArrayExpress is an international repository for gene expression data, which uses the MAGE-OM model. The MAGE-OM model is an (array) platform independent data model which can equally represent data from single and dual channel experiments. This means that data from various LIMS databases, manufacturers and public databases can be mapped to MAGE and data exchanged in the same format – MAGE-ML. As MAGE is now an adopted OMG standard there has been significant take-up of the format and SMD, TIGR, RZPD, Agilent, Affymetrix and others are now making data and array designs available in MAGE-ML format.

5.13 Submissions to ArrayExpress

ArrayExpress accepts submissions in two formats – pipeline submissions in MAGE-ML format from institutions and manufacturers and submissions from submitters with little or no bioinformatics support. MAGE-ML is a heavyweight format and requires a mapping of the source database to the MAGE-OM model. Therefore the EBI has developed a MIAME compliant online submission tool.

5.14 MIAMExpress and other MIAME Compliant Annotation Systems

MIAMExpress is essentially an implementation of the MIAME questionnaire as a series of web forms which write to an underlying MySQL database. It uses the MGED ontology to populate controlled vocabulary fields and allows users to define their own terms where appropriate. For example, users working outside the field of model organisms will not have appropriate ontologies from which to select terms and these can be submitted through MIAMExpress and collated by the curators who act as a point of reference for ontology advice. MIAMExpress is freely available as a standalone tool for those who wish to install it locally and it can be configured for use by a single community for their local needs with the addition of local controlled vocabulary terms.

There are many other annotation tools under development which are similar to MIAMExpress and which also use terms from the MGED ontology and are capable of exporting MAGE-ML, for example RAD from the University of Pennsylvania (Stoeckert *et al.*, 2001) is used by biologists working on a diverse set of organisms and uses the same web form approach as MIAMExpress. The take-up of MIAME and MAGE-ML and use of ontologies means that the annotation of these datasets will become very much easier for both users and curators and the potential for analysis is huge.

5.15 Databases of Protein Expression Patterns

The ability to analyse and store gene expression data from high throughput technologies is a relatively recent development. However, protein expression data have been available for many years from low throughput visualization methods such as immuno-histochemistry, radioactive labelling methods and beta-galactosidase staining. Proteomics is a term used to describe what are essentially biochemical methods (two dimensional gel electrophoresis, two hybrid interaction screening and mass spectroscopy). These techniques provide quantitative or semi-quantitative information about protein interactions and what proteins are present in a given sample.

All of these methods have attendant problems in data storage, quality and format. The approach taken by the proteomics community has been to divide up the problem by technique and data type. For example, the Intact project has a standard and a data model for protein interaction data. Other groups work with mass spectroscopy and 2D gel data. Databases for proteomics are typically less mature (with the exception of SwissProt) than those that deal with expression data obtained using visualization methods.

Visualization methods are useful as they provide an anatomical context for expression data. Experimental 'data' produced using visualization are typically a microscopic image of a tissue or organism, with some staining pattern that is associated with structures within the tissue or organism. Interpreting such images requires knowledge of the basic anatomy of the organism in question, and details of the 'probe' used. Comparison of images is particularly difficult as they can be of normal, mutant or diseased samples, are often in the form of serial sections and may be from different animals and are not necessarily in the same plane. Storing images is computationally expensive and good annotation of images is critical for efficient querying.

5.16 The Gene Expression Database (GXD)

GXD (Ringwald *et al.*, 2001) is an expression database for the mouse which integrates data from *in situ* hybridization, immuno-histochemistry, northern and western blotting and microarray data. It aims to integrate these disparate data types into a single resource, GXD. GXD in turn is integrated with the mouse gene model and gene sequence information.

GXD annotates anatomical data using the Mouse Anatomical Dictionary (MAD). The MAD is a dictionary of terms to describe mouse anatomy in the developing embryo organized in a hierarchical structure – or an ontology – and is used by other projects such as the Mouse Atlas Database (Davidson *et al.*, 1997), which combines the ontology with three dimensional models of the mouse to produce annotated images. The integration of GXD with other information on the mouse, including the annotation of GO terms to sequences, allows queries such as 'What genes annotated to GO term DNA binding are expressed in the CNS at Theiler stage 15?'. This combinatorial use of terms from different ontologies allows a complex query to be made efficiently across different data types.

GXD includes images from publications that are curated and annotated. However, in many experiments much of the primary data obtained are never published (in some fields this may be as high as 80 per cent of all data generated), and to obtain these data GXD has developed an annotation and submission tool, the Gene Expression Notebook (GEN). This tool is for use by bench biologists, is Excel based, and allows annotation of experiments such as *in situ* hybridizations when they are performed. These can then be later submitted to GXD. Development of simple tools such as GEN for biologists are critical if all the 'missing' data are to be accessed and made available to the research community. GXD, along with many other databases, is now using its experience of using and contributing to existing ontologies to develop a cross-organism phenotype ontology. Given that we are now using sequenced organisms to study human disease, controlled annotation of phenotype will be critical in making efficient use of forthcoming data.

5.17 Conclusion

This chapter has reviewed expression databases and the way that ontologies can be used to annotate them. The examples selected are only two of many relevant examples, and show how common annotation resources such as the Gene Ontology and the Mouse Anatomical Dictionary can be used to benefit users of different levels of expertise and different analysis needs. Use of ontologies in bioinformatics is a growing field and we are slowly moving towards the goal of automated data mining.

References

Blaschke, C., Hirschman, L. and Valencia, A. (2002). Information extraction in molecular biology. *Briefings Bioinformat.* **3**, 154–165.

Brazma, A. *et al.* (2001). Minimum information about a microarray experiment (MIAME)-toward standards for microarray data. *Nat Genet* **29**(4), 365–371.

Brazma, A. and Parkinson, H. *et al.* (2003). ArrayExpress – a public repository for microarray gene expression data at the EBI. *Nucleic Acids Res.* **31**(1), 68–71.

Brooksbank, C. and Camon, E. *et al.* (2003). The European Bioinformatics Institute's data resources. *Nucleic Acids Res.* **31**(1), 43–50.

Clamp, M. and Andrews, D. *et al.* (2003). Ensembl 2002: accommodating comparative genomics. *Nucleic Acids Res.* **31**(1), 38–42.

Davidson, D. and Bard, J. *et al.* (1997). The mouse atlas and graphical gene-expression database. *Semin. Cell Dev. Biol.* **8**(5), 509–517.

Dudoit, S. and Gentleman, R.C. *et al.* (2003). Open source software for the analysis of microarray data. *Biotechniques Suppl.* 45–51.

Orchard, S., Hermjakob, H. and Apweiler, R. (2003). The proteomics standards initiative. *Proteomics* **3**, 1374–1376.

Ringwald, M. and Eppig, J.T. *et al.* (2001). The Mouse Gene Expression Database (GXD). *Nucleic Acids Res.* **29**(1), 98–101.

Spellman, P. T. and Miller, M. *et al.* (2002). Design and implementation of microarray gene expression markup language (MAGE-ML). *Genome Biol.* **3**(9), RESEARCH0046.

Stoeckert, C.J. Jr. and Parkinson, H. (2002). The MGED Ontology: a framework for describing functional genomics experiments. *Comparative Functional Genom.* **4**, 127–132.

Stoeckert, C. and Pizarro, A. *et al.* (2001). A relational schema for both array-based and SAGE gene expression experiments. *Bioinformatics* **17**(4), 300–308.

II
The Basis of Annotation

6 Taxonomy: a Moving Target for Sequence Data

M. I. Krichevsky

Abstract

We report species diversity as species incidence. Molecular biologists want one species name per sequence. Taxonomists write conflicting treatments. Commonly, sequence database users utilize species annotation sequences as a gold standard. Often, the annotation violates a code of nomenclature. Five components of the International Council for Scientific Unions manage the current codes of nomenclature applying to all forms of life. Sometimes, ambiregnal names occur, i.e. organisms named under multiple codes. Conclusions are as follows.

Taxonomy is not exactly congruent with function.
Restating Darwin's conclusion: *clones vary*.
Sequences are not exactly congruent with taxonomy or function.
Species names are useful pointers to information.
Species names are *not* revealed truth or immutable.
Incidence of species is *not* a primary measure of diversity.
Scientific names and the sources of the names must be used to avoid ambiguity at the species level.
Adequate annotation must describe in detail all known attributes of the clone studied.

Keywords

taxonomy, nomenclature, species, zoology, botany, microbiology, codes, sequences, ambiregnal, ICSU

Database Annotation in Molecular Biology   Edited by Arthur M. Lesk
© 2005 John Wiley & Sons, Ltd.   ISBN: 0-470-85681-5

6.1 Introduction

'I am almost convinced... that species are not (it is like confessing to murder) immutable'.

'After describing a set of forms as distinct species, tearing up my M.S., and making them separate, and then making them one again. I have gnashed, my teeth, cursed species, and asked what sin I had committed to be so punished' (Darwin, 1905) (Murray, personal communication).

SPECIES (abbreviated to sp. or spp. (plural)).

1. A category, definable only in terms of position (below genus) in a hierarchical system.

2. A taxonomic group, definable in terms of the characters of the constituent members.

3. A concept; that it is useful cannot be denied, but the user must realize that the species does not exist and is not an entity.

'To summarize: a species is a group of organisms defined more or less subjectively by the criteria chosen by the taxonomist to show to best advantage and as far as possible put into practice his individual concept of what a species is' (Cowan, 1978) (Murray, personal communication).

The limiting factor in interdisciplinary communication is the ability of the persons involved to understand the vocabulary and nomenclature of all the disciplines included to the level needed to reason with the information. The user of information must receive input from disparate disciplines each of which has its own jargon. The practitioners of the various disciplines invent new words and give new meaning to old words as their disciplines advance. This inevitable practice facilitates communication locally but creates noise globally.

The most prevalent unit for describing biodiversity is the 'species'. The boundary delineating the definition of a species is critical to deciding whether a species is endangered, even though, as Erlich (1988) posits, 'The loss of genetically distinct populations within species is, at the moment, at least as an important a problem as the loss of entire species'. We report species diversity based on the incidence of species using informational content measures. However, the concept of what constitutes a species varies across the spectrum of life. In general, the larger the organism, the simpler the demarcation into species appears. An elephant or sequoia usually is identified with much more certainty, even when somewhat atypical, than a bacterium such as *E. coli*. A three-legged elephant would still be identified as an elephant even though both the elephant and the sequoia are described as having a 'trunk'.

People yearn for consistency in their intellectual pursuits. Consider a simple example of this dilemma. Biologists name organisms. They develop the concept of 'species'. Then the users of the names try to ignore the Darwinian principles of variability within and between species. The molecular biologist wants one species name for a biological specimen sequence. Taxonomists write conflicting (and valid) treatments and a corresponding rationale for each treatment. This pleases taxonomists, but the molecular biologists are confused and do not understand the distinctions. The converse is just as common. Yet, one or another of the conflicting opinions becomes part of the annotation data of the sequence.

As with polynomials, the data have multiple valid roots. As our knowledge of the diversity and classification of the biosphere increases, a form of Heisenberg uncertainty increases. The more tools for classification available, the less certain the 'truth'. Ultimately, rules, no matter how arbitrary, must develop for defining species in terms of the boundaries as well as their typical genetic and phenetic attributes. Even then, uncertainty reigns.

The English philosopher John Locke (29 August 1632–28 October 1704) argued that communication is the motivation for establishing species names and definitions. That is, nature does not make species. People do, as a mechanism to facilitate communication of a collection of ideas under one general term. In addition, Locke states that the boundaries of species are opinions rather than natural borders.

A wish for consistency is not confined to molecular biologists. Ecologists, environmentalists, lawyers, legislators and other groups seek stability as well. Biologists currently expend great effort in developing check-lists, official nomenclature lists and databases of names of species. The great utility of these is clear. However, these communication devices are necessarily in a state of flux because of varying classification methods and opinions.

Thus, a fundamental barrier to communication of information in biology is the lack of adequate information transfer bridges among the subdisciplines of biology. To carry the above example even further, many biologists will use the common name of an organism in recording and communicating their data without understanding the limitations of the common names. 'Mouse' covers either one or two genera of rodent, depending on the dictionary consulted. Peanuts are not nuts. Hospital records list 'atypical E. coli' without keeping the original observations justifying the designation of 'atypical'. All of this taxonomic imprecision creates serious problems for adequate searching and interpreting of data in biology.

Commonly, both sequence databases contributors and users utilize one or a few examples of sequences of a species as a gold standard for describing the species. They speak of the 'mouse genome'. As pointed out above, there cannot be a 'mouse genome'. In many cases, the various Codes of Nomenclature are violated. Further, different codes of nomenclature exist for various biota. Consider the codes of nomenclature in common use as well as some of those proposed.

6.2 Nomenclature

The International Council for Scientific Unions (ICSU), through various component organizations, maintains, modifies, and applies the currently active codes of nomenclature applying to all forms of life. In addition, proposals exist for additional codes to address issues such as lack of uniformity of rules among the existing codes and treatment of cladistic organization of biological information.

The following outline gives the organization and Internet addresses of the components of ICSU managing the current codes.

I. International Council for Scientific Unions (ICSU) (www.icsu.org)

   A. International Union of Biological Sciences (IUBS) (www.iubs.org)

      1. International Commission on Zoological Nomenclature (ICZN) (www. iczn.org)

         (a) International Code of Zoological Nomenclature

      2. International Association for Plant Taxonomy (IAPT) (www.botanik. univie. ac.at/iapt/)

         (a) International Code of Botanical Nomenclature

      3. International Commission for the Nomenclature of Cultivated Plants (ICNCP) (www.ishs.org/sci/icracpco.htm)

         (a) International Code of Nomenclature for Cultivated Plants

         (b) Code derived from the International Code of Botanical Nomenclature with specific elements relating to cultivated plants

   B. International Union of Microbiological Societies (IUMS) (www.iums.org)

      1. International Committee on Systematics of Prokaryotes (ICSP) (www.the-icsp.org)

         (a) International Code of Nomenclature of Bacteria

         (b) 'Bacteria' in the name of the code, rather than 'Prokaryotes', reflects the name of the official publication of the code

         (c) An earlier name of the code was the International Code of Nomenclature of Bacteria and Viruses

      2. International Committee on the Taxonomy of Viruses (ICTV) (http://www.mcb.uct.ac.za/ictv/ICTV.html) (www.ncbi.nlm.nih.gov/ICTV/ rules.html)

         (a) International Code of Virus Classification and Nomenclature.

Both a publication and the deposit of a type specimen or culture validates a new name for any biological entity (except a virus). The stringency of both the rules of publication and type specimen deposition vary with the individual codes. The original publication usually lists the place(s) of deposit.

The following outline lists the practices for deposit of nomenclatural types for codes. The outline elements are the code name, usual name for deposited material, physical nature of deposit and the stringency of the requirement for deposit.

(I) International Code of Zoological Nomenclature

- Type specimen: nature varies with organism – deposition in a recognized institution not required by the code, although most authors do, making specimens available. Type specimen may be deposited in a private collection.

- Now must be designated and clearly identified for any species described after 2000.

(II) International Code of Botanical Nomenclature

- Type: single plant, parts of one or several plants, or of multiple small plants – usually mounted on a single herbarium sheet or in an equivalent preparation, such as a box, packet, jar or microscope slide.

- Either a single specimen conserved in one herbarium or other collection or institution, or an illustration for any species described after 1990.

(III) International Code of Nomenclature of Bacteria

- Type culture: living culture.

- Publication in the *International Journal of Systematic and Evolutionary Microbiology* and deposition in two recognized culture collections in two different countries.

- Living pathogenic entities are exceptions to the principle of accessibility because of the risk of accidental or criminal release. Rules and laws regulating accessibility and transport are on the increase.

(IV) International Code of Virus Classification and Nomenclature

- Physical type not used.

- Nomenclatural type description serves this function.

- Accepted description maintained by ICTV.

With the exception of virus nomenclature, the biological codes do not allow for judgments as to the scientific validity of the application of the name of an organism.

(The ICTV does make such judgments through a system of specialist committees.) The only judgments made are on the etymological validity of a name. No judgment is made of the scientific basis of the new name. Thus, competing taxonomies, reflecting the views of differing scholarly taxonomists, are valid as long as they follow the rules for publication of the name. Only usage decides which of the alternative taxonomies will prevail.

Another source of nomenclatural confusion is the phenomenon of 'ambiregnal' nomenclature. That is, an organism may be validly published under the rules of more than one code. Most of the ambiregnal occurrences are microorganisms. Well known examples are the 'blue-green algae', which are prokaryotes. Under the Bacteriological Code, they are the *Cyanobacteria*. The cellular slime moulds are amoebae, which differentiate into a stalked fruiting body, which contains a form of cellulose. Upon differentiation, the cellular slime moulds resemble fungi.

Names can be 'ambiregnal' as well. Isaak (2004) lists a number of instances of names of plants and animals sharing the same name such as *Aotus* (pea or monkey) and *Bartramia* (moss or sandpiper). This reference contains discussion and lists of various unusual aspects of the naming of organisms.

6.3 Operational Definitions

The construct of species requires observation of the attributes of multiple biological objects. Usually, these objects start with a single organism or part thereof, be it a microbial cell, a tree or a rodent. The single object is the basic observational unit. Each object is viewed in isolation. At the individual level, terms used for single objects may be 'isolate' (in microbiology) or 'specimen' or 'sample'. A group of isolates comprises a 'strain', 'klone', 'cultivar' and so forth. (The term 'klone' in German appears to be equivalent to the English 'strain'.) Finally, a species emerges from the accumulated observations of multiple objects.

Consider the following operational definitions and attributes of 'isolate', 'strain' and 'species' for microorganisms. Here we do not considering the metaphysical definition of 'species'. We leave that to the biological philosophers. We want to manipulate data in a frame of reference that is consistent, even if arbitrary. This discussion uses the terminology and examples from microbiology. However, the issues pervade all of biology, albeit with varying terms and severity.

Simplest first. We can define the description of an isolate as a single assemblage of data (a record) resulting from the observations of a single, unique object. (The observations may be of phenotype, serotype, genotype, virulence, host range etc. All these methods have been used to define or describe isolates, strains and species.) There may be redundant observations of the properties of the singular object for error reduction. Each observation has only one 'true' value (either numerical or presence/ absence). Recording incidence is a trivial concept. An isolate can only occur once. However, recording the source of isolation is usually quite important.

Rampant confusion abounds in use of the term 'strain'. Often 'strain' and 'isolate' are used interchangeably. Nothing is wrong if clearly stated that the isolate definition is the one that obtains. However, a strain commonly is defined as a series of isolates that are 'identical' (as in the annual search for the new flu strain). Thus, at least two isolate records must be compared to establish identity. Since identity is required, any single isolate definition may be the definitive record. Describing incidence of the strain becomes a two step process. First, identity must be confirmed by exact match to the definition (allowing for some observational error). The result of this step can only be true or false (identity/no identity). Second, the time and place of isolation of the individual isolations must be recorded. Only the incidence data are further analysable.

Some would argue that isolates exhibiting 'small' differences should still belong to the same strain. However, a single change in a viral epitope or an amino acid on the haemoglobin molecule profoundly affects their biological activity. A flower cultivar that loses a pigment through a single base change may warrant a patent as a unique entity. Here again we have a boundary problem. How many nucleotide changes in an t-RNA molecule form the boundary condition between strains? Five? Four? Three? Two? One?

A species is described in terms of at least one record describing one or more isolates that are distinctly different from other isolates. The requirement of distinction implies some decision rule (either codified or personally operational) as to what is sufficient distinction. Between identity (strain) and distinction (species) lies the area of similarity. (For simplicity, this discussion omits consideration of decision planes for subspecies and other intermediate taxonomic levels between strain and species.) The same arguments with respect to the need for decision rules obtain. Only the level of required similarity differs. We speak of 'atypical' strains, variants (serovars, pathovars etc.). This verbal imprecision actually reflects the degree of similarity, ascertained by some distance measure, to the idealized strain description. Thus, the definition of a species has two components: the idealized strain description and the decision boundary of allowable variation.

Incidence of species in space and time is a statistical problem in that the incidence must be derived from the individual isolate records. First, the species 'identity' (actually similarity) must be computed or deduced from experience. Second, the distributions must be calculated or mapped. At this point, the raw data from which the species is determined are often discarded. One sees the aforementioned phrase 'atypical *E. coli*' on hospital patient records with no information as to what made them 'atypical'. Useful epidemiological studies are thus precluded.

An even more basic problem occurs when these distinctions are blurred. The logical difference between the concept of isolate and species impacts directly on the design of data structures. We find data elements for both in the same data structure. What is the 'habitat' of an isolate? What is the 'source of isolation' of a species? What is the virulence of a 'species'? The host range of an isolate can be determined experimentally. That of a species must be inferred from the data accumulated by test of the host ranges of a representative set of isolates or by inference based on source of isolation of many isolates.

Consequently, isolate and strain data can be recorded largely as presence/absence or continuous variables. Species data usually take the form of numerical data (frequencies, continuous variables, ratios, ranges, distributions etc.). Strain data can be calculated from isolate data. Species data are calculated from isolate or strain data. Species data cannot yield strain data and strain data cannot yield isolate data. These concepts are summarized in Boxes 6.1–6.3.

Box 6.1. Isolate

```
! OBSERVATIONS OF A CLONE
! A SINGLE ASSEMBLAGE OF DATA (A RECORD)
  " PHENOTYPE
  " SEROTYPE
  " GENOTYPE
  " VIRULENCE
  " HOST RANGE
! ONE 'TRUE' VALUE/OBSERVATION
! INCIDENCE = ISOLATE CAN ONLY OCCUR ONCE
SOURCE OF ISOLATION USUALLY QUITE IMPORTANT
```

Box 6.2. Strain

```
! SERIES OF ISOLATES THAT ARE 'IDENTICAL'
! ISOLATE RECORDS COMPARED TO ESTABLISH IDENTITY
! ANY SINGLE ISOLATE THE DEFINITIVE RECORD
! INCIDENCE OF STRAIN — TWO STEP PROCESS
  " IDENTITY = EXACT MATCH TO THE DEFINITION
  " TIME AND PLACE OF ISOLATION
ONLY THE INCIDENCE DATA ARE FURTHER ANALYSABLE
```

Box 6.3. Species

```
! 1 RECORD COMPUTED FROM MULTIPLE ISOLATES
! ISOLATES DIFFERENT, BUT NOT TOO DIFFERENT
! OPERATIONAL SPECIES DEFINITION — 2 COMPONENTS
  " IDEALIZED STRAIN DESCRIPTION
    —HYPOTHETICAL MEDIAN ORGANISM
  " DECISION BOUNDARY OF ALLOWABLE VARIATION
    —CODIFIED (COMPUTED STATISTIC)
    —PERSONALLY OPERATIONAL
# EXPERIENCE
# KEY
```

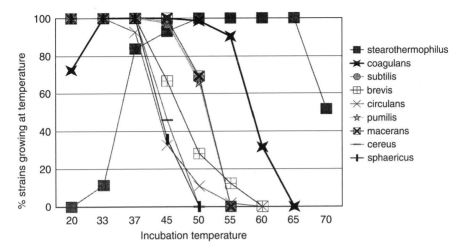

Figure 6.1 Growth of multiple strains of *Bacillus* species at various temperatures

Consider Figure 6.1. The ability to grow at various temperatures is at least partially under genetic control. Critical heat sensitive or resistant cellular components that confer the ability to grow at differing temperatures must differ in their chemical structures. Therefore, differing responses within the same species must reflect such structural differences. The temperature responses of multiple strains of these species of the genus *Bacillus* varied at the outer bounds of the tested temperatures (Mitchell, 1951).

The figure indicates clearly that there are no definitive extremes usable as a range at the species level. For example, the strains of *B. stearothermophilus* exhibit percentage levels that vary as the incubation temperatures increase from 33 to 45 °C. Not until 50 °C do all strains grow. At 70 °C approximately half the strains grew. The decline of the ability of *B. coagulans* to grow at higher temperatures is the approximate obverse of the *B. stearothermophilus* increase. Thus, the variability at the extremes for each species makes reporting a growth range at the species level confusing at best. A sequence analysis of the genes or proteins sensitive to the increased temperature levels should reflect an analogous distribution in fine structure.

6.4 Searching for the Taxonomic Gold Standard

A 1991 workshop (Krichevsky *et al.*, 1991) considered questions of establishing a taxonomy and the desired nature of the methodological 'gold standard' for taxonomy or identification in bacteria. The conclusion reached at that time was that no clear candidate exists. The method is question dependent. Conversely, the question is method dependent. The conclusion applies to later times and other organisms.

The following scheme illustrates the iterative nature of establishing a collection of biological objects from nature (or from other collections) and classifying the organisms thus obtained. This scheme describes the process for cultivatable micro-organisms. The scheme is largely method independent and applies to all organisms. With only minor modification of the protocol for data gathering it would apply to Darwin's finches (http://www.pnas.org/cgi/content/full/94/15/7768) (http://hometown.aol.com/darwinpage/darfinch1.htm).

Establishing strain population for accession and study

- sample econiche to classify predominant phenetic biotypes
- accumulate representatives of each major biotype
- assign biotypes to appropriate putative taxa
- establish minimum phenetic span for inclusion in each biotype.

Data gathering on isolates in each category

- collect data on physiology, biochemistry, morphology, serology, macromolecular sequences, DNA homology etc. of isolates.

Data management and quality control

- store and search data (simple bookkeeping)
- evaluate tests
- compare results of repeats as controls
- feed back results to investigator
- generate reports.

Analysis

- compare by direct matching with authentic strains
- evaluate tests for applicability and discriminatory power
- do statistical analysis
- determine feature frequencies
- choose taxonomy (by informational content for intended use).

Classify isolates

- establishment of identification methods
- construct keys
- construct probabilistic matrix.

As the collection grows, the above process is repeated and the taxonomy is updated. Why not use a 'standard' taxonomy? As stated above, there is no 'official' scientific definition of the boundaries of each taxon. Therefore, the individual taxonomists must use their best professional judgment to identify a new object.

Sneath and Sokal (1973) stated the possible informational states for placing an object into a species. These are as (a) a member of a particular existing species, (b) a member of another species, (c) a transitional organism between two species or (d) an outlier, thus a member of no known species. Implicit in this construct are decision boundaries distinctly separating these states. A mathematician colleague observed that the formulation by Sneath and Sokal is an example of what is now known as 'fuzzy logic'.

Commonly, the user of a sequence data bank asks for the nearest match to the sequence at hand. When a satisfactory closest match results, the user next asks for the the name of the organism associated with that match. The assumption is that the annotation is taxonomically correct and yields the identity of the user's sequence. Thus, a single sequence in the database becomes the reference standard for identification.

Under the codes of nomenclature, the type does not have to be typical. It is the object that was first associated with the name by valid publication. Thus the position of the sequence donor organism has an unknown position in the distribution of biological entities that make up the construct of the species. If the detected best match is from a donor on the periphery of the species, an error of only a small number of bases in either sequence could shift the identification from one species to another, closely related, species.

Further, the errors of nomenclature can propagate in the databank with time. Assume that the first instance of a reference sequence was taxonomically misidentified. A second sequence exhibiting the closest match to the erroneously identified sequence would also have erroneous taxonomic identification. One can imagine a (presumably rare) cascade of misidentifications, a virtual clade of erroneously identified sequences.

Changes in taxonomy due to new valid publication of names continue unabated. The annotation of organism names is a snapshot in time of the name of the sequence donor organism. The database user should consult the various sources for updated information in the taxonomic area of interest.

Placing a sequence in an existing taxonomy is as much art as science. The sequence data bank consists of a large set of single reference sequences which may or may not be at the 'centre' of the named taxon. In cases where probability or other statistical descriptions of the phenotypes in the taxon are available, the donor organism should be 'identified' in this way as well. If the two agree, the identification is satisfying and acceptable. That is the best possible outcome. There is no absolute gold standard for identification.

6.5 Conclusions

- Taxonomy is not exactly congruent with function

- Restating Darwin's conclusion: *clones vary*

- Sequences are not exactly congruent with taxonomy or function

- Species names are useful pointers to information

- Species names are *not* revealed truth or immutable

- Incidence of species is *not* a primary measure of diversity

- Scientific names and the sources of the names must be used to avoid ambiguity at the species level

- Adequate annotation must describe in detail all known attributes of the clone studied.

References

Cowan, S.T. (1978) *A Dictionary of Microbial Taxonomic Usage*, Cambridge University Press, Cambridge (as quoted by R. G. E. Murray, University of Western Ontario).

Darwin, C. (1905) C. Darwin to J.D. Hooker. Down, September 25th [1853]. In Darwin, F., ed., *The Life and Letters of Charles Darwin*, Appleton, New York (as quoted by R. G. E. Murray, University of Western Ontario).

Erlich, P.R. (1988). The Loss of Diversity: causes and consequences. In Wilson, E.O., ed., *Biodiversity*, National Academy Press, Washington, DC, p. 22.

Isaak, M. (2004) *Curiosities of Biological Nomenclature*. http://home.earthlink.net/~misaak/taxonomy.html

Krichevsky, M.I. and the Workshop Participants. (1991) Draft results of a workshop to develop guidelines for studies involving microbial incidence or populations in the oral cavity. *J. Dent. Res.* **70**, 226–232.

Locke, J. (1690) *An Essay Concerning Human Understanding: Book 3: Chapter V: Of the Names of Mixed Modes and Relations.*

Mitchell, P. (1951) Recalculated from the work of Gordon and Smith as reproduced by Mitchell, P. In Werkman, C.H. and Wilson, P.W., eds, *Bacterial Physiology*. Academic, New York, p. 135.

Sneath, P.H.A. and Sokal, R.R. (1973) *Numerical Taxonomy: the Principles and Practice of Numerical Classification*, Freeman, San Francisco.

7 Genomics and Proteomics: Design and Sources of Annotation

K. Mayer and **G. Mannhaupt**

Abstract

Sequencing and analysis of complete genomes has become a primary focus within modern biology. Analysis of small bacterial genomes is now fairly routine, but structuring the genomic sequences of complex organisms is still a considerable challenge. Powerful systems are available to exploit the data, extract coding information and attach biological information to genetic units.

This chapter outlines strategies to extract information, add biological knowledge to gene products and place them in a genome-wide and comparative frame.

Apart from key requirements in modern genome analysis, such as gene detection and modelling, we address the problem of continuously and consistently assigning functional information and attaching molecular cues to individual genetic units.

Finally, we address the problem of data standardization and connecting heterogenous data and databases.

Keywords

genome analysis, gene finding, annotation, functional association, domain detection, database interoperability, ontology, genome topology

Database Annotation in Molecular Biology   Edited by Arthur M. Lesk
© 2005 John Wiley & Sons, Ltd.   ISBN: 0-470-85681-5

7.1 Beyond the Sequence: the Challenge of Complete Genome Analysis

The last decade of the 20th century saw a paradigm shift in the biological sciences. The focus of research shifted away from the study of individual genes. Sequencing and analysis of complete genomes, study of complete genomes, the genetic networks governing molecular circuits, communication and responses have now become a primary focus within biology. The shift started with the sequencing of small viral or bacterial genomes, accelerated after complete genome sequences from insects (Adams *et al.*, 2000), yeast (Goffeau *et al.*, 1996) and worms (Anon., 1998) became available, and reached a peak with the publication of a draft sequence of the human genome (Lander *et al.*, 2001; Venter *et al.*, 2001).

Technology has developed considerably in a comparably short time period. Deciphering the complete sequence of smaller genomes such as those of bacteria is now fairly routine. However, determining and structuring the genomic sequences of complex organisms with enormous genome sizes and complexities is still a considerable challenge for research groups worldwide, and the successful determination of complete genomes of several mammals is an achievement of the greatest significance.

Notwithstanding the successes, a complete genome sequence does not easily reveal the information stored and the elements encoded. Powerful systems and strategies have recently been developed to exploit the data, to extract the information about the genomic inventory of the individual organisms and to attach biological information to individual units. In addition, it is widely accepted that a genomic 'part list' is only a starting point to learn about the biology of individual organisms. The highly orchestrated interplay of the individual components to form complex, highly flexible and interconnected molecular networks connects and integrates the individual jigsaw pieces (the proteins) into function on a whole-organism scale. Thus genome-wide functional analysis of the individual constituents is the logical follow-up to elucidate the molecular function of organisms and to gain insight into similarities and diversities between organisms.

In this chapter we focus on strategies to extract the information from genomic sequences and to add biological knowledge to individual genes and gene products, and highlight current strategies that attempt to analyse individual elements and place them in a genome-wide, contextual frame.

7.2 Extracting the Genes

Genome sizes range in order of magnitude from 10^3 basepairs for small viral genomes such as SV40 up to an over hundred gigabase range (10^{11} basepairs) (Table 7.1). Although superficially genome size seems to reflect the complexity of the

Table 7.1 Genome sizes and gene content of organisms within different taxa

Organism	Genome size	Gene number
Bacteriophage *Lambda* (Sanger *et al.*, 1982)	48 kb	70
Haemophilus influenzae (Fleischmann *et al.*, 1995)	1.8 Mb	1 850
Brewers' yeast (Goffeau *et al.*, 1996) (*Saccharomyces cerevisiae*)	12.5 Mb	6 200
E. coli (Blattner *et al.*, 1997)	4.6 Mb	4 300
Fruit fly (Adams *et al.*, 2000) (*Drosophila melanogaster*)	180 Mb	14 100
C. elegans (Anon., 1998)	97 Mb	19 100
Thale cress (Anon., 2000) (*Arabidopsis thaliana*)	125 Mb	26 000
Rice (Goff *et al.*, 2002; Yu *et al.*, 2002b) (*Oryza sativa*)	430 Mb	~40 000–60 000
Human (Lander *et al.*, 2001; Venter *et al.*, 2001) (*Homo sapiens*)	2900 Mb	~30 000–40 000
Mouse (Anon., 2002) (*Mus musculus*)	~2500 Mb	~30 000
Maize (Bennetzen, Chandler and Schnable, 2001) (*Zea mais*)	~2500 Mb	~50 000
Pufferfish (Aparicio *et al.*, 2002) (*Fugu rubripes*)	~365 Mb	~31 000
Wheat (*Triticum aestivum*)	16 500 Mb	~50 000 (?)

organism, huge genome size-range variations exist within taxa. For example, lilies or salamander genomes are far larger than the human genome. Moreover, in contrast to the exponential increase in genome size for multicellular and complex organisms, the number of genes encoded within the respective genomes does not increase in proportion to the genome sizes, although there is a pronounced increase in gene number with the increase in organism complexity, reaching approximately 35 000 genes for human and between 45 000 and 60 000 genes in rice (Table 7.1) (Goff *et al.*, 2002; Lander *et al.*, 2001; Venter *et al.*, 2001; Yu *et al.*, 2002a). Indeed, the pronounced differences in genome size are not directly related to the number of genes encoded but largely attributable to highly expanded repetitive regions (see below).

For genome analysis and gene annotation, it is not the number of genes that complicates the analysis and gene extraction in higher eukaryotes. Typically, genes encoded in lower eukaryote genomes contain only a few introns, whereas in higher eukaryotes multiple introns appear to be the rule. In vertebrates introns can reach several 100 kilobases in length, and additional genetic elements such as transposable elements can be located within them. In simple organisms, intergenic spaces are in general relatively small, and conserved features such as ribosome binding sites

(RBSs) appear to be tightly connected to transcription start sites and can thus be used to delineate gene borders by using the transcription initiation sites. As in bacterial genomes and lower eukaryotes genes are most often encoded as uninterrupted open reading frames, this allows effective gene identification by scanning the genomic sequence for open reading frames exceeding a given limit in size, and fulfilling additional criteria such as elevated GC content and coding potential.

Although in eukaryotes also coding regions usually differ from noncoding regions (such as introns and intergenic regions) by various features such as elevated GC content and coding potential, the more complex structure of eukaryotic genes poses a challenge for gene detection and modelling. Within genomes of higher eukaryotes split gene structure becomes the rule rather than the exception. This has severe implications for the detection and modelling of individual genes, for in addition to the detection of coding exons these have to be combined to complete genes. Thus correct splicing as well as 5′ and 3′ gene borders need to be detected and integrated into the output (see also below).

7.3 Organism Specific Peculiarities

Is there a generalizable recipe for the analysis of large genomic stretches for all organisms? There are huge differences between organisms in the composition and overall structure of genomes. Despite the general rule that intergenic and intronic sequences have a more or less pronounced difference in AT content compared to exons, AT contents in genomes vary over a wide range. For example, the genome of *Borrelia burgdorferi* has a GC content of only 20 per cent whereas *Streptomyces coelicolor* has 69 per cent GC content.

Even between organisms with comparable AT contents within coding regions, the usage of nucleotides often has pronounced differences. On the one hand, this allows us to distinguish DNA from different organisms based on hexanucleotide frequency, and on the other it complicates analysis procedures and gene detection. Thus, underlying parameters for gene detection, such as GC content and coding probability, differ among organisms. To achieve a maximum fidelity in gene detection, training and adjustment of the programs has to be done individually for each organism, as even subtle differences in individual peculiarities accumulate and contribute to errors in gene prediction.

A special case appears in the nucleotide and codon composition of genes in monocotyledonous plants, e.g., genes in grasses such as rice, maize, wheat or barley. Grass genes contain a gradient of GC content along most of their genes. In these genes a higher GC content is observed at the 5′ part of the gene compared with the 3′ part. Comparison of orthologous genes between dicotyledonous and monocotyledonous plants typically show a pronounced slope in GC content (Wong *et al.*, 2002). This peculiarity poses a challenge for gene identification and the correct delineation of gene structure, as the computer programs have to cope with a pronounced variation of both GC content and codon usage in the $5'$ to $3'$ course of the individual genes.

7.4 Topology of Genomes

Whereas smaller bacterial and lower eukaryotic genomes contain only very restricted intergenic regions, these regions can become very large in higher eukaryotes. In addition, in larger genomes the intergenic space (as well as intronic regions in vertebrates) often contain large amounts of repetitive sequences, transposable elements, and remnants of transposable elements. These are often highly enriched in, and around, centromeric regions, as well as in island-like regions that are often clearly recognizable on a cytological level (Fransz *et al.*, 2000; McCombie *et al.*, 2000). For grass genomes it has been found that transposon-enriched regions alternate with gene-rich islands. For the maize genome, which is in the same size range as the human genome, there are estimates that the genome is comprised of up to 80 per cent transposable elements of different type, which are arranged in a very complex manner (SanMiguel *et al.*, 1996). Transposons can also be located within individual genes, especially within introns.

As during the course of evolution the reading frame and gene structure of elements no longer active have been mutated, open reading frames frequently appear to be disrupted and often are detected as a mosaic of subframes of the respective element. In addition, for transposons located within introns of genes, as well as for transposons located in the close surroundings of genes, it is often difficult to distinguish the two closely located but separate genetic elements. In consequence, automated application of genefinding programs on genomic DNA stretches containing no longer active transposable elements often leads to models that contain exon – intron structures that do not reflect the actual structure of the element. These models reflect the mutated nature of no longer transposable elements by circumventing mutations causing frameshifts and stop codons by aberrant splicing. For transposable elements located within introns or the surroundings of genes, automated prediction methods often fail to distinguish the two different genetic elements, but instead report gene models that are concatenations or mosaics of the two elements.

Thus, for transposon-containing genomic regions it is important to have criteria to separate transposable elements from genic regions, that allow us to detect, classify and distinguish the two features. A popular and robust approach is to detect and mask transposable elements based on homology matches to known transposable elements. The regions harbouring these elements are masked and not considered in subsequent genefinding procedures. However, intrinsic limitations appear, as the approaches rely on already known classes of transposons, and the individual transposon borders are often blurred. Thus homology-driven methods for transposon detection and masking can potentially be complemented by methods that focus on structural features of individual transposon classes, such as tRNA-like structural features found in SINE elements and/or long terminal repeat stretches (LTRs) flanking the borders of LTR retrotransposons.

7.5 Gene Extraction Pipelines

As described above, various parameters have to be considered for distinguishing coding from non-coding stretches and combining individual exons into complete genes. Because of the complexity of both signals and genomic structure, multi-layered analysis pipelines (Figure 7.1) have been developed which allow integration of input from various programs. The scheme in Figure 7.1 shows the principal steps and workflow of individual modules involved in the initial analysis of genomic sequences. Several genefinding programs are widely used. They differ in the under-lying parameters used for gene and exon detection, and their assembly into gene models. Consequently, there are differences in performance accuracy at the exon, splice site and whole-gene level. Combinatorial approaches aim to combine the output of several genefinders by weighting their signals according to the performance of the individual programs. Programs having a relatively low accuracy for one parameter (e.g. delineation of 5′ ends) are assigned a lower weight for such features than others, but are assigned a higher weight for features for which they show a higher accuracy rate (e.g., detection of internal splice sites).

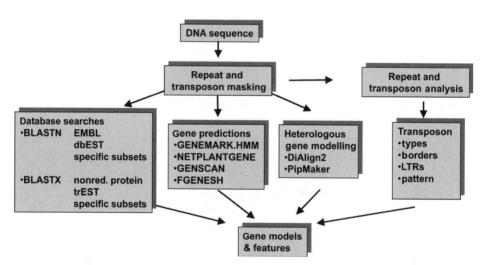

Figure 7.1   Schematic analysis pipeline for gene modelling and annotation

As already mentioned, it is of the highest importance to include only correctly parameterized and evaluated programs in analysis pipelines (Pavy *et al.*, 1999). Accuracy can dramatically change when faced with new species specific peculiarities. Usually the training and adjustment of programs for a new genome to be analysed requires a large set of experimentally known genes from the respective organism. For exotic organisms this can be a limiting factor, as frequently only too few experimentally characterized genes are publicly available.

Not only is the correct delineation of exons and introns of major importance, but the correct detection of acceptor and donor splice sites, as well as the detection of 5' and 3' borders of the genes and the correct separation of genetic elements, is also essential. For these purposes, specialized programs based on hidden Markov models, neural networks and support vector machines have been developed (see Table 7.2), which are now common components of large scale analysis pipelines.

Table 7.2 Programs for gene detection

	Specificity	Information and availability
Genscan (Burge and Karlin, 1997)	Detection of exons; modelling of complete genes	http://genes.mit.edu/GENSCAN.html
Genemark HMM (Lukashin and Borodovsky, 1998)	Detection of exons; modelling of complete genes; various species specific matrices available	http://opal.biology.gatech.edu/ GeneMark/hmmchoice.html
Genemark (Lukashin, and Borodovsky, 1998)	Detection of exons; modelling of complete genes; various species specific matrices available	http://opal.biology.gatech.edu/ GeneMark/genemark24.cgi
FGENESH (Salamov and Solovyev. 2000)	Detection of exons; modelling of complete genes; various species specific matrices available	http://www.softberry.com/berry.phtml
Glimmer (Delcher et al., 1999)	Detection of exons; modelling of complete genes	http://www.tigr.org/software/ glimmer/
Netplantgene (Hebsgaard et al., 1996)	Detection of splice sites	http://www.cbs.dtu.dk/services/ NetPGene/
Netstart (Pedersen and Nielsen, 1997)	Detection of transcription start sites; delineation of 5' borders	http://www.cbs.dtu.dk/services/ NetStart/
Eugene	Combination of different programs; weighting and generation of a combinatorial output	http://www-bia.inra.fr/T/EuGene/
PipMaker (Schwartz et al., 2000)	Homology-dependent gene modelling	http://bio.cse.psu.edu/pipmaker/
SGP-1 (Wiehe et al., 2001)	Homology-dependent gene modelling	http://195.37.47.237/sgp-1/
DiAlign2 & Agenda (Morgenstern et al., 2002)	Homology-dependent gene modelling	http://bibiserv.techfak.uni-bielefeld.de/cgi-bin/dialign_submit
TwinScan (Korf et al., 2001)	Combination of ab initio gene prediction and homology-driven gene modelling	http://genome.cs.wustl.edu/~bio/

So far we have focussed only on methods for the detection of intrinsic signals, e.g. signals embedded within the nucleotide sequence. However, with the exponential growth of publicly available sequence information, a vast amount of available extrinsic information can be applied to genome analysis. Although usually only a small fraction of genes of an organism have been detected experimentally, there are often rich resources of expressed sequence tags (ESTs), and orthologous and homologous sequences. For highly conserved genes, such sequence information can be used even across kingdom borders. For less conserved genes or gene families, present only in specific evolutionary lineages, such homology-dependent information can still be used between evolutionarily diverged organisms.

For purposes of genome analysis it is most practical to divide large sequence repositories like Genbank, EMBL or SWISSPROT into protein accessions, nucleotide sequence accessions and ESTs. Further subdividing these selections, into species specific collections, allows us to carry out homology searches against selected databases of evolutionarily related organisms. For example, for the analysis of a novel vertebrate genome comparison against a database or databases containing human, mouse, rat and/or cow, ESTs would be preferable to comparisons to plant or fungal sequences. As homology searches on the nucleotide level necessarily have a lower sensitivity than against three or six frame translations, or protein sequences, nucleotide-based homology searches (i.e. BlastN) commonly are complemented by comparisons with dynamic translations and protein sequences (i.e. BlastX and BlastP). Matches very often support pure *in silico* detections or allow correction and fine-tuning of predictions based on intrinsic data. A typical example of gene modelling is given in Figure 7.2. In the bottom panel the analysis output of several programs as well as the analysis for open reading frames (ORFs) are graphically

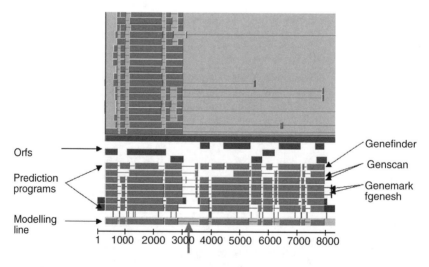

Figure 7.2 Gene modelling involves both extrinsic and intrinsic data

depicted. The filled bars depict individual exons/ORFs. Deviations in the prediction between different programs are apparent.

The top panel graphically shows the position of BlastX database matches. The arrow indicates that from extrinsic data it can be concluded that the region contains two genes and the proposed gene model has to be split. Only one program successfully predicts the presence of two genes.

The increasing amount of sequence and genomic information deposited in public databases also allows exploitation of evolutionary relationships between sequences. Coding sequences and encoded protein sequences tend to be more highly conserved than intronic sequences. Thus comparisons on the genomic sequence level allow detection of better conserved regions, which are likely to be functionally conserved (i.e. likely to represent exons), and distinguishing them from regions with a lower degree of conservation, i.e. regions that are intronic or that flank coding regions. Such systems have now been developed (Table 7.2) and, with the availability of appropriate reference genomes for comparison, are becoming an integral part of analysis pipelines. It should be noted that systems have been devised that aim to combine gene prediction on genomic DNA sequence with homology-dependent gene modelling, and indeed evaluation data show that combinatorial approaches are likely to be more accurate and powerful than *ab initio* or homology-driven approaches alone.

7.6 Added Value and Knowledge

Although gene modelling is a challenging topic, requiring sophisticated analytical tools, its goal is limited to elucidating the correct structure of individual genes. However, gene structure and primary peptide sequence do not instantly reveal information about the molecular role of the individual genetic elements. Additional analysis modules and systems have to be applied to retrieve information about the function, or at least the potential function, of genes. As already mentioned, typically only a small percentage of genes within organisms has been detected and experimentally characterized before genomic analysis. In fact the majority of assigned functional information found in today's databases arises from transferred knowledge. In the majority of cases, functional information attached to individual genes has not been gained by experimental analysis of the respective gene but has been transferred from a related gene.

The most commonly used approach to gain information and hints for the function of novel genes is homology search. Primary databases against which comparisons are carried out are Genbank (Benson *et al.*, 2002), EMBL (Stoesser *et al.*, 2002) and SWISS-PROT (Bairoch and Apweiler, 2000). Although the SWISS-PROT database does not reach the completeness achieved by Genbank and EMBL it has the advantage of being highly curated, a crucial advantage for any information transfer between homologous genes. When carrying out large scale genome annotation every group feels pressure to rationalize and speed up annotation by automatable procedures. However, there are no commonly used and accepted standards or thresholds for assigning or suggesting molecular function based on homology measures. Thus annotation and functional assignments done at different centres usually are not readily comparable, as different standards have been applied.

At best there is a grey area. As an example take a protein that has a considerable homology to others in a restricted region of the sequence, indicative of a conserved domain. One annotator may decide to name this an 'unknown protein' and state within the note the apparent similarity. A second annotator might decide that the conservation marks a functional domain, and that the molecular function can be transferred from the annotatory information associated with the matching protein sequence, and the title of the gene now reflects the homology match.

There are several problems associated with these procedures. Often there is no indication that the title and tentative functional assignment has been made based on detected homology rather than experimental verification. This bears the danger of transferring functional hints from one predicted protein to the next without requiring homologies to *experimentally characterized* genes. This blurs the transferred information. In addition, information on the thresholds used and the basis for assigning a molecular function are only rarely reported.

There are even more profound problems. Often the vocabulary used is uncontrolled, aggravating considerably the difficulty of reliable retrieval of annotation and of genes belonging to a particular family. Another problem is that any functional assignment depends on the version of the reference database. Thus assignments represent the state of knowledge at a particular time point.

A fundamental demand on genome and sequence databases however is to represent the most up-to-date information on the particular genes, a goal that can hardly be achieved by non-automated and non-recursive methodologies. Such methodologies are currently beginning to emerge. They include dynamically updated homology searches, and intelligent systems to analyse for family relationship – and thus functional relationship – against curated databases containing functional annotation.

A highly automated approach to assign function to new genes detected in genome projects is the analysis for conserved functional domains. An example is given in Figure 7.3. From top to bottom the panels show

- the probable secondary structure of the protein (alpha helices and beta sheets)

- detected PFAM and

- prosite domains

- BLASTP matches and the region they cover and

- the protein sequence of the analysed protein.

Numerous domain databases, created at least in part using different underlying methodologies, are available for the development of diagnostic domain signatures. The InterPro database marks a remarkable effort of most of the important domain

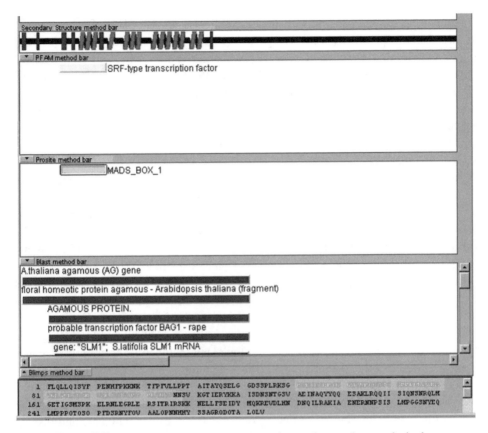

Figure 7.3 Display of summarized annotation and secondary analysis data

databases to develop a unified domain database which integrates various individual databases with different scientific focus and different methodology (Apweiler *et al.*, 2000). Screening of new genes against these databases allows scanning for the presence of characteristic sequence signatures. These signatures subsequently allow transfer of established knowledge from the highly curated and documented database entries to the respective new protein, and indicates a potential molecular function.

Another level of knowledge transfer, and an approach to structure and organize the biological knowledge associated with individual genes, is to use controlled vocabularies, or ontologies. Genes that carry out specific functions are retrievable within thousands of genes, and comparison of functions between organisms beyond the sequence homology level is facilitated. Common levels of classification include

molecular function, e.g. the tasks performed by individual gene products,

biological process and

cellular component, e.g. subcellular structures, location, and macromolecular complexes.

Among the most prominent classification schemes are the MIPS Funcat (Mewes *et al.*, 2002), the TIGR role categories (Peterson *et al.*, 2001) and the GO (Gene Ontology) classification scheme (Ashburner *et al.*, 2000), an effort carried out by a collaboration of various different genome databases. The first two classification schemes are hierarchically organized, which facilitates their use as an additional data axis to structure and analyse large scale genomic data, such as expression arrays. The GO classification schema is based on directed acyclic graphs, which allow higher resolution, and more easily cope with the complexity of biological functions.

Among the increasing armoury of analytical tools and databases, a basic repertoire of analysis is being carried out within large scale genome sequence analysis. This includes comparison with the *Kyoto Encyclopaedia of Genes and Genomes* (KEGG) (Kanehisa *et al.*, 2002) to assign enzyme classification, comparison against the *Protein Data Bank* (PDB) (Laskowski, 2001) tentatively to assign three dimensional structure, and against the COG database (Tatusov *et al.*, 2001), which contains phylogenetic classification of proteins encoded in complete genomes. Analytical tools to analyse for secondary structure (Heringa, 2000), transmembrane domains (Krogh *et al.*, 2001) or localization signals (Emanuelsson, Nielsen and von Heijne, 1999) complete the repertoire of standard analytical tools applied to individual genes. Workbenches to apply a suite of selected tools automatically to large sets of genes have been developed (Frishman *et al.*, 2001) (a cutout is shown in Figure 7.3). They generate a comprehensive analysis summary for each individual tool and gene. Such workbenches have become an indispensable component within large scale genome annotation workflows, and constitute a convenient way to communicate and display the results of highly complex analysis, and to pave the way to elucidating the function of the individual genes.

7.7 Beyond the Parts List

Classification into ontology classes, assigning enzyme-nomenclature codes to individual genes, or analysis for localization signals, already goes beyond the isolated analysis of individual genes. It is widely accepted that the initial sequencing, analysis for gene content and exhaustive analysis of the individual genetic units can be only a starting point for the molecular understanding of the lifestyle of individual organisms. The list of genetic elements contained within genomes has been compared to a parts list. Everybody who ever tried to assemble a piece of furniture that has been delivered in individual parts without using the assembly instructions has experienced the difficulty of constructing the object. Usually only for a few parts is it obvious which function they carry out. For most it is mysterious where they fit in, and which function they serve.

In the analysis of genomes we face a very similar problem. Only a few genes have clear hints (by homologies, domain signatures etc.) that let us identify their molecular function and functional role. Most, unfortunately, provide only vague or no hints towards their functional role that can be deduced from the primary sequence information.

Bacterial genomes however contain additional information, that is encoded within the coappearance of genes within the same operon. As it is known that genes located in the same operon carry out related functions, this can be exploited in the analysis. By analysing for genomic colocalization between functionally uncharacterized genes and genes with attached functional information, and comparison of detected associations between different genomes, it is possible to assign potential function to previously functionally uncharacterized genes (Kolesov, Mewes and Frishman, 2001).

A characteristic of biological systems is that the individual components are organized in complex networks and pathways that often resemble a scale-free network (Koonin, Wolf and Karev, 2002). Current genome analysis can cope with this in only a rudimentary way. Usually, even genes with clear functional indications do not appear to be connected with genes that take part in the same pathway or functional module. Future directions of development of genome analysis will necessarily aim at integrative analysis strategies that utilize contextual information, and apply functional associations such as signalling, metabolic or regulatory networks and pathways. In addition to development and refinement of bioinformatic analysis strategies (i.e. regulatory elements and the embedding of detected element combinations into regulatory networks), the integration of large scale experimental data into genomic analysis backbones are logical steps towards getting insight into how to assemble the individual parts. Examples include large scale analysis for protein interactions, whole genome expression analysis or large scale experimental analysis for protein localization.

Integration of a large variety of heterogeneous data into a centralized database has been shown to be impractical. Database schemes to cope with diverse and heterogeneous data sets, often with ambiguous definitions of different data types, are extremely difficult to establish. Novel developments therefore are focussing on distributed database approaches and forging technical links among different databases. One example is the SRS system (Etzold, Ulyanov and Argos, 1996) that allows searching and retrieving information in and from different databases. Within specified data fields in selected databases, specific queries can be carried out and information of interest selected. Future genome databases probably will be less centralized repositories, but instead will follow a distributed schema with different, in part highly specific, contributing databases, that will allow us to carry out complex queries across multiple databases without the need to navigate between them. This will have a major impact on our understanding of genomes and of the underlying molecular principles of life. Once we meet the challenge of analysing the enormous amount of genomic and experimental data in a genomic context and integrating them into functional modules, we shall be able to look at the molecular basis of life on a more systematic level.

References

Adams, M.D., Celniker, S.E., Holt, R.A., Evans, C.A., Gocayne, J.D., Amanatides, P.G., Scherer, S.E., Li, P.W., Hoskins, R.A., Galle, R.F., George, R.A., Lewis, S.E., Richards, S., Ashburner, M., Henderson, S.N., Sutton, G.G., Wortman, J.R., Yandell, M.D., Zhang, Q., Chen, L.X., Brandon, R.C., Rogers, Y.H.C., Blazej, R.G., Champe, M., Pfeiffer, B.D., Wan, K.H., Doyle, C., Baxter, E.G., Helt, G., Nelson, C.R., Miklos, G.L.G., Abril, J.F., Agbayani, A., An, H.J., Andrews-Pfannkoch, C., Baldwin, D., Ballew, R.M., Basu, A., Baxendale, J., Bayraktaroglu, L., Beasley, E.M., Beeson, K.Y., Benos, P.V., Berman, B.P., Bhandari, D., Bolshakov, S., Borkova, D., Botchan, M.R., Bouck, J., Brokstein, P., Brottier, P., Burtis, K.C., Busam, D.A., Butler, H., Cadieu, E., Center, A., Chandra, I., Cherry, J.M., Cawley, S., Dahlke, C., Davenport, L.B., Davies, A., de Pablos, B., Delcher, A., Deng, Z.M., Mays, A.D., Dew, I., Dietz, S.M., Dodson, K., Doup, L.E., Downes, M., Dugan-Rocha, S., Dunkov, B.C., Dunn, P., Durbin, K.J., Evangelista, C.C., Ferraz, C., Ferriera, S., Fleischmann, W., Fosler, C., Gabrielian, A.E., Garg, N.S., Gelbart, W.M., Glasser, K., Glodek, A., Gong, F.C., Gorrell, J.H., Gu, Z.P., Guan, P., Harris, M., Harris, N.L., Harvey, D., Heiman, T.J., Hernandez, J.R., Houck, J., Hostin, D., Houston, D.A., Howland, T.J., Wei, M.H., Ibegwam, C., Jalali, M., Kalush, F., Karpen, G.H., Ke, Z.X., Kennison, J.A., Ketchum, K.A., Kimmel, B.E., Kodira, C.D., Kraft, C., Kravitz, S., Kulp, D., Lai, Z.W., Lasko, P., Lei, Y.D., Levitsky, A.A., Li, J.Y., Li, Z.Y., Liang, Y., Lin, X.Y., Liu, X.J., Mattei, B., McIntosh, T.C., Mcleod, M.P., McPherson, D., Merkulov, G., Milshina, N.V., Mobarry, C., Morris, J., Moshrefi, A., Mount, S.M., Moy, M., Murphy, B., Murphy, L., Muzny, D.M., Nelson, D.L., Nelson, D.R., Nelson, K.A., Nixon, K., Nusskern, D.R., Pacleb, J.M., Palazzolo, M., Pittman, G.S., Pan, S., Pollard, J., Puri, V., Reese, M.G., Reinert, K., Remington, K., Saunders, R.D.C., Scheeler, F., Shen, H., Shue, B.C., Siden-Kiamos, I., Simpson, M., Skupski, M.P., Smith, T., Spier, E., Spradling, A.C., Stapleton, M., Strong, R., Sun, E., Svirskas, R., Tector, C., Turner, R., Venter, E., Wang, A.H.H., Wang, X., Wang, Z.Y., Wassarman, D.A., Weinstock, G.M., Weissenbach, J., Williams, S.M., Woodage, T., Worley, K.C., Wu, D., Yang, S., Yao, Q.A., Ye, J., Yeh, R.F., Zaveri, J.S., Zhan, M., Zhang, G.G., Zhao, Q., Zheng, L.S., Zheng, X.Q.H., Zhong, F.N., Zhong, W.Y., Zhou, X.J., Zhu, S.P., Zhu, X.H., Smith, H.O., Gibbs, R.A., Myers, E.W., Rubin, G.M. and Venter, J.C. (2000). The genome sequence of *Drosophila melanogaster*. *Science* **287**, 2185–2195.

Anon. (1998). Genome Sequence of the Nematode *C. elegans*: a platform for investigating biology. *Science* **282**, 2012–2018.

Anon. (2000). Analysis of the genome sequence of the flowering plant *Arabidopsis thaliana*. *Nature* **408**, 796–815.

Anon. (2002). The mouse genome. *Nature* **420**, 510.

Aparicio, S., Chapman, J., Stupka, E., Putnam, N., Chia, J.M., Dehal, P., Christoffels, A., Rash, S., Hoon, S., Smit, A., Gelpke, M.D., Roach, J., Oh, T., Ho, I.Y., Wong, M., Detter, C., Verhoef, F., Predki, P., Tay, A., Lucas, S., Richardson, P., Smith, S.F., Clark, M.S., Edwards, Y.J., Doggett, N., Zharkikh, A., Tavtigian, S.V., Pruss, D., Barnstead, M., Evans, C., Baden, H., Powell, J., Glusman, G., Rowen, L., Hood, L., Tan, Y.H., Elgar, G., Hawkins, T., Venkatesh, B., Rokhsar, D. and Brenner, S. (2002). Whole-genome shotgun assembly and analysis of the genome of *Fugu rubripes*. *Science* **297**, 1301–1310.

Apweiler, R., Attwood, T.K., Bairoch, A., Bateman, A., Birney, E., Biswas, M., Bucher, P., Cerutti, L., Corpet, F., Croning, M.D.R., Durbin, R., Falquet, L., Fleischmann, W., Gouzy, J., Hermjakob, H., Hulo, N., Jonassen, I., Kahn, D., Kanapin, A., Karavidopoulou, Y., Lopez, R., Marx, B., Mulder, N.J., Oinn, T.M., Pagni, M., Servant, F., Sigrist, C.J.A. and Zdobnov, E.M. (2000). InterPro – an integrated documentation resource for protein families, domains and functional sites. *Bioinformatics* **16**, 1145–1150.

Ashburner, M., Ball, C.A., Blake, J.A., Botstein, D., Butler, H., Cherry, J.M., Davis, A.P., Dolinski, K., Dwight, S.S., Eppig, J.T., Harris, M.A., Hill, D.P., Issel-Tarver, L., Kasarskis, A., Lewis, S.,

Matese, J.C., Richardson, J.E., Ringwald, M., Rubin, G.M. and Sherlock,G. (2000). Gene Ontology: tool for the unification of biology. The gene ontology consortium. *Nat. Genet.* **25**, 25–29.

Bairoch, A. and Apweiler, R. (2000). The SWISS-PROT protein sequence database and its supplement TrEMBL in 2000. *Nucleic Acids Res.* **28**, 45–48.

Bennetzen, J.L., Chandler, V.L. and Schnable, P. (2001). National Science Foundation-sponsored workshop report. Maize genome sequencing project. *Plant Physiol.* **127**, 1572–1578.

Benson, D.A., Karsch-Mizrachi, I., Lipman, D.J., Ostell, J., Rapp, B.A. and Wheeler, D.L. (2002). GenBank. *Nucleic Acids Res.* **30**, 17–20.

Blattner, F.R., Plunkett, G., Bloch, C.A., Perna, N.T., Burland, V., Riley, M., ColladoVides, J., Glasner, J.D., Rode, C.K., Mayhew, G.F., Gregor, J., Davis, N.W., Kirkpatrick, H.A., Goeden, M.A., Rose, D.J., Mau, B. and Shao, Y. (1997). The complete genome sequence of *Escherichia coli* K-12. *Science* **277**, 1453–1474.

Burge, C. and Karlin, S. (1997). Prediction of complete gene structures in human genomic DNA. *J. Mol. Biol.* **268**, 78–94.

Delcher, A.L., Harmon, D., Kasif, S., White, O. and Salzberg, S.L. (1999). Improved microbial gene identification with GLIMMER. *Nucleic Acids Res.* **27**, 4636–4641.

Emanuelsson, O., Nielsen, H. and von Heijne, G. (1999). ChloroP, a neural network-based method for predicting chloroplast transit peptides and their cleavage sites. *Protein Sci.* **8**, 978–984.

Etzold, T., Ulyanov, A. and Argos, P. (1996). SRS: information retrieval system for molecular biology data banks. *Methods Enzymol.* **266**, 114–128.

Fleischmann, R.D., Adams, M.D., White, O., Clayton, R.A., Kirkness, E.F., Kerlavage, A.R., Bult, C.J., Tomb, J.F., Dougherty, B.A., Merrick, J.M. *et al.* (1995). Whole-genome random sequencing and assembly of *Haemophilus influenzae* Rd. *Science* **269**, 496–512.

Fransz, P.F., Armstrong, S., de Jong, J.H., Parnell, L.D., van Drunen, G., Dean, C., Zabel, P., Bisseling, T. and Jones, G.H. (2000). Integrated Cytogenetic Map of Chromosome Arm 4S of *A. thaliana*: structural organization of heterochromatic knob and centromere region. *Cell* **100**, 367–376.

Frishman, D., Albermann, K., Hani, J., Heumann, K., Metanomski, A., Zollner, A. and Mewes, H.W. (2001). Functional and structural genomics using PEDANT. *Bioinformatics* **17**, 44–57.

Goff, S.A., Ricke, D., Lan, T.H., Presting, G., Wang, R.L., Dunn, M., Glazebrook, J., Sessions, A., Oeller, P., Varma, H., Hadley, D., Hutchinson, D., Martin, C., Katagiri, F., Lange, B.M., Moughamer, T., Xia, Y., Budworth, P., Zhong, J.P., Miguel, T., Paszkowski, U., Zhang, S.P., Colbert, M., Sun, W.L., Chen, L.L., Cooper, B., Park, S., Wood, T.C., Mao, L., Quail, P., Wing, R., Dean, R., Yu, Y.S., Zharkikh, A., Shen, R., Sahasrabudhe, S., Thomas, A., Cannings, R., Gutin, A., Pruss, D., Reid, J., Tavtigian, S., Mitchell, J., Eldredge, G., Scholl, T., Miller, R.M., Bhatnagar, S., Adey, N., Rubano, T., Tusneem, N., Robinson, R., Feldhaus, J., Macalma, T., Oliphant, A. and Briggs, S. (2002). A draft sequence of the rice genome (*Oryza sativa* L. ssp japonica). *Science* **296**, 92–100.

Goffeau, A., Barrell, B.G., Bussey, H., Davis, R.W., Dujon, B., Feldmann, H., Galibert, F., Hoheisel, J.D., Jacq, C., Johnston, M., Louis, E.J., Mewes, H.W., Murakami, Y., Philippsen, P., Tettelin, H. and Oliver, S.G. (1996). Life with 6000 genes. *Science* **274**, 546, 563–567.

Hebsgaard, S.M., Korning, P.G., Tolstrup, N., Engelbrecht, J., Rouze, P. and Brunak, S. (1996). Splice site prediction in *Arabidopsis thaliana* pre-mRNA by combining local and global sequence information. *Nucleic Acids Res.* **24**, 3439–3452.

Heringa, J. (2000). Computational methods for protein secondary structure prediction using multiple sequence alignments. *Curr. Protein Pept. Sci.* **1**, 273–301.

Kanehisa, M., Goto, S., Kawashima, S. and Nakaya, A. (2002). The KEGG databases at GenomeNet. *Nucleic Acids Res.* **30**, 42–46.

Kolesov, G., Mewes, H.W. and Frishman, D. (2001). SNAPping up Functionally Related Genes Based on Context Information: a collinearity-free approach. *J. Mol. Biol.* **311**, 639–656.

Koonin, E.V., Wolf, Y.I. and Karev, G.P. (2002). The structure of the protein universe and genome evolution. *Nature* **420**, 218–223.

Korf, I., Flicek, P., Duan, D. and Brent, M.R. (2001). Integrating genomic homology into gene structure prediction. *Bioinformatics* **17**, (Suppl. 1) S140–S148.

Krogh, A., Larsson, B., von Heijne, G. and Sonnhammer, E.L.L. (2001). Predicting Transmembrane Protein Topology with a Hidden Markov Model: application to complete genomes. *J. Mol. Biol.* **305**, 567–580.

Lander, E.S., Linton, L.M., Birren, B., Nusbaum, C., Zody, M.C., Baldwin, J., Devon, K., Dewar, K., Doyle, M., FitzHugh, W., Funke, R., Gage, D., Harris, K., Heaford, A., Howland, J., Kann, L., Lehoczky, J., Levine, R., McEwan, P., McKernan, K., Meldrim, J., Mesirov, J.P., Miranda, C., Morris, W., Naylor, J., Raymond, C., Rosetti, M., Santos, R., Sheridan, A., Sougnez, C., Stange-Thomann, N., Stojanovic, N., Subramanian, A., Wyman, D., Rogers, J., Sulston, J., Ainscough, R., Beck, S., Bentley, D., Burton, J., Clee, C., Carter, N., Coulson, A., Deadman, R., Deloukas, P., Dunham, A., Dunham, I., Durbin, R., French, L., Grafham, D., Gregory, S., Hubbard, T., Humphray, S., Hunt, A., Jones, M., Lloyd, C., McMurray, A., Matthews, L., Mercer, S., Milne, S., Mullikin, J.C., Mungall, A., Plumb, R., Ross, M., Shownkeen, R., Sims, S., Waterston, R.H., Wilson, R.K., Hillier, L.W., McPherson, J.D., Marra, M.A., Mardis, E.R., Fulton, L.A., Chinwalla, A.T., Pepin, K.H., Gish, W.R., Chissoe, S.L., Wendl, M.C., Delehaunty, K.D., Miner, T.L., Delehaunty, A., Kramer, J.B., Cook, L.L., Fulton, R.S., Johnson, D.L., Minx, P.J., Clifton, S.W., Hawkins, T., Branscomb, E., Predki, P., Richardson, P., Wenning, S., Slezak, T., Doggett, N., Cheng, J.F., Olsen, A., Lucas, S., Elkin, C., Uberbacher, E., Frazier, M., Gibbs, R.A., Muzny, D.M., Scherer, S.E., Bouck, J.B., Sodergren, E.J., Worley, K.C., Rives, C.M., Gorrell, J.H., Metzker, M.L., Naylor, S.L., Kucherlapati, R.S., Nelson, D.L., Weinstock, G.M., Sakaki, Y., Fujiyama, A., Hattori, M., Yada, T., Toyoda, A., Itoh, T., Kawagoe, C., Watanabe, H., Totoki, Y., Taylor, T., Weissenbach, J., Heilig, R., Saurin, W., Artiguenave, F., Brottier, P., Bruls, T., Pelletier, E., Robert, C., Wincker, P., Rosenthal, A., Platzer, M., Nyakatura, G., Taudien, S., Rump, A., Yang, H.M., Yu, J., Wang, J., Huang, G.Y., Gu, J., Hood, L., Rowen, L., Madan, A., Qin, S.Z., Davis, R.W., Federspiel, N.A., Abola, A.P., Proctor, M.J., Myers, R.M., Schmutz, J., Dickson, M., Grimwood, J., Cox, D.R., Olson, M.V., Kaul, R., Raymond, C., Shimizu, N., Kawasaki, K., Minoshima, S., Evans, G.A., Athanasiou, M., Schultz, R., Roe, B.A., Chen, F., Pan, H.Q., Ramser, J., Lehrach, H., Reinhardt, R., McCombie, W.R., de la Bastide, M., Dedhia, N., Blocker, H., Hornischer, K., Nordsiek, G., Agarwala, R., Aravind, L., Bailey, J.A., Bateman, A., Batzoglou, S., Birney, E., Bork, P., Brown, D.G., Burge, C.B., Cerutti, L., Chen, H.C., Church, D., Clamp, M., Copley, R.R., Doerks, T., Eddy, S.R., Eichler, E.E., Furey, T.S., Galagan, J., Gilbert, J.G.R., Harmon, C., Hayashizaki, Y., Haussler, D., Hermjakob, H., Hokamp, K., Jang, W.H., Johnson, L.S., Jones, T.A., Kasif, S., Kaspryzk, A., Kennedy, S., Kent, W.J., Kitts, P., Koonin, E.V., Korf, I., Kulp, D., Lancet, D., Lowe, T.M., McLysaght, A., Mikkelsen, T., Moran, J.V., Mulder, N., Pollara, V.J., Ponting, C.P., Schuler, G., Schultz, J.R., Slater, G., Smit, A.F.A., Stupka, E., Szustakowki, J., Thierry-Mieg, D., Thierry-Mieg, J., Wagner, L., Wallis, J., Wheeler, R., Williams, A., Wolf, Y.I., Wolfe, K.H., Yang, S.P., Yeh, R.F., Collins, F., Guyer, M.S., Peterson, J., Felsenfeld, A., Wetterstrand, K.A., Patrinos, A. and Morgan, M.J. (2001). Initial sequencing and analysis of the human genome. *Nature* **409**, 860–921.

Laskowski, R.A. (2001). PDBsum: summaries and analyses of PDB structures. *Nucleic Acids Res.* **29**, 221–222.

Lukashin, A.V. and Borodovsky, M. (1998). GeneMark.hmm: new solutions for gene finding. *Nucleic Acids Res.* **26**, 1107–1115.

McCombie, W.R., de la Bastide, M., Habermann, K., Parnell, L., Dedhia, N., Gnoj, L., Schutz, K., Huang, E., Spiegel, L., Yordan, C., Sehkon, M., Murray, J., Sheet, P., Cordes, M., Threideh, J., Stoneking, T., Kalicki, J., Graves, T., Harmon, G., Edwards, J., Latreille, P., Courtney, L., Cloud, J., Abbott, A., Scott, K., Johnson, D., Minx, P., Bentley, D., Fulton, B., Miller, N., Greco, T., Kemp, K., Kramer, J., Fulton, L., Mardis, E., Dante, M., Pepin, K., Hillier, L., Nelson, J., Spieth, J., Simorowski, J., May, B., Ma, P., Preston, R., Vil, D., See, L.H., Shekher, M., Matero, A., Shah, R.,

Swaby, I., O'Shaughnessy, A., Rodriguez, M., Hoffman, J., Till, S., Granat, S., Shohdy, N., Hasegawa, A., Hameed, A., Lodhi, M., Johnson, A., Chen, E., Marra, M., Wilson, R.K. and Martienssen, R. (2000). The complete sequence of a heterochromatic island from a higher eukaryote. *Cell* **100**, 377–386.

Mewes, H.W., Frishman, D., Guldener, U., Mannhaupt, G., Mayer, K., Mokrejs, M., Morgenstern, B., Munsterkotter, M., Rudd, S. and Weil, B. (2002). MIPS: a database for genomes and protein sequences. *Nucleic Acids Res.* **30**, 31–34.

Morgenstern, B., Rinner, O., Abbeddaim, S., Haase, D., Mayer, K.F.X., Dress, A.W.M. and Mewes, H.W. (2002). Exon discovery by genomicy sequence alignment. *Bioinformatics* **18**, 777–787.

Pavy, N., Rombauts, S., Dehais, P., Mathe, C., Ramana, D.V., Leroy, P. and Rouze, P. (1999). Evaluation of Gene Prediction Software Using a Genomic Data Set: application to *Arabidopsis thaliana* sequences. *Bioinformatics* **15**, 887–899.

Pedersen, A.G. and Nielsen, H. (1997). Neural Network Prediction of Translation Initiation Sites in Eukaryotes: perspectives for EST and genomye analysis. *Proc. Int. Conf. Intell. Syst. Mol. Biol.* **5**, 226–233.

Peterson, J.D., Umayam, L.A., Dickinson, T., Hickey, E.K. and White,O. (2001). The Comprehensive Microbial Resource. *Nucleic Acids Res.* **29**, 123–125.

Salamov, A.A. and Solovyev, V.V. (2000). Ab initio gene finding in *Drosophila* genomic DNA. *Genome Res.* **10**, 516–522.

Sanger, F., Coulson, A.R., Hong, G.F., Hill, D.F. and Petersen, G.B. (1982). Nucleotide sequence of bacteriophage lambda DNA. *J. Mol. Biol.* **162**, 729–773.

SanMiguel, P., Tikhonov, A., Jin, Y.K., Motchoulskaia, N., Zakharov, D., MelakeBerhan, A., Springer, P.S., Edwards, K.J., Lee, M., Avramova, Z. and Bennetzen, J.L. (1996). Nested retrotransposons in the intergenic regions of the maize genome. *Science* **274**, 765–768.

Schwartz, S., Zhang, Z., Frazer, K.A., Smit, A., Riemer, C., Bouck, J., Gibbs, R., Hardison, R. and Miller,W. (2000). PipMaker – a web server for aligning two genomic DNA sequences. *Genome Res.* **10**, 577–586.

Stoesser, G., Baker, W., van den, B.A., Camon, E., Garcia-Pastor, M., Kanz, C., Kulikova, T., Leinonen, R., Lin, Q., Lombard, V., Lopez, R., Redaschi, N., Stoehr, P., Tuli, M.A., Tzouvara, K. and Vaughan, R. (2002). The EMBL nucleotide sequence database. *Nucleic Acids Res.* **30**, 21–26.

Tatusov, R.L., Natale, D.A., Garkavtsev, I.V., Tatusova, T.A., Shankavaram, U.T., Rao, B.S., Kiryutin, B., Galperin, M.Y., Fedorova, N.D. and Koonin, E.V. (2001) The COG Database: new developments in phylogenetic classification of proteins from complete genomes. *Nucleic Acids Res.* **29**, 22–28.

Venter, J.C., Adams, M.D., Myers, E.W., Li, P.W., Mural, R.J., Sutton, G.G., Smith, H.O., Yandell, M., Evans, C.A., Holt, R.A., Gocayne, J.D., Amanatides, P., Ballew, R.M., Huson, D.H., Wortman, J.R., Zhang, Q., Kodira, C.D., Zheng, X.Q.H., Chen, L., Skupski, M., Subramanian, G., Thomas, P.D., Zhang, J.H., Miklos, G.L.G., Nelson, C., Broder, S., Clark, A.G., Nadeau, C., McKusick, V.A., Zinder, N., Levine, A.J., Roberts, R.J., Simon, M., Slayman, C., Hunkapiller, M., Bolanos, R., Delcher, A., Dew, I., Fasulo, D., Flanigan, M., Florea, L., Halpern, A., Hannenhalli, S., Kravitz, S., Levy, S., Mobarry, C., Reinert, K., Remington, K., Abu-Threideh, J., Beasley, E., Biddick, K., Bonazzi, V., Brandon, R., Cargill, M., Chandramouliswaran, I., Charlab, R., Chaturvedi, K., Deng, Z.M., Di Francesco, V., Dunn, P., Eilbeck, K., Evangelista, C., Gabrielian, A.E., Gan, W., Ge, W.M., Gong, F.C., Gu, Z.P., Guan, P., Heiman, T.J., Higgins, M.E., Ji, R.R., Ke, Z.X., Ketchum, K.A., Lai, Z.W., Lei, Y.D., Li, Z.Y., Li, J.Y., Liang, Y., Lin, X.Y., Lu, F., Merkulov, G.V., Milshina, N., Moore, H.M., Naik, A.K., Narayan, V.A., Neelam, B., Nusskern, D., Rusch, D.B., Salzberg, S., Shao, W., Shue, B.X., Sun, J.T., Wang, Z.Y., Wang, A.H., Wang, X., Wang, J., Wei, M.H., Wides, R., Xiao, C.L., Yan, C.H., Yao, A., Ye, J., Zhan, M., Zhang, W.Q., Zhang, H.Y., Zhao, Q., Zheng, L.S., Zhong, F., Zhong, W.Y., Zhu, S.P.C., Zhao, S.Y., Gilbert, D., Baumhueter, S., Spier, G., Carter, C., Cravchik, A., Woodage, T., Ali, F., An, H.J., Awe, A., Baldwin, D., Baden, H., Barnstead, M., Barrow, I., Beeyson, K., Busam, D., Carver, A., Center, A., Cheng, M.L., Curry, L., Danaher, S., Davenport, L., Desilets, R., Dietz, S., Dodson, K., Doup, L., Ferriera, S., Garg, N.,

Gluecksmann, A., Hart, B., Haynes, J., Haynes, C., Heiner, C., Hladun, S., Hostin, D., Houck, J., Howland, T., Ibegwam, C., Johnson, J., Kalush, F., Kline, L., Koduru, S., Love, A., Mann, F., May, D., McCawley, S., McIntosh, T., McMullen, I., Moy, M., Moy, L., Murphy, B., Nelson, K., Pfannkoch, C., Pratts, E., Puri, V., Qureshi, H., Reardon, M., Rodriguez, R., Rogers, Y.H., Romblad, D., Ruhfel, B., Scott, R., Sitter, C., Smallwood, M., Stewart, E., Strong, R., Suh, E., Thomas, R., Tint, N.N., Tse, S., Vech, C., Wang, G., Wetter, J., Williams, S., Williams, M., Windsor, S., Winn-Deen, E., Wolfe, K., Zaveri, J., Zaveri, K., Abril, J.F., Guigo, R., Campbell, M.J., Sjolander, K.V., Karlak, B., Kejariwal, A., Mi, H.Y., Lazareva, B., Hatton, T., Narechania, A., Diemer, K., Muruganujan, A., Guo, N., Sato, S., Bafna, V., Istrail, S., Lippert, R., Schwartz, R., Walenz, B., Yooseph, S., Allen, D., Basu, A., Baxendale, J., Blick, L., Caminha, M., Carnes-Stine, J., Caulk, P., Chiang, Y.H., Coyne, M., Dahlke, C., Mays, A.D., Dombroski, M., Donnelly, M., Ely, D., Esparham, S., Fosler, C., Gire, H., Glanowski, S., Glasser, K., Glodek, A., Gorokhov, M., Graham, K., Gropman, B., Harris, M., Heil, J., Henderson, S., Hoover, J., Jennings, D., Jordan, C., Jordan, J., Kasha, J., Kagan, L., Kraft, C., Levitsky, A., Lewis, M., Liu, X.J., Lopez, J., Ma, D., Majoros, W., McDaniel, J., Murphy, S., Newman, M., Nguyen, T., Nguyen, N. and Nodell, M. (2001). The sequence of the human genome. *Science* **291**, 1304–1351.

Wiehe, T., Gebauer-Jung, S., Mitchell-Olds, T. and Guigo, R. (2001). SGP-1: prediction and validation of homologous genes based on sequence alignments. *Genome Res.* **11**, 1574–1583.

Wong, G.K.S., Wang, J., Tao, L., Tan, J., Zhang, J.G., Passey, D.A. and Yu, J. (2002). Compositional gradients in *Gramineae* genes. *Genome Res.* **12**, 851–856.

Yu, J., Hu, S.N., Wang, J., Wong, G.K.S., Li, S.G., Liu, B., Deng, Y.J., Dai, L., Zhou, Y., Zhang, X.Q., Cao, M.L., Liu, J., Sun, J.D., Tang, J.B., Chen, Y.J., Huang, X.B., Lin, W., Ye, C., Tong, W., Cong, L.J., Geng, J.N., Han, Y.J., Li, L., Li, W., Hu, G.Q., Huang, X.G., Li, W.J., Li, J., Liu, Z.W., Li, L., Liu, J.P., Qi, Q.H., Liu, J.S., Li, L., Li, T., Wang, X.G., Lu, H., Wu, T.T., Zhu, M., Ni, P.X., Han, H., Dong, W., Ren, X.Y., Feng, X.L., Cui, P., Li, X.R., Wang, H., Xu, X., Zhai, W.X., Xu, Z., Zhang, J.S., He, S.J., Zhang, J.G., Xu, J.C., Zhang, K.L., Zheng, X.W., Dong, J.H., Zeng, W.Y., Tao, L., Ye, J., Tan, J., Ren, X.D., Chen, X.W., He, J., Liu, D.F., Tian, W., Tian, C.G., Xia, H.G., Bao, Q.Y., Li, G., Gao, H., Cao, T., Wang, J., Zhao, W.M., Li, P., Chen, W., Wang, X.D., Zhang, Y., Hu, J.F., Wang, J., Liu, S., Yang, J., Zhang, G.Y., Xiong, Y.Q., Li, Z.J., Mao, L., Zhou, C.S., Zhu, Z., Chen, R.S., Hao, B.L., Zheng, W.M., Chen, S.Y., Guo, W., Li, G.J., Liu, S.Q., Tao, M., Wang, J., Zhu, L.H., Yuan, L.P. and Yang, H.M. (2002). A draft sequence of the rice genome (*Oryza sativa* L. ssp indica). *Science* **296**, 79–92.

8 Annotation of Protein Sequences

W. C. Barker and **C. H. Wu**

Abstract

Protein sequence databases with accurate, comprehensive and up-to-date information on proteins are fundamental resources for a wide range of researchers, educators and students. Inaccurate annotations in these databases have led to erroneous conclusions and to propagation of errors into other databases and into the literature. The relatively few annotations in these databases that are based on direct experimental data are the most reliable and should be well identified, with citations to the sources of the information. Conversely, it must also be very clear which annotations are based, implicitly or explicitly, on sequence similarity or predictive algorithms. Such predictions are more reliable when applied within groups of closely related proteins in which one or more members have been experimentally characterized. UniProt, the Universal Protein Resource, strives to assist users to judge the quality of the data by clearly distinguishing experimental from predicted annotations, by using reliable and multiple prediction methods, by providing clear evidence attribution and by using standardized terminology. PIR protein family and superfamily classification serve as one basis for rule-based procedures that perform integrity checks and provide rich automatic functional annotation among homologous sequences.

Keywords

database annotation, protein sequence databases, UniProt, Protein Information Resource (PIR), protein family classification, protein superfamilies, rule-based annotation, automated annotation, annotation errors, evidence attribution

Database Annotation in Molecular Biology   Edited by Arthur M. Lesk
© 2005 John Wiley & Sons, Ltd.   ISBN: 0-470-85681-5

8.1 Introduction

With the recent accumulation of genome sequences of many organisms, notably including the human sequence, attention has turned to the identification of all of the different proteins in cells and to the comprehensive study of protein interactions, modifications and functions, defining the field of proteomics. In addition, structural genomics initiatives are generating new protein structures that will elucidate the mechanistic details of protein function. Inevitably, the experimental determination of protein functions and properties lags far behind the current avalanche of sequence data.

Identification of all of the genes encoding functional proteins in the genome of an organism is essential but not sufficient for understanding how these proteins function in making up a living cell. The number of different functional proteins in an organism often substantially exceeds the number of genes due to the generation of protein isoforms by alternative RNA processing as well as by covalent modifications of the precursor proteins. To cope with the complexity of protein sequence and functional information, annotated databases of protein sequence and function, with high interoperability to the multitude of related biomolecular databases, provide a cornerstone for a wide range of scientists active in modern biological research, especially in the field of proteomics. The major protein sequence databases are the most comprehensive sources of information on proteins. In addition to these universal databases that cover proteins from all species, there are collections storing information about specific families or groups of proteins, or about the proteins of a specific organism. Regardless of the scope and size of the database or whether it is intended for public, commercial or in-house use, the extent and quality of the annotation that accompanies the sequence data will be critical in determining the utility of the database for scientific investigations.

8.2 What is Annotation?

In a database of protein sequences, annotation generally refers to all information other than the sequence. This information can include (but is not limited to)

- Database unique identifiers
- Protein name and synonyms
- Protein source (organism, tissue, cell type, organelle)
- Dates of accession and modification
- Citations for the sequence and annotation data

- Classifications

- Genetics

- Function and activities

- Secondary, tertiary and quaternary structure

- Covalent modifications and other position specific features

- Sequence variants

- Cross-references to other databases

- Keywords.

To make the data readable, searchable and retrievable, annotations are structured into labelled records and fields, which are presented in a database-defined order in each entry. They also usually follow a defined syntax and often employ a controlled vocabulary. Although data structure, syntax and semantics vary significantly among databases, there are ways for database designers to maximize interoperablility with related databases. These include, for example, adopting widely used ontologies and classifications and providing PubMed cross-references for citations. Here we will discuss some practical aspects of protein sequence annotation, drawing examples from the databases of the UniProt and InterPro consortiums.

8.3 UniProt: Universal Protein Resource

UniProt (Apweiler *et al.*, 2004) joins the experience and expertise of the three major annotated and comprehensive protein sequence databases, PIR-PSD, Swiss-Prot and TrEMBL. The Protein Information Resource (PIR) (Wu *et al.*, 2003) provides an integrated public resource of protein informatics to support genomic and proteomic research and scientific discovery. PIR produces the Protein Sequence Database (PSD) of functionally annotated protein sequences, which grew out of the *Atlas of Protein Sequence and Structure* edited by Margaret Dayhoff (1965–1978). Swiss-Prot (Boeckmann *et al.*, 2003) is a protein knowledgebase established in 1986 and maintained collaboratively by the Swiss Institute of Bioinformatics (SIB) and the European Bioinformatics Institute (EBI). It strives to provide a high level of annotation, a minimal level of redundancy, a high level of integration with other biomolecular databases and extensive external documentation. Because maintaining Swiss-Prot is a time-consuming process involving extensive sequence analysis and detailed curation, a supplement to Swiss-Prot was created in 1996. This supplement, TrEMBL (Translation of EMBL nucleotide sequence database) (Apweiler *et al.*, 1997), contains computer-annotated protein sequences not yet integrated into Swiss-Prot, including entries derived from the translation of coding sequences in the DDBJ/

EMBL/GenBank nucleotide sequence database, sequences extracted from the literature and sequences submitted to Swiss-Prot. Together, PIR, EBI and SIB maintain and provide UniProt, a stable, comprehensive, fully classified, richly and accurately annotated protein sequence knowledgebase, with extensive cross-references and querying interfaces as the central hub for the collection of functional information on proteins (http://www.uniprot.org). The three groups continue to maintain web sites (http://pir.georgetown.edu, http://www.ebi.ac.uk and http://expasy.org) that provide many useful sequence analysis tools and databases.

8.4 Protein Family Classification

Classification of proteins provides valuable clues to structure, activity and metabolic role. Protein family classification has several advantages as a basic approach for large-scale genomic annotation: (i) it improves the identification of proteins that are difficult to characterize based on pairwise alignments; (ii) it assists database maintenance by promoting family-based propagation of annotation and making annotation errors apparent; (iii) it provides an effective means to retrieve relevant biological information from vast numbers of data and (iv) it reflects the underlying gene families, the analysis of which is essential for comparative genomics and phylogenetics.

A number of different classification systems, some highly automated and others curated, have been developed in recent years to organize proteins. Among the variety of classification schemes are (i) hierarchical families of proteins, such as the superfamilies/families (Barker, Pfeiffer and George, 1996) in the PIR-PSD, and protein groups in ProtoNet (Sasson et al., 2003), (ii) families of protein domains, such as those in Pfam (Bateman *et al.*, 2002) and ProDom (Corpet *et al.*, 2000), (iii) sequence motifs or conserved regions, such as in PROSITE (Falquet *et al.*, 2002) and PRINTS (Attwood *et al.*, 2003), (iv) structural classes, such as in SCOP (Lo Conte *et al.*, 2002) and CATH (Pearl *et al.*, 2003) and (v) integrations of various family classifications, such as iProClass (Huang *et al.*, 2003) and InterPro (Mulder *et al.*, 2003). While each of these databases is useful for particular needs, no classification scheme is by itself adequate for addressing all protein annotation needs.

8.5 InterPro: Integrated Resource of Protein Families, Domains and Sites

Databases of domain and motif signatures are essential tools for identifying distant relationships in novel sequences and hence for inferring protein function. Several publicly available signature databases, including PROSITE, PRINTS, Pfam, ProDom,

SMART (Letunic *et al.*, 2002) and TIGRFAMs (Haft *et al.*, 2001), collaborate to produce InterPro (Mulder *et al.*, 2003), an integrated documentation resource for protein families, domains and functional sites. Each InterPro entry contains signatures from one or more of the member databases describing the same group of proteins. Each entry includes a unique name and short name; an abstract, which provides annotation about the proteins matching the entry; literature references and links back to the relevant member database(s) and a list of precomputed matches against the whole of Swiss-Prot and TrEMBL. PIR protein superfamilies have been included in InterPro starting in 2003.

The InterPro database is maintained at the EBI with close collaboration with the member databases. It is updated regularly to coincide with new releases of the member databases. All data are stored in a relational database and direct web access via Java servlets is provided. The InterPro database is also distributed as flat files in XML format via FTP. On the web server (http://www.ebi.ac.uk/interpro/) the data are available for text or sequence searches. The sequence search package, InterProScan (Zdobnov and Apweiler, 2001), combines the search methods from each of the databases into a single package and provides an output with all results in a single format. In this way, researchers can submit their sequences using a web interface and obtain results of hits in InterPro in both a graphical and tabular view.

8.6 PIR Protein Families and Superfamilies

PIR defines 'closely related' proteins as having at least 50 per cent sequence identity; such sequences are automatically assigned to the same family. The families produced by automatic clustering can be refined during curation to produce groups that make biological sense, for example to include somewhat more distantly related members that are clearly orthologous and functionally equivalent. A PIR superfamily is a collection of families. Sequences in different families in the same superfamily may have as little as 15–20 per cent sequence identity. The PIR superfamily/family concept (Dayhoff, 1976), which is the earliest classification based on sequence similarity, is unique in providing comprehensive and non-overlapping clustering of protein sequences into a hierarchical order to reflect their evolutionary relationships. Proteins are assigned to the same superfamily/family only if they share end-to-end sequence similarity, including common domain architecture (i.e. similar number, order and types of domains), and do not differ excessively in overall length (unless they are fragments or result from alternative splicing or initiators). Other major family databases are organized based on similarities of domain or motif regions alone, as in Pfam and PRINTS, or consist of mixtures of domain families and families of whole proteins, such as SCOP and TIGRFAMs. However, in these the protein-to-family relationship is not necessarily one to one, as in PIR superfamily/family, but can also be one to many. The PIR superfamily classification is useful to discriminate among multidomain proteins where functional differences are associated with the presence or absence of one or more domains.

Family and superfamily classification frequently allow identification or probable function assignment for uncharacterized ('hypothetical') sequences. To assure correct functional assignments, protein identifications must be based on both global (whole protein, e.g. PIR superfamily) and local (domain and motif) sequence similarities.

8.7 Ontologies

The use of non-standardized vocabularies to name proteins, genes or organisms or to describe protein function can hinder searching across multiple proteins and species in different databases for common characteristics. Compiling a dictionary or thesaurus of biological terms is a major project that is most effectively done by a consortium of interested and expert parties, with the visibility needed to assure widespread adoption. In order to maximize interoperability and take advantage of the work of others, databases are well advised to minimize the use of in-house controlled vocabularies and instead rely on established external ontologies. Useful examples of these are the Enzyme Commission categorization, naming and description of enzyme functions (http://www.chem.qmul.ac.uk/iubmb/enzyme/), the taxons and their hierarchical arrangement from the NCBI Taxonomy Browser (Wheeler *et al.*, 2003), the RESID Database of Protein Modifications (Garavelli, 2003), gene designations from various sources, ontologies for molecular function, biological process and intracellular location from the Gene Ontology Consortium (2000, 2001) and authoritative sources for gene names, such as HUGO (http://www.gene.ucl.ac.uk/hugo/) or FlyBase (FlyBase Consortium, 2003).

For example, to provide standardization for enzyme names, activities, pathways and associated keywords, PIR compiled an electronic database of enzyme activities from the publications of the Enzyme Nomenclature Commission before an official electronic version was available. Now enzyme entries in PIR-PSD and iProClass are linked to the official IUBMB Enzyme Nomenclature which serves as the standard for classification and naming of enzymes and a source for representation of the reaction catalysed. The EC numbers (e.g. 1.1.1.1 designates alcohol dehydrogenase) provide a hierarchical organization of enzyme activities and can also be used to establish links to other enzyme and pathway databases such as the BRENDA collection of enzyme functional data (http://www.brenda.uni-koeln.de) (Schomburg *et al.*, 2002) and KEGG, the Kyoto Encyclopedia of Genes and Genomes (http://www.genome.jp/kegg/) (Kanehisa *et al.*, 2002). The PIR also maintains an in-house relational database implementation of the Enzyme Commission data, which contains EC numbers, nomenclature, reaction and other information. Such relational implementations can contain the hierarchical relationships of terms, as well as synonyms, usage guide and other associated information.

8.8 Protein Names, Source Information and Unique Identifiers

Databases typically assign a name to each protein. These names are characterized by their great variety. Like people, proteins can have the equivalent of nicknames as well as official or formal or full names. The same protein can be called by different names. It is extremely common to have a plethora of variations of spelling, capitalization, punctuation and spacing, especially for the nicknames. Some protein names are single words: trypsin, myosin, tropomyosin, insulin, haemoglobin, collagen. Even these, however, are more properly understood to refer to a fairly specific class or type of protein that may be further differentiated by additional modifiers. More often protein names contain several terms and mix uppercase and lowercase letters, numerical figures and non-alphabetical characters. Common examples are enzyme names, well established or ad hoc abbreviations (the equivalent of nicknames), gene symbols and arbitrary designations. These names can include simple protein names, nicknames, common English words (even including 'and' and 'of'), words that describe some general or specific property or activity of the protein and indications of the source of the protein (organism, tissue, organelle). Curated databases typically impose some conventions of syntax and semantics and provide a list of other names (including misnomers as well as synonyms) that have been used so that users can search using terminology with which they are familiar.

Organism names in the UniProt databases have been mapped to NCBI taxons and linked to the descriptions in the NCBI Taxonomy Browser (Wheeler *et al.*, 2003), which include synonymous names, lineages, and genetic codes. Although this source is not a taxonomic authority, it is compiled from many sources and is widely used for macromolecular sequence data. Relational database implementation of the NCBI taxonomy at PIR is used to map organism names from different source databases and to provide the taxonomy hierarchical tree. This implementation allows easy query and term alignment among related databases.

The Gene Ontology Consortium (2000, 2001) has developed ontologies for molecular function, biological process and cellular component (location of action) to describe gene products and to allow the annotation and comparison of molecular characteristics across species. Each vocabulary is structured so that any term may have more than one parent as well as zero, one or more children. This makes attempts to describe biology much richer than would be possible with a strictly hierarchical structure. Currently the GO vocabulary consists of over 17 000 terms, which will, in time, all have strict definitions for their usage. The Swiss-Prot/TrEMBL/InterPro group at EBI belongs to the Gene Ontology Consortium and will use its standard vocabulary to characterize the activities of proteins in the UniProt knowledgebase. The EBI will provide assignments of GO terms to gene products for all organisms with completely and incompletely sequenced proteomes and will contribute to the expansion of the ontologies by requesting new terms when necessary, thus extending the scope of the GO ontologies beyond those terms necessary to describe the proteins of the model organism databases.

Because protein names in databases may be complex and are often changed as the proteins become better characterized, it is very important also to assign database specific unique identifiers to each protein. These are of two types: entry identifiers and accession numbers. Entry identifiers can be suggestive mnemonics (e.g. HBB_HUMAN), though it can become tedious to keep up with this practice, or arbitrary combinations of letters and/or numbers (B91637 or Q9UNL6). Accession numbers are arbitrary, permanent, machine-generated combinations of letters and/or numbers assigned to a reported sequence. Both PIR-PSD and TrEMBL initially use the same token for the entry identifier and accession number. Entry identifiers can be changed, which may happen when two reports of the same protein are merged into one entry or when a meaningful identification is made for a previously poorly characterized protein.

8.9 Common Identification Errors

The usual approach for naming of proteins translated from genomic sequences is to infer protein characteristics based on sequence similarity to annotated proteins in sequence databases. This process is error prone (Bork and Koonin, 1998) and has produced many genome annotation errors (Brenner, 1999; Devos and Valencia, 2001), many of which have been propagated to other molecular databases. There are several sources of errors. Usually the sequence will be searched against a single comprehensive dataset, such as PIR-NREF (Wu *et al.*, 2003) or Swiss-Prot/TrEMBL, and the sequence will be assigned the name of the highest-scoring sequence(s). The common sequence searching algorithms, BLAST or PSI-BLAST (Altschul *et al.*, 1997) and FASTA (Pearson and Lipman, 1988) find best-scoring similarities; however, the similarity may involve only parts of the query and target molecules. The retrieved similarity may be to a known domain that is tangential to the main function of the protein or to a region with compositional similarity, e.g. a region containing several transmembrane domains. Since many proteins are multifunctional, the assignment of a single function, which is common in genome projects, results in incomplete or incorrect information. Before making or accepting identification, users should examine the domain structure in comparison to the pairwise alignments and determine whether the similarity is local, perhaps associated with a common domain, or extends convincingly over the entire sequences.

Second, annotation in the searched databases is at best inconsistent and incomplete and at worst misleading or erroneous, having been based on partial or weak similarity. The major nucleotide sequence databases GenBank (Benson *et al.*, 2003), EMBL (Stoesser *et al.*, 2003), and DDBJ (Miyazaki *et al.*, 2003) are 'archival' databases, recording the original identifications as submitted by the sequencers unless a revision is submitted by the same group. Therefore, the protein identifications in GenPept, which are taken directly from GenBank annotations, may never be updated in light of more recent knowledge. In many databases, it may not be evident when identification is based on solid experimental evidence, inference from properties of a closely related protein or simply the best partial match in a database search.

Over-identification is a common error when similarity is not strong over the entire lengths of the query and target sequences. Sequences in different families in the same superfamily may have different activities, though often falling within the same general class. For example, the long chain alcohol dehydrogenase superfamily contains alcohol dehydrogenase (EC 1.1.1.1), L-threonine 3-dehydrogenase (EC 1.1.1.103), L-iditol 2-dehydrogenase (EC 1.1.1.14), D-xylulose reductase (EC 1.1.1.9), galactitol-1-phosphate 5-dehydrogenase (EC 1.1.1.251) and others. Of five sequences from the recently sequenced genome of *Brucella melitensis* (DelVecchio *et al.*, 2002) that were identified specifically as alcohol dehydrogenase (EC 1.1.1.1), only two are closely related (60 per cent identity) to well characterized alcohol dehydrogenases. For the others, the functional assignment may be overly specific, as they are more distantly related (less than 40 per cent identity). For the most part, users will need to inspect database entries and read at least the abstracts of published reports to ascertain whether a functional assignment is based on experimental evidence or only on sequence similarity. Users should also ascertain that any residues critical for the ascribed activity (e.g. active site residues) are conserved.

In many cases a more thorough and time-consuming analysis is needed to reveal the most probable functional assignments. Factors that may be relevant, in addition to presence or absence of domains, motifs or functional residues, include similarity or potential similarity of three-dimensional structures (when known), proximity of genes (may indicate that their products are involved in the same pathway), metabolic capacities of the organisms and evolutionary history of the protein as deduced from aligned sequences. Bork and Koonin (1998) discuss additional effective strategies. Iyer *et al.* (2001) analyse several additional examples of misidentifications and their subsequent correction.

8.10 Evidence Attribution

To prevent propagation of annotation errors and improve information content, protein annotations ideally should include, for both experimental and computational data, the types of evidence and methods for the annotation along with attribution of their sources. Evidence attribution is of growing importance since the comprehensive biomolecular databases combine data from a broad variety of sources. Data in TrEMBL, for example, may be automatically imported from the underlying DDBJ/EMBL/GenBank coding sequences, imported from other databases, partially curated by EBI staff, generated from specific programs, or added by automatic annotation systems. Although every effort is made to ensure correct and consistent data, data quality is limited by the quality of the input data. Currently, it is difficult for database users to recognize where individual data items come from and whether they are well founded, reasonably inferred or highly speculative. Too often users assume that all data in the major databases are accurate and authoritative.

Attribution of protein annotations to validated experimental sources provides effective means to avoid propagation of errors that may have resulted from large scale genome annotation. This is already possible, in part, both in Swiss-Prot/TrEMBL (http://expasy.org/cgi-bin/lists?annbioch.txt) (Junker, Apweiler and Bairoch, 1999) and in PIR, through the use of a number of qualifiers or status tags which differentiate between experimental and non-experimental data. To distinguish experimentally verified from computationally predicted data, PIR entries are labelled with status tags of 'validated', 'similarity' or 'imported' in protein title, function and complex annotations (Figure 8.1(a)). The validated function or complex annotation includes hypertext-linked PubMed unique identifiers for the articles in which the experimental determinations are reported. The entries are also tagged with 'experimental', 'absent', 'atypical' or 'predicted' in feature annotations (Figure 8.1(b)). The first two tags are used to indicate the experimentally determined presence or absence of features. To appropriately attribute bibliographic data to features with experimental evidence, we are conducting a retrospective bibliography mapping. Literature citations within each protein entry are computationally filtered based on titles and abstracts, using controlled terms describing the experimental

		(a)
ENTRY	T48678	
TITLE	proteasome alpha-1 chain (**validated**) - Haloferax volcanii	
COMPLEX	heterodimer; alpha-1 and beta-1 (PIR:T48677) chain (**validated; PMID:99412283**)	
FUNCTION	#description the predominant peptide-hydrolyzing activity of the alpha (1)beta(1)-proteasome is cleavage carboxyl to hydrophobic residues (**validated; PMID:99412283**)	

		(b)
ENTRY	XNHUSP #type complete	
TITLE	serine--pyruvate transaminase (EC 2.6.1.51), peroxisomal - human	
FEATURE		
2-392	#product serine--pyruvate transaminase, peroxisomal #status **experimental** #label MAT\	
390-392	#region peroxisome/glyoxysome location signal #status **atypical**\	
2	#modified_site acetylated amino end (Ala) (in mature form) #status **experimental** (**PMID:7798168**)\	
209	#binding_site pyridoxal phosphate (Lys) (covalent) #status **predicted**\	
367	#binding_site carbohydrate (Asn) (covalent) #status **absent**	

Figure 8.1 PIR evidence attribution for (a) title, complex and function annotation and (b) feature annotation

features. Subsequently, the filtered papers are manually curated and added to the feature lines as literature attributions.

Evidence tags will be added to UniProt records by computer programs and during the literature-based curation process, allowing users to view the source of all data items in each record and to distinguish between experimental and computationally derived data. During the annotation process, curators will assess any information that has been added by a program, and if it is correct they will confirm it using the appropriate evidence tag. This will increase the reliability of all program-added information and will also allow for improvements to programs through feedback from curators to programmers. It will also prevent the overwriting by a program of any data that have been edited by a curator so that it will be possible to use programs to add information to a curated entry without touching manually curated data items. As each piece of data may have more than one evidence tag, this system is appropriate for data items that are derived from multiple sources. This system has been used internally at EBI for some time and a large number of data items in the TrEMBL database have already been tagged. The UniProt consortium will build on this method and extend it to allow tagging of known false information, e.g. if a keyword generated by an automated annotation system is known to be wrong by curator judgment. This will allow the incorporation of feedback from users and curators to improve the rules for automatic annotation. All data items tagged with a 'negative' evidence tag will be removed from the entry before publication.

8.11 Position Specific Annotations

Position specific annotations appear in the 'feature table' sections of database entries and are of several types, including amino acids that are post-translationally modified, unusual encoded amino acids (selenocysteine being the most common), active or inhibitory sites and binding sites. These are annotated with reference to a specific residue (position) or to a short list of residues (e.g. 34, 52). Properly speaking, a 'site' should not be designated by a range (e.g. 32–38) of residues.

An important class of post-translational modifications comprises those amino acids that are chemically changed in such a way that they could not be restored by physiological processes of hydrolysis, ammonolysis or simple reduction, including chemical changes involving the alpha amino group (e.g. N-formylmethionine), or the alpha-carboxyl group of the carboxyl terminal residue, and selenocysteine and other rare amino acids that are translationally incorporated but for historical reasons are represented as modified residues. Active site residues are those known or thought to function in the actual catalytic reaction of an enzyme. Similarly, inhibitory site residues are those residues in enzyme inhibitors that serve as pseudo-substrates to block enzymatic activity.

Binding sites may be either covalent of non-covalent. Covalent changes may occur transiently or more or less permanently, but the original amino acid could in principle be recovered and detected by typical methods of sequence analysis, whereas modified residues could not be. Non-covalent bonds may be ionic, ligand, Van der Waals or donative or receptive hydrogen bonds with ions, cofactors or other molecules (excluding the protein constituting the entry).

The RESID Database (Garavelli, 2003), originally compiled at the NBRF to support PIR databases, is the most comprehensive collection of annotations and structures for protein modifications, including amino-terminal, carboxyl-terminal and peptide chain cross-link post-translational modifications. It has been publicly accessible since 1995 and currently contains more than 300 entries. The current version (http://www.ncifcrf.gov/RESID/) maps post-translational modifications to both PIR and Swiss-Prot feature table representations. Ideally, post-translational modifications appearing in feature tables will be linked to the corresponding entries in RESID.

8.12 Rule-based Annotation

For large databases of protein sequences, the time and effort involved in thorough curation by a staff annotator dictates that only a small fraction of entries can be carefully annotated by hand. One strategy is to carefully choose representative entries for hand curation. Often this is paired with a strategy of automatic carry-over of annotations from a curated entry to other closely related entries. PIR family and superfamily classification serves as the basis for rule-based procedures that perform integrity checks and provide rich automatic functional annotation among homologous sequences. Integrity checks are based on controlled vocabulary, standard nomenclature and other ontologies. For example, the IUBMB Enzyme Nomenclature is used to detect obsolete EC numbers, misspelled enzyme names or inconsistent EC number and enzyme name.

Combining the classification information and sequence patterns or profiles, rules have been defined to predict position specific sequence features such as active sites, binding sites, modification sites and sequence motifs. For example, when a new sequence is classified into a superfamily containing a 'ferredoxin (2Fe–2S) homology domain', that sequence is automatically searched for the pattern for the 2Fe–2S cluster and, if the pattern is found, the feature 'Binding site: 2Fe–2S cluster (Cys) (covalent)' is added. Such sequence features are most accurately predicted if based on patterns or profiles derived from sequences closely related to those that are experimentally verified. For example, within the cytochrome c domain (PF00034), the 'CXXCH' pattern, containing three annotatable residues, is easily identified, and the ligands (haem and haem iron) are invariant; however, there is no single pattern derivable for identifying the Met that is the second axial ligand of the hame iron. In contrast, within the many superfamilies containing the calcineurin-like phosphoesterase domain (PF00149), the metal chelating residues, the identity of the bound metal

Table 8.1 Classification-driven and rule-based approach for automated and quality annotation

Action	Process	Rule	Description[*]
1	Protein classification	Superfamily	Superfamily: SF000460, phosphorylase Domain: PF00343, Carbohydrate phosphorylase Motif: PS00102, Phosphorylase pyridoxal-phosphate attachment site
2	Site identification	Feature Rule 1	IF pattern: EASG(QT)(GS)NM^KXXXN(GR) THEN add feature: 'Binding site: pyridoxal phosphate (Lys) (covalent)'
3	Site identification	Feature Rule 2	IF superfamily member + animal (Metazoa) And IF pattern: (KR)(KR)(KR)QI^S(VIL)RG THEN add feature: 'Binding site: phosphate (Ser) (covalent) (by phosphorylase kinase) (in phosphorylase a)'
4	Protein name checking	Protein name rule	IF: superfamily member + feature rule 1 THEN use name: 'phosphorylase (EC 2.4.1.1)' IF: superfamily member + feature rule 1 + plant (Viridiplantae) THEN use name: 'starch phosphorylase (EC 2.4.1.1)'
5	Keyword checking	Keyword rule	IF protein name includes: EC 2.4.1.1 THEN add keywords: 'glycosyltransferase', 'phosphorylase', 'hexosyltransferase'
6	Keyword checking	Keyword rule	IF: feature rule 1 THEN add keyword: 'pyridoxal phosphate'
7	Keyword checking	Keyword rule	IF: feature rule 2 THEN add keywords: 'phosphoprotein', 'allosteric regulation'

[*]The quoted texts are terms in PIR controlled vocabularies.

ion and the catalytic activity are variable. In such a case, automated annotation must be superfamily or family specific in order to be accurate.

Table 8.1 illustrates how an integrated set of rules can be triggered by family classification to produce dynamic annotation of protein entries. After classification, all SF000460 superfamily members containing positive identifications of Pfam domain PF00343 and PROSITE motif PS00102 are automatically tested (Action 2) for the superfamily-tailored pyridoxal-phosphate binding site 'EASG(QT)(GS) NM^KXXXN(GR)' (where K is the residue covalently binding the cofactor) and instructions are generated to add the appropriate feature. If all essential sequence and site features are present, the entry title is checked for the string 'phosphorylase (EC 2.4.1.1)' or, even more specifically, 'starch phosphorylase (EC 2.4.1.1)' if the organism is a plant (Action 4). Then, enzyme-associated keywords such as 'glycosyltransferase' and 'hexosyltransferase' are added (Action 5). Superfamily members from animals are tested for the phosphorylase kinase phosphorylation site and the appropriate feature is added (Action 3). The two new features trigger the addition of keywords 'pyridoxal phosphate' (Action 6), and 'phosphoprotein' and 'allosteric regulation' (Action 7), respectively.

Family specific patterns for such features are derived from alignments of closely related sequences for which some of the sequences have experimentally determined properties. The rule may further specify other topological constraints for the pattern, such as restricting the annotation of the P-loop feature to the ABC transporter domain regions for the excinuclease ABC chain A superfamily. Looking for expected active site and binding site sequence motifs and disulfide bonds only by homology within the family or superfamily prevents errors such as annotation of signal sequences for nuclear proteins, myristylation sites internally in sequences, phosphorylation sites when there is no evidence that the protein is phosphorylated, carbohydrate-binding sites in cytosolic proteins etc. Sometimes the concatenation of predicted features in a sequence is so plausible as to justify a functional classification and feature annotation even if there is no family or superfamily member with validated function. For example, a eukaryotic protein containing a predicted signal sequence, followed by several predicted immunoglobulin-like domains, followed by a predicted transmembrane domain, followed by a predicted protein kinase or protein phosphatase domain is very likely a receptor involved in a signal transduction pathway.

8.13 Conclusions

A diverse community, including students and professors of biochemistry and bioinformatics, researchers in structural biology and cancer therapeutics, scientists at patent offices and regulatory agencies, statisticians and ontologists, depends on general or specialized protein sequence databases. Inaccurate annotation in these databases will lead to erroneous conclusions and propagation of errors (Wu and Barker, 2004). Although relatively few of the annotations in these databases are based on direct experimental data, these are the most important and reliable of the annotations. Consequently, they should be well identified, with citations to the sources of the information. Conversely, it must also be very clear which annotations are based, implicitly or explicitly, on sequence similarity or predictive algorithms. Such predictions are more reliable when applied within groups of closely related proteins (families and some superfamilies) in which one or more members have been experimentally characterized. Although, in the final analysis, it is the responsibility of the user to judge the credibility of the data, the databases must strive to make this feasible by distinguishing experimental from predicted annotations, using reliable prediction methods, giving clear evidence attribution and using standardized terminology.

Acknowledgements

The PIR is supported by grant U01 HG02712 from the National Institutes of Health. The iProClass database is supported by DBI-9974855 and DBI-0138188 from the National Science Foundation.

References

Altschul, S.F., Madden, T.L., Schaffer, A.A., Zhang, J., Zhang, Z., Miller, W. and Lipman, D.J. (1997). Gapped BLAST and PSI-BLAST: a new generation of protein database search programs. *Nucleic Acids Res.* **25**, 3389–3402.

Apweiler, R., Bairoch, A., Wu, C.H., Barker, W.C., Boeckmann, B., Ferro, S., Gasteiger, E., Huang, H., Lopez, R., Magrane, M., Martin, M.J., Natale, D.A., O'Donovan, C., Redaschi, N. and Yeh, L.S. (2004). UniProt: the Universal Protein knowledgebase. *Nucleic Acids Res.* **32**, D115–D119.

Apweiler, R., Gateau, A., Contrino, S., Martin, M.J., Junker, V., O'Donovan, C., Lang, F., Mitaritonna, N., Kappus, S. and Bairoch, A. (1997). Protein Sequence Annotation in the Genome Era: the annotation concept of SWISS-PROT + TREMBL. In Gaasterland, T., Karp, P., Karplus, K., Ouzonis, C., Sander, C. and Valencia, A., eds, *Proceedings of the Fifth International Conference on Intelligent Systems for Molecular Biology (ISMB)*, Halkidiki, pp. 33–43.

Attwood, T.K., Bradley, P., Flower, D.R., Gaulton, A., Maudling, N., Mitchell, A.L., Moulton, G., Nordle, A., Paine, K., Taylor, P., Uddin, A. and Zygouri, C. (2003). PRINTS and its automatic supplement, prePRINTS. *Nucleic Acids Res.* **31**, 400–402.

Barker, W.C., Pfeiffer, F. and George, D.G. (1996). Superfamily classification in PIR – International Protein Sequence Database. *Methods Enzymol.* **266**, 59–71.

Bateman, A., Birney, E., Cerruti, L., Durbin, R., Etwiller, L., Eddy, S.R., Griffiths-Jones, S., Howe, K.L., Marshall, M., and Sonnhammer, E. (2002). The Pfam protein families database. *Nucleic Acids Res.* **30**, 276–280.

Benson, D.A., Karsch-Mizrachi, I., Lipman, D.J., Ostell, J. and Wheeler, D.L. (2003). GenBank. *Nucleic Acids Res.* **31**, 23–27.

Boeckmann, B., Bairoch, A., Apweiler, R., Blatter, M.-C., Estreicher, A. Gasteiger, E. Martin, M.J., Michoud, K., O'Donovan, C., Phan, I., Pilbout, S. and Schneider, M. (2003). The SWISS-PROT protein knowledge base and its supplement TrEMBL in 2003. *Nucleic Acids Res.* **31**, 365–370.

Bork, P. and Koonin, E.V. (1998). Predicting functions from protein sequences – where are the bottlenecks? *Nat. Genet.* **18**, 313–318.

Brenner, S.E. (1999). Errors in genome annotation. *Trends Genet.* **15**, 132–133.

Corpet, F., Servant, F., Gouzy, J. and Kahn, D. (2000). ProDom and ProDom-CG: tools for protein domain analysis and whole genome comparisons. *Nucleic Acids Res.* **28**, 267–269.

Dayhoff, M.O. (1965–1978) *Atlas of Protein Sequence and Structure*, National Biomedical Research Foundation, Washington, DC, Vols 1–5, Suppls 1–3.

Dayhoff, M.O. (1976). The origin and evolution of protein superfamilies. *Fed. Proc.* **35**, 2132–2138.

DelVecchio, V.G., Kapatral, V., Redkar, R.J., Patra, G., Mujer, C., Los, T., Ivanova, N., Anderson, I., Bhattacharyya, A., Lykidis, A., Reznik, G., Jablonski, L., Larsen, N., D'Souza, M., Bernal, A., Mazur, M., Goltsman, E., Selkov, E., Elzer, P.H., Hagius, S., O'Callaghan, D., Letesson, J.J., Haselkorn, R., Kyrpides, N. and Overbeek, R. (2002). The genome sequence of the facultative intracellular pathogen *Brucella melitensis. Proc. Natl Acad. Sci. USA* **99**, 443–448.

Devos, D. and Valencia, A. (2001). Intrinsic errors in genome annotation. *Trends Genet.* **17**, 429–431.

Falquet, L., Pagni, M., Bucher, P., Hulo, N., Sigrist, C.J.A., Hofmann, K. and Bairoch, A. (2002). The PROSITE database, its status in 2002. *Nucleic Acids Res.* **30**, 235–238.

FlyBase Consortium. (2003). The FlyBase database of the *Drosophila* genome projects and community literature. *Nucleic Acids Res.* **31**, 172–175.

Garavelli, J.S. (2003). The RESID Database of Protein Modifications: 2003 developments. *Nucleic Acids Res.* **31**, 499–501.

Gene Ontology Consortium. (2000). Gene Ontology: tool for the unification of biology. *Nature Genet.* **25**, 25–29.

Gene Ontology Consortium. (2001). Creating the Gene Ontology Resource: design and implementation. *Genome Res.* **11**, 1425–1433.

Haft, D. H., Loftus, B.J., Richardson, D. L., Yang, F., Eisen J.A., Paulsen, I. T. and White O. (2001). TIGRFAMs: a protein family resource for the functional identification of proteins. *Nucleic Acids Res.* **29**, 41–43.

Huang, H., Barker, W.C., Chen, Y. and Wu, C.H. (2003). iProClass: an integrated database of protein family, function, and structure information. *Nucleic Acids Res.* **31**, 390–392.

Iyer, L.M., Aravind, L., Bork, P., Hofmann, K., Mushegian, A.R., Zhulin, I.B. and Koonin, E.V. (2001). Quod erat demonstrandum? The mystery of experimental validation of apparently erroneous computational analyses of protein sequences. *Genome Biol.* **2**, research0051.

Junker, V., Apweiler, R. and Bairoch, A. (1999). Representation of functional information in the SWISS-PROT data bank. *Bioinfomatics* **15**, 1066–1067.

Kanehisa, M., Goto, S., Kawashima, S. and Nakaya, A. (2002). The KEGG databases at GenomeNet. *Nucleic Acids Res.* **30**, 42–46.

Letunic, I., Goodstadt, L., Dickens, N.J., Doerks, T., Schultz, J., Mott, R., Ciccarelli, F., Copley, R.R., Ponting, C.P. and Bork, P. (2002). Recent improvements to the SMART domain-based sequence annotation resource. *Nucleic Acids Res.* **30**, 242–244.

Lo Conte, L., Brenner, S.E., Hubbard, T.J. P, Chothia, C. and Murzin, A.G. (2002). SCOP Database in 2002: refinements accommodate structural genomics. *Nucleic Acids Res.* **30**, 264–267.

Miyazaki, S., Sugawara, H., Gojobori, T. and Tateno, Y. (2003). DNA Data Bank of Japan (DDBJ) in XML. *Nucleic Acids Res.* **31**, 13–16.

Mulder, N.J., Apweiler, R., Attwood, T.K., Bairoch, A., Barrell, D., Bateman, A., Binns, D., Biswas, M., Bradley, P., Bork, P., Bucher, P., Copley, R.R., Courcelle, E., Das, U., Durbin, R., Falquet, L., Fleischmann, W., Griffiths-Jones, S., Haft, D., Harte, N., Hulo, N., Kahn, D., Kanapin, A., Krestyaninova, M., Lopez, R., Letunic, I., Lonsdale, D., Silventoinen, V., Orchard, S.E., Pagni, M., Peyruc, D., Ponting, C.P., Selengut, J.D., Servant, F., Sigrist, C.J.A., Vaughan, R. and Zdobnov, E.M. (2003). The InterPro database, 2003 brings increased coverage and new features. *Nucleic Acids Res.* **31**, 315–318.

Pearl, F.M.G., Bennett, C.F., Bray, J.E., Harrison, A.P., Martin, N., Shepherd, A., Sillitoe, I., Thornton, J. and Orengo, C.A. (2003). The CATH Database: an extended protein family resource for structural and functional genomics. *Nucleic Acids Res.* **31**, 452–455.

Pearson, W.R. and Lipman, D.J. (1988). Improved tools for biological sequence comparison. *Proc. Natl Acad. Sci. USA* **85**, 2444–2448.

Sasson, O., Vaaknin, A., Fleischer, H., Portugaly, E., Bilu, Y., Linial, N. and Linial, M. (2003). ProtoNet: hierarchical classification of the protein space. *Nucleic Acids Res.* **31**, 348–352.

Schomburg, I., Chang, A., Hofmann, O., Ebeling, C., Ehrentreich, F. and Schomburg, D. (2002). BRENDA: a resource for enzyme data and metabolic information. *Trends Biochem Sci.* **27**, 54–56.

Stoesser, G., Baker, W., van den Broek, A., Garcia-Pastor, M., Kanz, C., Kulikova, T., Leinonen, R., Lin, Q., Lombard, V., Lopez, R., Mancuso, R., Nardone, F., Stoehr, P., Tuli, M.A., Tzouvara, K. and Vaughan, R. (2003). The EMBL Nucleotide Sequence Database: major new developments. *Nucleic Acids Res.* **31**, 17–22.

Wheeler, D.L., Church, D.M., Federhen, S., Lash, A.E., Madden, T.L., Pontius, J.U., Schuler, G.D., Schriml, L.M., Sequeira, E., Tatusova, T.A. and Wagner, L. (2003). Database resources of the National Center for Biotechnology. *Nucleic Acids Res.* **31**, 28–33.

Wu, C.H. and Barker, W.C. (2004). Information flow and data integration of databanks (in this volume).

Wu, C.H., Yeh, L-S., Huang, H., Arminski, L., Castro-Alvear, J., Chen, Y., Hu, Z., Kourtesis, P., Ledley, R.S., Suzek, B.E., Vinayaka, C.R., Zhang, J. and Barker, W.C. (2003). The Protein Information Resource. *Nucleic Acids Res.* **31**, 345–347.

Zdobnov, E.M. and Apweiler R. (2001). InterProScan – an integration platform for the signature-recognition methods in InterPro. *Bioinformatics* **17**, 847–848.

9 Issues in the Annotation of Protein Structures

G. J. Swaminathan, J. Tate, R. Newman, A. Hussain, J. Ionides, K. Henrick and **S. Velankar**

Abstract

With structural genomics initiatives taking off all around the world, it is now more important than ever that there are systems in place to handle the large number of expected depositions in an efficient and consistent manner. With the tools designed and implemented by the E-MSD for the annotation of depositions, the stage is set for high throughput curation of PDB entries deposited at EBI. Our collaborations with various scientific programmers and users have already led to major advancements in the ease with which new structures and the information associated with them can be deposited at the E-MSD. We believe that the deposition and curation tools produced by the E-MSD group will be instrumental in creating a richer and more consistent database of protein structures.

Keywords

macromolecular structure database, protein structure curation, annotation, data harvesting, quaternary structure, geometry validation, ligand chemistry, protein databank, wwPDB

The European Bioinformatics Institute (http://www.ebi.ac.uk) was established in 1995 as a home for a large set of biological databases covering a broad range of topics from nucleotide sequence through to protein function. From its inception the EBI has hosted the EMBL nucleotide sequence database (Hamm and Cameron, 1986) and SWISS-PROT (Bairoch and Boeckmann, 1994). The E-MSD (EBI-Macromolecular

Database Annotation in Molecular Biology   Edited by Arthur M. Lesk
© 2005 John Wiley & Sons, Ltd.   ISBN: 0-470-85681-5

Structure Database (Boutselakis *et al.*, 2003; Golovin *et al.*, 2004) (http://www.ebi.ac.uk/msd/) was set up in 1996 to give Europe an autonomous facility to collect, organize and make available data about macromolecular structures and to integrate biological macromolecular co-ordinate data with the other databases already at the EBI. Since then, the E-MSD group has been working in three main areas:

- Accepting and processing depositions to the Protein Data Bank (PDB) (Berman *et al.*, 2002)

- Transforming the PDB flat file archive to a relational database system

- Developing services to search the PDB.

The E-MSD, together with the Research Collaboratory for Structural Biology (RCSB) and PDB Japan (PDBj) form the single repository for macromolecular structures called the Worldwide Protein Data Bank (wwPDB) (http://www.wwpdb.org). All three organizations serve as deposition, data processing and distribution sites of the PDB archive. Structures are deposited with the RCSB and PDBj using the ADIT deposition interface (Berman *et al.*, 2002), whereas the E-MSD uses a new deposition system called autodep4 (http://www.ebi.ac.uk/msd-srv/autodep4). This system has some superficial similarity with AutoDep (Lin *et al.*, 2000) but is a completely re-written software package. New depositions at the E-MSD are generated by autodep4 and are processed locally into complete PDB entries. The finished PDB files are then forwarded to the RCSB for inclusion in the weekly public release. Mechanisms are also put in place to ensure that the archive maintains its unity despite originating from different deposition streams worldwide.

The E-MSD deposition and annotation tools are designed to implement a consistent approach in the handling and curation of deposition data. The new version of our in-house deposition system, autodep4, has drastically reduced the time it takes to complete a deposition; a deposition will typically take 45 minutes, and for 95 per cent of depositions a processed review copy and a report on the processing procedure is sent back to the depositor in less than one working day and often within a few hours. It has also ensured that certain mandatory fields defined by the PDB format are handled in exactly the same way for all new structures that are deposited with the E-MSD.

The annotation of the deposited entry, which occurs at the post-AutoDep stage, is difficult to automate fully given the diverse range of structural data that can be deposited with the PDB. However, using a large set of in-house programs (around 270 perl scripts and 110 legacy fortran programs, comprising over 200 000 lines of code) and some third party software, many of the mundane tasks in the annotation of the PDB entry are automated. Despite this, there are many issues concerning the annotation of PDB entries that need to be addressed on a case-by-case basis. These include

- Data harvesting

- Assembly identification

- Taxonomy

- Sequence identification

- Secondary structure

- Structure validation

- Residue and ligand identification

- Solvent handling.

9.1 Data Harvesting

The concept of data harvesting for macromolecular data involves the automatic or semi-automatic communication of relevant data from the software used during structure determination and analysis to the deposition software. The most time-consuming step in the deposition process for structural data was previously the manual entry of various data fields required by the PDB format. In order to simplify this task, data harvesting was first incorporated in X-PLOR, a refinement program for both crystallography and NMR (Brünger, 1992). At the end of the refinement process, the program would write out a PDB file suitable for deposition with many mandatory PDB fields filled in. Data harvesting was incorporated into the latest release of AutoDep at the E-MSD for the task of making deposition simpler and more automated. As a result, the new deposition software no longer requires authors to provide manually any information that can be derived from the co-ordinates (e.g. secondary structure and disulfide bonds) and the vast majority of the data fields may be populated directly from uploaded CNS (Brünger *et al.*, 1998) and CCP4 (CCP4, 1994) harvest files. This approach greatly reduces the occurrence of typing and cutting/pasting errors, allows more information to be archived without placing additional burden on the depositor and has also simplified the process of manual annotation of the deposited entries. In addition to the benefits to the depositor, this approach has resulted in the generation of a database that is richer in the volume of data and its accuracy, as well as being more consistent between various PDB entries that are deposited with harvest files. A generalized scheme of the data harvesting process is shown in Figure 9.1. The aim of the harvesting is to make it as painless as possible for the depositor to provide details about the structure in question. This is achieved by automatically extracting information from various harvest files produced by refinement and data processing programs during the course of structure determination.

Data Harvesting

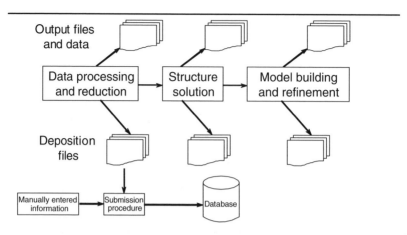

Figure 9.1   A general scheme for the data harvesting process

9.2 Identification of the Biologically Relevant Assembly

Quaternary structure is defined as that level of form in which units of tertiary structure aggregate to form homo- or hetero-multimers. Consideration of the presence of a quaternary state is important in the understanding of a protein's biological function. For a PDB entry determined using X-ray crystallography, the deposited co-ordinates typically consist of the contents of the asymmetric unit (ASU). The deposited co-ordinates may, therefore, contain one or more complete macromolecule(s), some parts of which may require crystallographic symmetry operations to be applied to each part in order to generate the complete macromolecule(s). Algorithms (Henrick and Thornton, 1998; Ponstingl, Henrick and Thornton, 2000) have been developed to determine the most likely oligomeric state, taking into account the symmetry related chains. These algorithms form the basis of the Protein Quaternary Structure (PQS) server (http://www.ebi.ac.uk/msd-srv/pqs).

In simple terms, these algorithms calculate the overall loss of accessible surface area from an isolated chain to that in the assembly predicted by the crystal symmetry operations (Example 1 below). As a rule of thumb, a buried surface area of about 15 per cent of the total accessible surface area of an isolated chain indicates the possibility of an oligomeric state. However, since crystal structures often make many contacts with other protein molecules from neighbouring unit cells, the prediction from the PQS algorithm can never be 100 per cent accurate. In some cases, true physiological dimers may also have a buried interface area less than 15 per cent. It is, therefore, necessary to incorporate information from other sources, including bio-chemical data and visual inspection of surface complementarity at the oligomeric interface to determine the biological assembly (Example 2 below). The occurrence of super-secondary structures formed by the association of monomers, for example, the formation of a large beta-sheet by the alignment of individual beta-sheets from each monomer, could also provide important information regarding the nature of an assembly. Additionally, the effects of a single amino acid substitution in a functionally important region of a protein can also cause changes in the oligomerization state (Example 3 below). Another category that is problematic in the correct annotation of the assembly information involves the structures that constitute only a small fragment of a larger protein. In these cases, the assembly information for a fragment can be substantially different from the true quaternary structure of the full-length protein (Example 4 below).

Example 1. Figure 9.2(a) shows the structure of ascorbate oxidase as deposited with the PDB (PDB entry 1aoz) (Messerschmidt *et al.*, 1992). The two arms, at the top and the bottom left, are well ordered and PQS finds an alternative dimer in which these two arms interlock at the dimer interface as shown in Figure 9.2(b). Interestingly, ascorbate oxidase is also found in higher oligomeric states and so both the interfaces shown in Figure 9.2(a) and (b) are likely to be biologically significant.

Example 2. Figure 9.2(c) shows the structure of arginase (PDB entry 5cev) (Bewley *et al.*, 1999). The asymmetric unit contains two tightly packed trimers arranged around a three-fold axis. PQS analysis of this entry suggested that the oligomeric structure could be a tightly packed hexamer, a claim also supported by biochemical information for this protein from BRENDA (Schomburg, Chang and Schomburg, 2002) (http://www.brenda.uni-koeln.de/). The hexameric assembly generated by PQS is shown in Figure 9.2(d).

Example 3. The native structure of human importin alpha-fragment (PDB entry 1bk5) (Conti *et al.*, 1998), under conditions required for crystallization, forms a homodimer that prevents the study of peptide binding (Figure 9.2(e)). Tyr 397 triggers dimer formation even though it is distant from binding site. On the other hand, the structure of importin mutant Tyr397Asp (PDB entry 1ee5) (Conti and Kuriyan, 2000) shows that this mutant does not form a homodimer, allowing peptide complex formation (Figure 9.2(f)).

Example 4. The human mannose-binding protein exists as a trimeric or hexameric assembly, as documented by crystallographic and functional studies (PDB entry 1rtm) (Weis, Drickamer and Hendrickson, 1992), but the lectin domain of the protein (PDB entry 2msb) (Weis and Drickamer, 1994) forms a dimer, as predicted by PQS. However, since the fragment of the protein has little biological relevance when it exists in its true physiological state, the quaternary structure of the domain itself is not a significant biological oligomeric state for mannose-binding protein.

In addition to the automatic and manual procedures described above, depositor input is often crucial in annotating the correct oligomeric state of the protein in the PDB file.

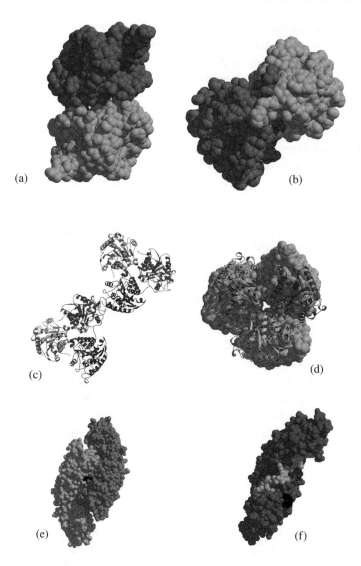

Figure 9.2   Examples of generating the PQS assembly from deposited coordinates

9.3 Taxonomy

The correct identification of the organism from which the deposited structure originates is a critical step in the annotation of the PDB entry. For any given entry, this step determines the subsequent annotation and identification of the sequence. The data regarding the organism is annotated in the ORGANISM_SCIENTIFIC section of the SOURCE records. During the annotation process, the species name is checked

against the EBI NEWT database[1] (http://www.ebi.ac.uk/newt) for consistent nomenclature. Where one particular species has many synonyms, the official name is used
instead. For example, the bacterial species *Cellvibrio japonicus* is also known as
Cellvibrio cellulosa, and *Pseudomonas fluorescens cellulosa*, but is corrected to the
former official name in any entry that refers to this species. Similarly, for entries that
derive from related sub-species for which there is no individual taxonomy identifier,
the nearest parent (species) or grandparent (genus) taxonomical definition is chosen
for annotation purposes. This follows the rationale that related proteins from closely
related organisms would have almost identical structures without necessarily having a
100 per cent sequence identity between them. In circumstances where a species does
not exist in the NEWT database or the NCBI taxonomy database (Wheeler *et al.*,
2001) (http://www.ncbi.nlm.nih.gov/taxonomy), the information regarding this species is sent to the NCBI in order to generate a new taxonomy identifier.

9.4 Sequence Recognition and Cross-reference

In structural study, the sequence is the basic chemical description of the system under
study, which is not necessarily the same as an entry in a sequence database. For a
PDB entry the coordinates contain only the observed atom positions and in many
cases the atom sites do not necessarily represent the complete sequence of the protein
studied, especially in cases where only an extracellular fragment or a structural
domain was used in the experiment. In addition, there are often additional residues at
the terminal ends of the protein arising from cloning or purification procedures in the
form of an artificial construct such as histidine tags. The problem in the correct
assignation of a sequence cross-reference is further exacerbated when artificial fusion
protein structures are described. Gaps in the protein structure (i.e. residues that were
disordered in the crystal and therefore not observed in electron density maps) are
often not reflected in the sequence information provided. In each case, determination
of the correct sequence database reference is vital, as information obtained from the
UNIPROT cross-reference is used to generate appropriate HEADER, COMPND,
DBREF, SEQADV, MODRES and SOURCE records in the PDB entry. UNIPROT is
a central repository of protein sequence and function created by joining the
information contained in Swiss-Prot, TrEMBL and PIR (Apweiler *et al.*, 2004).
Furthermore, correct assignment of a UNIPROT cross-reference allows the database
entry to be mapped to various other sequence and sequence-related databases. In
consultation with the depositor, we determine the exact sequence of the protein that
was used in the experiment, taking into account any expression constructs, unobserved residues and insertions including the usually flexible N- and C-termini.
Knowledge of the exact crystallized sequence is essential for the correct alignment

---

[1]The taxonomy database maintained by the Swiss-Prot group. It integrates taxonomy data compiled in the NCBI
database and data specific to the Swiss-Prot protein knowledgebase.

of the sequence from the PDB entry to the sequence database, in order for the generation of REMARK 465 and 470 PDB records, and their equivalent database records, which describe residues that were not observed in the structure.

The sequence of the protein under study is described in the SEQRES records, with one entry for each polypeptide or nucleotide chain described in the entry. The PDB file is also annotated with DBREF records that map the sequence of the protein studies with the appropriate UNIPROT (Apweiler et al., 2004) (http://www.ebi. uniprot.org/) cross-reference, including the numbering scheme from the sequence database. Where the protein contains artificial constructs, these regions are not mapped to a sequence database cross-reference. In cases where there are discrepancies between the sequences derived from the PDB file and that present in the appropriate sequence database, SEQADV records are added to the PDB file to indicate the nature of the conflict. These lines could indicate actual engineered mutations, variants or splice variants. However, this is not always an easy task, as many residues are regularly truncated to alanine in co-ordinate records when electron density for a particular residue side-chain is not unambiguously visible. Such matters are usually resolved in consultation with the depositor.

Deposition and annotation steps are taken to ensure that the data are not only consistent within a PDB entry and across the PDB archive but also consistent with other databases that contain related information. The E-MSD group works closely with UNIPROT in the development of procedures that match atom records to the experiment sequences and to the sequence databases. Information on chains, fragment sequences and journal references that are obtained during the curation of a PDB entry are passed back to the UNIPROT database at EBI, in order to maintain consistency between the structure and protein sequence archives. In cases where the protein sequence deposited with the structure is new to the UNIPROT, a new UNIPROT database entry for that sequence is generated in consultation with the UNIPROT group and the depositor.

9.5 Recognition of Secondary Structure Elements

In the PDB the HELIX, SHEET and TURN records represent secondary structure. In previous versions of AutoDep, the depositor was asked to provide secondary structure assignments, but these assignments were frequently found to be inconsistent with the co-ordinates, either due to typing errors or inappropriate cutting/pasting from other entries. The latest version of our deposition software does not ask for secondary structure and instead secondary structure assignments are generated during processing, using a single program that integrates DSSP (Kabsch and Sander, 1983) and the Promotif suite (Hutchinson and Thornton, 1996). The assignments are included in the copy of the PDB entry the depositor is sent for review and any changes to the secondary structure that the depositor wishes to make are incorporated at this stage, and are recorded in REMARK 650 to 700 as having been determined by the depositor. The PDB format also allows for the identification of bifurcated beta-sheets, which are also annotated in REMARK 700.

9.6 Validation of Structures

A key aspect of making the PDB useful to a diverse community of researchers is that the data should be accurate, consistent and machine-readable and carry clear indicators of quality. Data are more useful if they are associated with meaningful confidence criteria and if they can be retrieved in a form that indicates the degree of confidence that can be placed on any observation.

Both AutoDep and the subsequent processing stages contain a validation component that is primarily targeted at determining deviations from what is normally observed. This is achieved by comparison with a knowledgebase to identify unusual features. A validation report that follows the recommendations of Hooft *et al.*, 1996, is prepared as part of the AutoDep4 procedures and is made available to depositors. Deviations from standard geometry and expected backbone torsion angles are detected using in-house software. REMARK 500 records in PDB format files are used for describing such information. This section also includes information about close contact between atoms in the same asymmetric unit, close contacts between atoms of symmetry-related molecules and unusual deviations in bond lengths and bond angles in covalently linked atoms, as well as residues whose backbone torsion angles lie outside predicted Ramachandran (Kleywegt and Jones, 1996; Ramachandran and Sasisekharan, 1968) plot regions. As part of the validation and annotation process, atoms that lie on crystallographic axis are marked as being in 'special positions' and described in REMARK 375. Unusually high deviations from the standard statistical values are brought to the attention of the depositor and in many cases the depositor will provide a set of revised co-ordinates with corrected geometry, and this is used as a replacement for the initially deposited structure.

It is anticipated that validation during deposition will become more important as high throughput approaches for structure determination are developed and the determination of structures becomes separated from the analysis. The E-MSD works closely with the European software groups such as CCP4 (http://www.ccp4.ac.uk) (CCP4, 1994), for X-ray structure determination, and CCPN (Fogh *et al.*, 2002), for NMR techniques, as well as the EU-funded NMRQUAL (Spronk *et al.*, 2003) project for developing validation criteria for structure determined using NMR.

Increasingly, structure factors, which are the reduced raw data for an X-ray crystallographic experiment, are being deposited with the PDB. The raw data from these experiments are deposited in a wide variety of formats, depending on the programs used for refinement of the structure. As part of the annotation process, we automatically convert these into the format described by the PDB and run the CCP4 validation program SFCHECK (Vaguine, Richelle and Wodak, 1999) to calculate the goodness of fit between the deposited model and the data. We also run an in-house version of the Uppsala Electron Density Server (EDS) program (Kleywegt *et al.*, 2004) to calculate electron density maps, graphs and structure factor statistics that are made available to the depositor for their perusal. Unusually low values for the goodness of fit are brought to the attention of the depositor. Ideally all the validation checks that are run during deposition would have been run before the deposition process starts. To encourage this, the E-MSD runs the CRITQUAL validation service (http://www.ebi.ac.uk/msd-srv/biotech). CRITQUAL (Dodson, 1998; Dodson *et al.*, 1998; Wilson *et al.*, 1998) is the European 3D Validation Network, and has devised a series of geometrical and structure factor tests that may be used to assess how well a crystal structure fits the observed data and how well its geometry agrees with target values.

9.7 Residue Identification

This step comprises a major computational chunk of the annotation process. The process of residue identification not only involves a consistent standard in the nomen-clature of amino acids, nucleic acids and solvent molecules but also the recognition and classification of other chemically distinct species such as bound ligands, modified amino acids or nucleic acids and metal ions. PDB conventions dictate that each chemical entity is identified by a three-letter code that is consistent across the entire archive. In addition, each residue in a PDB entry is described by a chain identifier, a sequence number and an insert code, which may vary from one entry to another. The process of residue identification is the major part of the deposition and is a pre-requisite before properties for the chemical identities in a PDB entry can be derived for the annotation process. The problems inherent in the process of residue identification for standard amino acids are exacerbated by the occurrence of many topological variants of the same amino acid. For example, the standard PDB topology dictionary for L-histidine contains 12 distinct variants, which differ in their proto-nation states or their position within a polypeptide chain, and the nature of any termini with which they may be associated. As part of making the PDB globally consistent, it is important that all chemical species found in the PDB have atom names that match for each occurrence of the same, and that similar atoms have similar atom names for molecules related by chemistry. In order to achieve this goal in an automated fashion, the E-MSD has designed tools that implement both the recognition and matching of chemical identity as well as the comparison and matching of atoms names against reference data. Where an exact structural match for a residue is found in the reference database, the residue is renamed according to the database entry, and the constituent atoms of that residue are reordered and renamed to fit with PDB conventions. These tools are an extremely important component of the PDB curation and annotation process at E-MSD, especially in the identification of non-standard amino or nucleic acids or bound ligands, also known as heterogens or hetgroups.

9.8 Hetgroup Identification

Of the about 18 000 entries in the PDB, at least half contain metal ions or other non-polypeptide groups. These chemical entities include substrates, products, inhibitors and prosthetic groups. As in the case of standard residues, PDB conventions require that each chemically unique identity be assigned a unique identifier for each occurrence of the same in the whole archive. For example, every occurrence of beta-glucose should be labelled GLC. The PDB requires the additional check that the atom names for all residues must be compliant with the PDB hetgroup dictionary and are presented in a set order defined in that same dictionary.

The correct recognition of the chemistry for each of these entities is a complicated procedure, not least because the methods used to determine macromolecular structures often do not give accurate structures for the bound small molecules, but also because the deposited hetgroup may comprise only a small portion of the whole chemical used in the experiment. In addition, the deposited PDB entry may also contain chemical species that were not part of the experiment but which were observed to be associated with the protein; the chemical identity of these unknown compounds is frequently a mystery. The E-MSD has put in place a system for matching all the chemical constituents of the entry against the PDB hetgroup dictionary. Graph isomorphism approaches are used to match against a compound against a version of the PDB hetgroup dictionary that has been significantly extended to include stereochemical detail such as chirality, ring atom definition and *cis/trans* double bond information.

In addition, algorithms have been developed for matching fragments of molecules against fragments of the molecules in the PDB hetgroup dictionary (subgraph–subgraph isomorphism). A schematic diagram describing the logical flow of this process is shown in Figure 9.3. In short, graph representations for each of the chemical compounds present in the PDB archive are contained in an Oracle database, which is compiled into rapidly accessible binary files. The graph-matching utility allows a query hetgroup to be compared against the whole database of small molecules and individual precompiled compounds at a rate of 4000 reference compounds/minute. The graph matching utility can automatically differentiate between different stereoisomers of compounds and renames the residues deposited to the PDB hetgroup identifier for that compound. For example, both α-D-mannose (hetgroup code MAN) and β-D-mannose (hetgroup code BMA) are present in the PDB hetgroup dictionary (Figure 9.4) and occur in many PDB entries. When a new entry contains a residue described as XYZ, the graph-matching algorithm will compare the deposited hetgroup with its precompiled list of compounds. If the

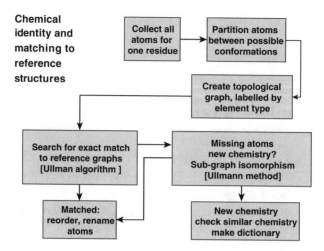

Figure 9.3 Schematic diagram illustrating the various steps involved in the graph-matching algorithm used for determining the correct identity of bound molecules/heterogens during the annotation process

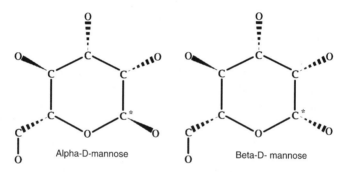

Figure 9.4 Schematic diagram showing the detailed chemical structures of α-D-mannose (MAN) and β-D-mannose (BMA), highlighting the stereochemical differences around position C1 (marked with *)

deposited compound matches BMA on stereochemistry and geometry, the name of the deposited hetgroup XYZ will be automatically changed to BMA with the atoms renamed to match that of BMA.

For new ligands, where no match could be obtained against the hetgroup database, procedures are in place to automatically generate the new dictionary entry. Generating a new dictionary entry automatically from the deposited co-ordinates is not always a simple matter since bond orders and protons must be correctly assigned.

In addition, procedures are in place for the automatic assignment of R and S stereochemistry on atoms and E or Z on double bonded atoms. Many of the procedures are built around the CACTVS software suite (Ihlenfeldt *et al.*, 1994, 2002), into which the co-ordinates of a new ligand are input via hydrogen-additive step. The new hetgroup dictionary entry also allows for the description of leaving groups/atoms.

The whole process of hetgroup identification and curation is under the control of a single in-house program called DOHLC. This script identifies any hetgroup in a PDB entry and matches atom names for known residues. The program also creates the necessary LINK, CONECT, HET, HETNAM, MODRES, FORMUL records and REMARK 600 with angles for metal coordination. For new residues the program also creates a new hetgroup dictionary. All new ligands are also visually inspected by annotators to flag any obvious errors or omissions in the deposited hetgroup, before choosing a new hetgroup identifier for the ligand. The hetgroup dictionary is also sent to the depositors for inspection and any problems or concerns are resolved in consultation with them. These procedures are extremely useful for ensuring that families of compounds are handled in a consistent manner. The completed chemical descriptions are exchanged with the RCSB on a daily basis to maintain PDB consistency between entries processed at the different sites.

9.9 Solvent Handling

Most entries deposited to the PDB that have been determined by X-ray crystallography contain within them a number of water molecules associated with the polypeptide or nucleotide chain. As part of making the PDB archive consistent in its approach in the handling of solvent molecules, a strict naming convention is usually enforced. All water molecules are assigned the residue name HOH (even if submitted as WAT, OH2 etc) and assigned chain identifiers depending on the polypeptide or nucleotide chain they are associated with. For example, for an entry that contains protein chains labelled from A to D, the corresponding water molecules will be assigned chain identifiers from Z to W, with chain Z corresponding to waters bound to chain A etc. A remark in the PDB file (REMARK 525) is used solely for describing the mapping relationships of macromolecular chains with solvent chains. The processing scripts used for annotation flag solvent molecules if they are found more than 4.0 Å from the nearest protein atom but could be transformed using crystallographic symmetry to a new location that would place them within 4.0 Å of a protein atom. A list of such solvent molecules is provided in a temporary addendum to REMARK 525 for the information of the depositor. If the depositor agrees that these solvent molecules can be moved to new locations or removed from the deposited entry, the necessary changes are applied to the PDB entry before its release.

9.10 Miscellaneous Annotation Issues

In addition to the various issues described in detail above, the annotation of structural data involves multifarious tasks, which are discussed in brief below.

HEADER records

The HEADER record in any PDB entry is the first data field of that entry. As part of the annotation process, the HEADER records are made extremely generic rather than entry specific. The header record describes the functional class of the entry under description. For example, enzymes which are a lyase or a ribonuclease are both marked as hydrolase in the header, as this best describes the functional class and activity of the protein.

Complex hetgroups

In cases where an entry contains a large hetgroup, submitted as a single chemical entity but the single hetgroup is really composed of a collection of covalently bound smaller hetgroups, the hetgroup matching algorithm will fail to find a match for the whole hetgroup. In such a case, the annotator must split the hetgroup into chemically sensible parts and match each separately against the database. This allows for greater flexibility in the use of the same hetgroup in other depositions and not merely specific to one entry alone. This also ensures that the hetgroup database consists of various building blocks and remains broadly generic. For example, where entries are deposited with N-acetyl-lactosamine (GlcNaC), we split the entry into its two component parts D-galactose (GAL) and N-acetyl-D-glucosamine (NAG) and match each one independently against our database. A similar approach is used for standard amino acids which have hetgroups covalently attached to their side-chain. For example, LYR (pyridoxal phosphate attached to lysine) is split into the amino acid lysine and pyridoxal phosphate before the latter is matched against our hetgroup database.

Terminal residues

In crystal structures where the electron density representing the last few C-terminal residues is ambiguous or uninterruptible, it is common practice to add a terminal oxygen to the last visible residue of a chain and treat the remaining residues as unobserved. Although this is a convenient way of simplifying the description of the protein for refinement programs, it leads to an incorrect description of the structure of the final observed residue, since the last observed residue is not actually the end of the polypeptide chain. To correct this problem we routinely convert atom OXT in the final observed residue into atom N from the following unobserved residue. This means that the final observed residue is assigned the correct chemical structure.

Journal citations

As structures are usually deposited at the PDB before the paper describing this is actually published, a series of perl scripts monitor the PubMed database

(Macleod, 2002) (http://www.ncbi.nlm.nih.gov/pubmed), looking for citations that match the JRNL record in the PDB entry. The list of positive hits is analysed on a weekly basis, and the correct citation information included in the PDB file. This process also impacts on the release status of the entry if the structure was initially deposited as HPUB (release on publication).

Correspondence

In order that the PDB entry is as accurate and globally consistent as possible, contact with the depositor is maintained on a regular basis during the initial stages of annotation following deposition. Any concerns and questions from both the depositor and the PDB are resolved in consultation with the depositor. This ensures that the data that are archived in the PDB meet the approval of the depositor and the high standards desired for the database. Great care is taken to ensure that any annotation steps that have been agreed with the depositor are documented by a paper-trail of email correspondence.

9.11 Conclusions

With structural genomics initiatives taking off all around the world, it is now more important than ever that there are systems in place to handle the large number of expected depositions in an efficient and consistent manner. With the tools designed and implemented by the E-MSD for the annotation of depositions, the stage is set for high throughput curation of PDB entries deposited at EBI. Our collaborations with various scientific programmers and users have already led to major advances in the ease with which new structures and information associated with them can be deposited at the E-MSD. It is hoped that the curation and deposition tools produced by us will go a long way in contributing to a richer protein database.

References

Apweiler, R., Bairoch, A., Wu, C.H., Barker, W.C., Boeckmann, B., Ferro, S., Gasteiger, E., Huang, H., Lopez, R., Magrane, M., Martin, M.J., Natale, D.A., O'Donovan, C., Redaschi, N. and Yeh, L.S. (2004). UniProt: the universal protein knowledgebase. *Nucleic Acids Res.* **32**, 115–119.

Bairoch, A. and Boeckmann, B. (1994). The SWISS-PROT Protein Sequence Data Bank: current status. *Nucleic Acids Res.* **22**, 3578–3580.

Berman, H.M., Battistuz, T., Bhat, T.N., Bluhm, W.F., Bourne, P.E., Burkhardt, K., Feng, Z., Gilliland, G.L., Iype, L., Jain, S., Fagan, P., Marvin, J., Padilla, D., Ravichandran, V., Schneider, B., Thanki, N., Weissig, H., Westbrook, J.D. and Zardecki, C. (2002). The protein data bank. *Acta Crystallogr.* **D 58**, 899–907.

Bewley, M.C., Jeffrey, P.D., Patchett, M.L., Kanyo, Z.F. and Baker, E.N. (1999). Crystal structures of *Bacillus caldovelox* arginase in complex with substrate and inhibitors reveal new insights into activation, inhibition and catalysis in the arginase superfamily. *Structure* **7**, 435–448.

Boutselakis, H., Dimitropoulos, D., Fillon, J., Golovin, A., Henrick, K., Hussain, A., Ionides, J., John, M., Keller, P.A., Krissinel, E., McNeil, P., Naim, A., Newman, R., Oldfield, T., Pineda, J., Rachedi, A., Copeland, J., Sitnov, A., Sobhany, S., Suarez-Uruena, A., Swaminathan, J., Tagari, M., Tate, J., Tromm, S., Velankar, S. and Vranken, W. (2003). E-MSD: the european bioinformatics institute macromolecular structure database. *Nucleic Acids Res.* **31**, 458–462.

Brünger, A.T. (1992). *X-PLOR Version 3.1 Manual: A System for X-Ray Crystallography and NMR*, Yale University Press, New Haven, CT.

Brünger, A.T., Adams, P.D., Clore, G.M., DeLano, W.L., Gros, P., Grosse-Kunstleve, R.W., Jiang, J.S., Kuszewski, J., Nilges, M., Pannu, N.S., Read, R.J., Rice, L.M., Simonson, T. and Warren, G.L. (1998). Crystallography & NMR System: a new software suite for macromolecular structure determination. *Acta Crystallogr.* **D 54**, 905–921.

CCP4. (1994). The CCP4 Suite: programs for protein crystallography. *Acta Crystallogr.* **D 50**, 760–763.

Conti, E. and Kuriyan, J. (2000). Crystallographic analysis of the specific yet versatile recognition of distinct nuclear localization signals by karyopherin alpha. *Structure* **8**, 329–338.

Conti, E., Uy, M., Leighton, L., Blobel, G. and Kuriyan, J. (1998). Crystallographic analysis of the recognition of a nuclear localization signal by the nuclear import factor karyopherin alpha. *Cell* **94**, 193–204.

Dodson, E. (1998). The role of validation in macromolecular crystallography. *Acta Crystallogr.* **D 54**, 1109–1118.

Dodson, E.J., Davies, G.J., Lamzin, V.S., Murshudov, G.N. and Wilson, K.S. (1998). Validation Tools: can they indicate the information content of macromolecular crystal structures? *Structure* **6**, 685–690.

Fogh, R., Ionides, J., Ulrich, E., Boucher, W., Vranken, W., Linge, J.P., Habeck, M., Rieping, W., Bhat, T.N., Westbrook, J., Henrick, K., Gilliland, G., Berman, H., Thornton, J., Nilges, M., Markley, J. and Laue, E. (2002). The CCPN Project: an interim report on a data model for the NMR community. *Nat. Struct. Biol.* **9**, 416–418.

Golovin, A., Oldfield, T.J., Tate, J.G., Velankar, S., Barton, G.J., Boutselakis, H., Dimitropoulos, D., Fillon, J., Hussain, A., Ionides, J.M., John, M., Keller, P.A., Krissinel, E., McNeil, P., Naim, A., Newman, R., Pajon, A., Pineda, J., Rachedi, A., Copeland, J., Sitnov, A., Sobhany, S., Suarez-Uruena, A., Swaminathan, G.J., Tagari, M., Tromm, S., Vranken, W. and Henrick, K. (2004). E-MSD: an integrated data resource for bioinformatics. *Nucleic Acids Res.* **32**, 211–216.

Hamm, G.H. and Cameron, G.N. (1986). The EMBL data library. *Nucleic Acids Res.* **14**, 5–9.

Henrick, K. and Thornton, J.M. (1998). PQS: a protein quaternary structure file server. *Trends Biochem. Sci.* **23**, 358–361.

Hooft, R.W., Vriend, G., Sander, C. and Abola, E.E. (1996). Errors in protein structures. *Nature* **381**, 272.

Hutchinson, E.G. and Thornton, J.M. (1996). PROMOTIF – a program to identify and analyze structural motifs in proteins. *Protein Sci.* **5**, 212–220.

Ihlenfeldt, W.D., Takahashi, Y., Abe, H. and Sasaki, J. (1994). Computation and Management of Chemical Properties in CACTVS: an extensible networked approach toward modularity and flexibility. *J. Chem. Inf. Comput. Sci.* **34**, 109–116.

Ihlenfeldt, W.D., Voigt, J.H., Bienfait, B., Oellien, F. and Nicklaus, M.C. (2002). Enhanced CACTVS browser of the Open NCI Database. *J. Chem. Inf. Comput. Sci.* **42**, 46–57.

Kabsch, W. and Sander, C. (1983). Dictionary of Protein Secondary Structure: pattern recognition of hydrogen-bonded and geometrical features. *Biopolymers* **22**, 2577–2637.

Kleywegt, G.J., Harris, M.R., Zou, J.Y., Taylor, T.C., Wahlby, A. and Jones, T.A. (2004). The uppsala electron density server. *Acta. Crystallogr.*, in press.

Kleywegt, G.J. and Jones, T.A. (1996). Phi/psi-chology: Ramachandran revisited. *Structure* **4**, 1395–1400.

Lin, D., Manning, N.O., Jiang, J., Abola, E.E., Stampf, D., Prilusky, J. and Sussman, J.L. (2000). AutoDep: a web-based system for deposition and validation of macromolecular structural information. *Acta. Crystallogr.* **D 56**, 828–841.

Macleod, M.R. (2002). PubMed: http://www.pubmed.org. *J. Neurol. Neurosurg. Psychiatry* **73**, 746.

Messerschmidt, A., Ladenstein, R., Huber, R., Bolognesi, M., Avigliano, L., Petruzzelli, R., Rossi, A. and Finazzi-Agro, A. (1992). Refined crystal structure of ascorbate oxidase at 1.9 Å resolution. *J. Mol. Biol.* **224**, 179–205.

Ponstingl, H., Henrick, K. and Thornton, J.M. (2000). Discriminating between homodimeric and monomeric proteins in the crystalline state. *Proteins* **41**, 47–57.

Ramachandran, G.N. and Sasisekharan, V. (1968). Conformation of polypeptides and proteins. *Adv. Protein Chem.* **23**, 283–438.

Schomburg, I., Chang, A. and Schomburg, D. (2002). BRENDA, enzyme data and metabolic information. *Nucleic Acids Res.* **30**, 47–49.

Spronk, C.A., Nabuurs, S.B., Bonvin, A.M., Krieger, E., Vuister, G.W. and Vriend, G. (2003). The precision of NMR structure ensembles revisited. *J. Biomol. NMR* **25**, 225–234.

Vaguine, A.A., Richelle, J. and Wodak, S.J. (1999). SFCHECK: a unified set of procedures for evaluating the quality of macromolecular structure-factor data and their agreement with the atomic model. *Acta Crystallogr.* **D 55**, 191–205.

Weis, W.I. and Drickamer, K. (1994). Trimeric structure of a C-type mannose-binding protein. *Structure* **2**, 1227–1240.

Weis, W.I., Drickamer, K. and Hendrickson, W.A. (1992). Structure of a C-type mannose-binding protein complexed with an oligosaccharide. *Nature* **360**, 127–134.

Wheeler, D.L., Church, D.M., Lash, A.E., Leipe, D.D., Madden, T.L., Pontius, J.U., Schuler, G.D., Schriml, L.M., Tatusova, T.A., Wagner, L. and Rapp, B.A. (2001). Database resources of the national center for biotechnology information. *Nucleic Acids Res.* **29**, 11–16.

Wilson, K.S., Butterworth, S., Dauter, Z., Lamzin, V.S., Walsh, M., Wodak, S.J., Pontius, J.U., Richelle, J., Vaguine, A.A., Sander, C., Hooft, R.W., Vriend, G., Thornton, J., Laskowski, R.A., MacArthur, M.W., Dodson, E., Murshudov, G.N., Oldfield, T., Kaptein, R. and Rullmann, J.A.C. (1998). Who checks the checkers? Four validation tools applied to eight atomic resolution structures. EU 3-D Validation Network. *J. Mol. Biol.* **276**, 417–436.

10 Classification of Protein Function

A. M. Lesk, H. Parkinson and J. C. Whisstock

Abstract

Annotation of a genome requires assignment of functions to gene products, in most cases on the basis of amino acid sequence alone. The goal of structural genomics projects is to make three dimensional information available, which is invaluable in assessing inferences from amino acid sequences. Nevertheless, prediction of protein function, even if sequence and structure are known, is in many cases a difficult problem. Comparative genomics and patterns of interaction sometimes provide essential clues. Some methods provide reasonable guesses at function, but none is foolproof. An underlying problem is that function is in many cases an ill defined concept. In this article we review the state of the art in function prediction.

Keywords

function prediction, function classification, phylogeny, homology, orthology, protein structure, interaction patterns

10.1 Introduction

The sequence of a genome contains the information required to build an organism, but the decoding and implementation of genetic information depends on the functions of the proteins and nucleic acids that it encodes. Assignment of functions to gene products, in most cases based on the analysis of amino acid sequence alone, is a crucial component of annotating a genome. Three-dimensional structure can aid the

Database Annotation in Molecular Biology   Edited by Arthur M. Lesk
© 2005 John Wiley & Sons, Ltd.   ISBN: 0-470-85681-5

assignment of function, motivating the challenge of structural genomics projects to make structural information available for novel uncharacterized proteins.

To reason from sequence and structure to function is to step onto shaky ground. Many procedures described in the literature on function prediction do not specify function exactly, but provide general hints. For instance, a protein known to contain a TIM barrel is likely to be a hydrolytic enzyme. Such evidence is very useful in guiding experimental investigations of function, and indeed a sufficient accumulation of evidence – based on sequence, structure, genomics, co-expression and interaction patterns – may well allow an expert to propose a specific function. However, such an approach, relying on human expertise, is difficult to automate for high throughput full genome analysis.

A common way to assign function to a protein is to identify a putative homologue of known function and guess that the function is shared. Many families of proteins do contain homologues with the same function, widely distributed among species. However, the assumption that homologues share function is less and less safe as the sequences progressively diverge. Moreover, even closely related proteins can change function, either through divergence to a related function or by recruitment for a very different function (Ganfornia and Sánchez, 1999). In such cases, assignment of function on the basis of homology can lead to misannotation in databanks. In the end there is no substitute for experiment.

An aspect of divergence important for its implications about function is the distinction between orthologues and paralogues. Any two proteins that are related by descent from a common ancestor are *homologues*. Two proteins in different species descended from the same protein in an ancestral species are *orthologues*. Two proteins related via a gene duplication within one species (and the respective descendants of the duplicates) are *paralogues*. After gene duplication, one of the resulting pairs of proteins can continue to provide its customary function, releasing the other to diverge to develop new functions. Therefore, inferences of function from homology are more secure for orthologues than for paralogues. The database, Clusters of Orthologous Groups (COGs), is a collection of proteins encoded in fully sequenced genomes, organized into families (Natale *et al.*, 2000). The COG database shows how this approach has successfully been applied to analysis of function and genome annotation.

It is becoming clear from the various genome-sequencing projects that there is likely to be a limited number of genes and proteins whose structure and function may be conserved across species. This means that knowledge of a protein function in one organism may be informative for the same protein in a related species. However, annotation systems and nomenclature in different species are very different, and the naming of genes and their products is often inconsistent even within a single organism, so one must also consider sources of data and their reliability. It is also common in prokaryote genomes to use the same gene name in different species even though the genes are not necessarily orthologous. At worst, gene names are simply human-readable identifiers. This complicates cross-species comparisons to infer function.

10.2 Mechanisms of Divergence of Protein Function

How much must a protein change its sequence before its function changes? The answer is 'not at all'! There are numerous examples of proteins with multiple functions.

1. Eye lens proteins in the duck are identical to active lactate dehydrogenase and enolase in other tissues, although they do not encounter the substrates in the eye. They have been recruited to provide a completely unrelated function based on the optical properties of their assembly. Several other avian eye lens proteins are identical or similar to enzymes. In some cases residues essential for catalysis have mutated, proving that the function of these proteins in the eye is not an enzymatic one (Wistow and Piatigorsky, 1987).

2. Some proteins interact with different partners to produce oligomers with different functions. In *E. coli*, a protein that functions on its own as lipoate dehydrogenase is also an essential subunit of pyruvate dehydrogenase, 2-oxoglutarate dehydrogenase and the glycine cleavage complex (Riley, 1997).

3. Proteinase Do functions as a chaperone at low temperatures and as a proteinase at high temperatures (Spiess, Beil and Ehrmann, 1999).

4. Phosphoglucose isomerase (= neuroleukin = autocrine motility factor = differentiation and maturation mediator) functions as a glycolytic enzyme in the cytoplasm, but as a nerve growth factor and cytokine outside the cell (Jeffery, 1999; Jeffery *et al.*, 2000). (We shall see that the Gene Ontology Consortium tracks cellular location, making it possible to disentangle certain cases of location-dependent functions.)

These cases show that *even if* experiments do identify a function, we cannot be sure that we know the protein's full repertoire of biological activities. As additional functions are discovered, it is important to pass the emended annotations on to derived databanks.

To understand the variety of functions shown by individual proteins and by close relatives, we must understand how proteins develop new functions during their evolution. Observed mechanisms of protein evolution that produce altered or novel functions include (1) *divergence*, (2) *recruitment* and (3) 'Mixing and matching' of domains.

Divergence

In families of closely related proteins, mutations usually conserve function but modulate specificity. For example, the trypsin family of serine proteinases contains a specificity pocket: a surface cleft complementary in shape and charge distribution to the side-chain adjacent to the scissile bond. Mutations affect the shape and charge of its lining, altering the specificity.

This theme is typical: homologous proteins show a general drifting apart of their sequences, but often only a few specific mutations account for functional divergence (Golding and Dean, 1998), as initially proposed by Perutz (1983) for haemoglobin. In some cases very large divergence has led to very different function. Murzin (1998) and Grishin (2001) have discussed how far divergence can push the relationships between homology, structure and sequence divergence, and functional change.

Recruitment

The application of enzymes as lens crystallins illustrated another route of evolution: a novel function *preceding* divergence. Divergence and recruitment are at the ends of a spectrum of changes in sequence and function. Aside from cases of 'pure' recruitment such as the duck eye lens proteins or phosphoglucose isomerase, there are examples on the one hand of relatively small sequence changes correlated with very small function changes (relatively pure divergence) and relatively small sequence changes with quite large changes in function (recruitment), but also many cases in which there are large changes in both sequence and function.

'Mixing and matching' of domains, including duplication/ oligomerization, and domain swapping or fusion

Many large proteins contain tandem assemblies of domains that appear in different contexts and orders in different proteins.[1]

Censuses of genomes suggest that many proteins are multimodular. Serres *et al.* (2001) report that, of 4401 genes in *E. coli*, 287 correspond to proteins containing two, three or four modules. Teichmann *et al.* (2001a, 2001b) have analysed, for enzymes involved in metabolism of small molecules, the distribution and redistribution of domains. The structural patterns of 510 enzymes could be accounted for in total or in part by 213 families of domains. Of the 399 which could be entirely divided into known domains, 68 per cent were single domain proteins, 24 per cent comprised two domains and seven per cent three domains. Only four of the 399 had four, five or six domains. Teichmann *et al.* also showed that there are marked preferences for pairing of different families of domains.

---

[1]The reader must be warned that there is no universal agreement about how to define a domain or a module; one traditional definition is that a domain is a compact subunit of a protein that looks as if it should have independent stability. Some authors refer to a compact unit as a module, and reserve the term domain for a unit that stays together as an evolutionary unit, appearing in partnership with different sets of other domains, or in different orders along the chain. These authors describe the serine protease structure as a single domain comprising two modules.

Multidomain proteins present particular problems for functional annotation, because domains may possess independent functions, modulate one another's function or act in concert to provide a single function. On the other hand, in some cases the presence of a particular domain or combinations of domains is associated with a specific function. For example, NAD-binding domains appear almost exclusively in dehydrogenases. Annotators have access to resources such as Interpro and Swiss-Prot to assist them (http://www.ebi.ac.uk/interpro, http://www.expasy.org/sprot).

10.3 Classification of Protein Functions

General classes

Andrade *et al.* (1999) distinguished the functional classes of proteins involved in energy, information, and communication and regulation (Table 10.1).

Table 10.1   General classification of protein functions (Andrade *et al.*, 1999)

- Energy
  - Biosynthesis of cofactors, amino acids
  - Central and intermediary metabolism
  - Energy metabolism
  - Fatty acids and phospholipids
  - Nucleotide biosynthesis
  - Transport

- Information
  - Replication
  - Transcription
  - Translation

- Communication and regulation
  - Regulatory functions
  - Cell envelope/cell wall
  - Cellular processes

The enzyme commission classification

The best known detailed classification of protein functions is that of the Enzyme Commission (EC) (http://www.chem.qmul.ac.uk/iubmb/enzyme/). The EC classification originated in the action taken by the General Assembly of the International Union of Biochemistry (IUB) and the International Union of Pure and Applied Chemistry (IUPAC), in 1955, to establish an International Commission on Enzymes.

EC numbers (looking suspiciously like IP numbers) contain four fields, corresponding to a four-level hierarchy. For example, EC 1.1.1.1 corresponds to alcohol dehydrogenase, catalysing the general reaction

$$\text{an alcohol} + \text{NAD} = \text{the corresponding aldehyde or ketone} + \text{NADH}$$

Several reactions, involving different alcohols, would share this number; but the same dehydrogenation of one of these alcohols by an enzyme using the alternative cofactor NADP would be assigned EC 1.1.1.2. The Commission has emphasized that 'It is perhaps worth noting, as it has been a matter of long-standing confusion, that enzyme nomenclature is primarily a matter of naming reactions catalysed, not the structures of the proteins that catalyse them'. The EC merges nonhomologous enzymes that catalyse similar reactions.

The first number indicates one of six main divisions:

Class 1. Oxidoreductases

Class 2. Transferases

Class 3. Hydrolases

Class 4. Lyases

Class 5. Isomerases

Class 6. Ligases.

The significance of the second and third numbers depends on the class. The fourth number gives the specific enzymatic activity.

Granting its groundbreaking achievement, there is consensus that the EC classification has many drawbacks that limit its utility for contemporary work.

Specialized classifications are available for some families of enzymes; for instance, the MEROPS database by N.D. Rawlings and A.J. Barrett provides a structure-based classification of peptidases and proteinases (http://www.merops.sanger.ac.uk/).

Given the goal of mapping a functional classification onto sequence and structure classifications, several problems associated with current functional categorizations are generally recognized. Gerlt and Babbitt (2000), who are among the most thoughtful writers on the subject, pointed out that 'no structurally contextual definitions of enzyme function exist'. They propose a general hierarchical classification of function better integrated with sequence and structure. For enzymes they define the following.

- *Family:* homologous enzymes that catalyse the same reaction (same mechanism same substrate specificity). These can be hard to detect at the sequence level if the sequence similarity becomes very low.

- *Superfamily:* homologous enzymes catalysing similar reaction with either (a) different specificity or (b) different overall reactions with common mechanistic attribute (partial reaction, transition state, intermediate) that share conserved active-site residues.

- *Suprafamilies:* different reactions with no common feature. Proteins belonging to the same suprafamily would not be expected to be detectable from sequence information alone.

There is also a 'culture clash': the traditional biochemist's view of function arises from the study of isolated proteins in dilute solutions; to a molecular biologist, an adequate definition of function must recognize the biological role of a molecule in the living context of a cell (or intracellular compartment) or the complete organism, and its role in a network of metabolic or control processes (Lan, Jansen and Gerstein, 2002; Lan, Montelione and Gerstein, 2003). There is a generic problem with all attempts to force functional classifications into a hierarchical format (see comments of Riley, 1998, and Shrager, 2003).

The Gene Ontology Consortium™

A more general approach to the *logical* structure of a functional classification has been adopted by The Gene Ontology™ Consortium (2000) (http://www.geneontology.org). Its goal is a systematic attempt to classify function, by creating a dictionary of terms and their relationships for describing molecular functions, biological processes and cellular context of proteins and other gene products.

The gene ontology (GO) consists of three orthogonal (non-overlapping) vocabularies, which describe *molecular function*, *biological process* and *cellular compartment*.

The organizing concepts of the gene ontology project include the following.

- *Molecular function:* a function associated with an activity performed by a protein or RNA molecule itself; either a general description such as 'enzyme', or a specific one such as 'alcohol dehydrogenase'. This is function from a biochemist's point of view.

- *Biological process:* a component of the activities of a living system, mediated by a protein or RNA, possibly in concert with other proteins or RNA molecules; either a general term such as signal transduction, or a particular one such as cyclic AMP synthesis. This is function from the cell's point of view.

Because many processes take place at specific locations within a cell or organism, gene ontology also tracks the following.

- *Cellular component:* the assignment of site of activity or partners; this can be a general term such as nucleus or a specific one such as ribosome.

Content of the gene ontology

The current number of defined terms across all three vocabularies is ∼16 000. GO is a resource that describes biology and that can be used to annotate gene products (RNAs and proteins). It is a very valuable resource for annotation of gene products and is now very widely used, even though it cannot yet claim to be complete.

GO has two types of term relationship: *is-a* and *part-of*. The ontology is structured as a directed acyclic graph (DAG). In the GO all paths to the root must be biologically true. If the terms are concatenated with the relationship types we can see the truth 'ATP dependent helicase IS_A helicase IS_A enzyme'. The biological 'truth' holds whichever way the DAG is navigated back to the root and however many branches the ontology has. Each term can have one or more parents and children in this structure and as the DAG is traversed down from the root granularity increases.

A full list of GO terms and current statistics can be found at http://www.geneontology.org/doc/GO.current.annotations.shtml. The GOA (Gene Ontology Annotation) project at the EBI is one of many contributors of mappings between GO terms and gene products. It uses a mixture of electronic and manual curation to assign GO terms to database records such as the human non-redundant proteome set. Data are made available in the GO flat file format. The files contain information on the originating database, identifiers for objects from that database (genes, gene products etc.) and GO and PubMed identifiers. Evidence codes indicate how the GO terms were assigned, and are an indicator of relative quality. For example, terms assigned on the basis of sequence similarity (IEA code) are typically less granular and less reliable.

Tools which use the gene ontology

Tools built around GO include editors, browsers, query services and analysis (http://www.geneontology.org/doc/GO.tools.html). Here we will consider just one category of these tools, which can be used to analyse microarray data. The EP:GO browser is built into Expression Profiler, http://ep.ebi.ac.uk/EP/GO, a suite of analysis tools for microarray data at the EBI. Microarray analysis often results in clusters of genes, which, as they are co-expressed, may be functionally related, 'a guilt by association' approach (Quackenbush, 2002). EP:GO allows a cluster to be associated with a GO term. This is a particularly useful approach when genes of unknown function within a cluster are to be analysed in future experiments.

GO is an important resource for discovery as well as for annotation. Pattern discovery in budding and fission yeast annotated by common GO terms reveals that proteins annotated by a common term can show putative regulatory patterns upstream of the initiator site.

10.4 Methods for Assigning Protein Function

Detection of protein homology from sequence

If there is a standard method for predicting protein function, it is the detection of similarity of amino acid sequence by database similarity searching, and assuming that the molecules identified are homologues with similar functions. However, the transfer of function assignment becomes less reliable as the similarity between the unknown sequence and its (putative) homologue falls.

Wilson, Kreychman and Gerstein (2000) conclude that for pairs of single domain proteins, at levels of sequence identity ≥40 per cent, precise function is conserved, and for levels of sequence identity ≥25 per cent broad functional class is conserved (according to a functional classification that uses the EC hierarchy for enzymes, and supplements it with material from FLYBASE (Ashburner and Drysdale, 1994) for nonenzymes). Todd, Orengo and Thornton (2001) found that for pairs of proteins, both known to be enzymes, slightly fewer than 90 per cent of pairs with sequence identity ≥40 per cent conserve all four EC numbers. Even at ≥30 per cent sequence identity they found conservation of three levels of the EC hiererchy for 70 per cent of homologous pairs of enzymes. Devos and Valencia (2000) reached very similar conclusions.

Having identified putative homologues, multiple sequence alignments enable identification of conserved residues. The literature may provide crucial information about the family as a whole and the role of conserved residues, and phylogenetic trees can provide information as to whether an unknown clusters with a particular functional grouping (Hannenhalli and Russell, 2000; Gu and Vander Velden, 2002). If an unknown protein shares significant sequence similarity with a family of known function, and possesses the 'essential conserved residues' (e.g., active site residues), then a prediction of function (proteinase, exonuclease etc.) can be proposed. In addition, if the unknown also forms part of a well supported functional cluster or clade within a phylogenetic tree, a more detailed level of functional prediction may be possible.

Detection of homologues may provide one or more relatives for which the three dimensional structure is known. This may permit construction of a molecular model. Even an approximate model may allow the compatibility of the unknown sequence with the fold to be assessed (Schonbrun, Wedemeyer and Baker, 2002). Furthermore, because the active sites of enzymes are often the most highly structurally conserved regions, it may be possible to build a detailed model around the active site, even if overall sequence similarity is low. If the results of an experimental structure determination are not available, theoretical methods of structure prediction may be useful in identifying putative remote homology (Schonbrun, Wedemeyer and Baker, 2002; Kinch *et al.*, 2003; Tramontano, 2003).

In some cases it is possible to bypass this type of reasoning and to recognize the residues comprising the active site from a specific signature pattern or motif within the sequence. However, although many motifs do reflect functional active sites, others reflect positions for post-translational modification (e.g. glycosylation sites), or structural signals (e.g. N and C caps of α-helices), or signal sequences, with no direct functional implications.

Attwood (2000) has described general methods for deducing sequence patterns. All start with (or produce) a multiple sequence alignment, and seek to identify common distinctive features of particular positions of the sequence. These features may involve the following.

1. A motif describing a single consecutive set of residues.

2. Multiple motifs – a combination of several motifs involving separate consecutive sets of residues.

3. Profile methods, based on entire sequences and weighting different residue positions according to the variability of their contents. Extensions and generalizations of profile methods, including hidden Markov models, are among the most sensitive detectors of distant homology based entirely on sequence data that we have.

Databases of profiles

PROSITE contains a compendium of profiles characterizing entire domains (Falquet *et al.*, 2002). Because matching of such profiles is sensitive to the sequences of entire domains, it is less likely to return false positives; but because the information contained in the most conserved part of the sequences is eroded, it may lose sensitivity relative to motif matching.

An alternative approach to describing a set of homologous sequences is hidden Markov models (HMMs) (Eddy, 1996). HMMs represent successive positions in a probabilistic way. They are more general than simple profiles, and do a better job of discriminating homologues from non-homologues, provided that they are trained with correct alignments. HMMs currently provide the most sensitive methods for detecting distant homologues given only the amino acid sequence of a query protein. Pfam is a database of multiple alignments of protein domains, and the hidden Markov models built from them (Bateman *et al.*, 2002). Search software permits detection of whether a query sequence belongs to any of the families in Pfam. The Superfamily database is a library of hidden Markov models for all proteins of known structure (Gough *et al.*, 2001). Its goal is to identify, from protein sequences, domains with folds corresponding to one or more known structures.

A weakness of single motif patterns is that an active site of a protein may be defined by regions that are distant in the sequence although nearby in space. Single motif patterns are also necessarily based on characteristics of single domains, whereas it may be useful to identify proteins by the presence of more than one domain. Multiple motif databases aim to remedy these problems. BLOCKS (Henikoff *et al.*, 2001) and PRINTS (Attwood, 2002; Attwood *et al.*, 2002, 2003) are databases of multiple motifs, typically ~20 residues long, presented in the form of ungapped multiple sequence alignments.

Profiles or HMMs are sensitive to overall folding pattern, sometimes at the expense of focus on specific active-site residues. Conversely, some motifs are sensitive to active-site residues but in their insensitivity to features of the sequence as a whole may pick up non-homologous proteins as false positives.

Among these classes of method, a combination of a profile and motif match would therefore seem to be the most reliable criterion for function assignment (see Chen and Jeong, 2000). This is the approach of InterPro, an umbrella database built from Pfam, PRINTs and PROSITE (http://www.ebi.ac.uk/interpro).

Detection of structural similarity, protein structure classifications and structure/function correlations

It is well known that structure changes more conservatively than sequence during evolution. Several authors have applied the known structures to infer homology among proteins too distantly related to be identified as homologues from the sequences alone (Holm and Sander, 1999; Aloy *et al.*, 2002).

Most classification schemes for sequences and structures are expressed as hierarchical clusterings. For instance, the Structural Classification of Proteins (SCOP) database has as its basis individual domains of proteins (Murzin *et al.*, 1995; LoConte *et al.*, 2002).

Several groups have attempted to correlate protein structure and function. For example, Hegyi and Gerstein (1999) correlated the enzymes in the yeast genome between their fold classification in SCOP and their EC functional categories, via the annotation in Swiss-Prot. They identified 8937 single domain proteins that could be assigned both a fold and a function. The broadest categories of structure were from the top of the SCOP hierarchy. The broadest categories of function were from the top of the EC hierarchy. There are therefore 6 (structural classes) × 7 (functional classes) = 42 possible combinations of highest level correlates. By using finer classifications of structure and function (down to the third level of EC numbers) there are a total of 21 068 potential fold–function combinations. Only 331 of these are observed, among the 8937 proteins analysed.

The observed distribution is highly non-random. Non-enzymatic functions account for 59 per cent of the sequences, of which well over half are in the all-α or all-β fold category. Of the enzymes, the most popular combinations were α/β folds among oxidoreductases and transferases, and all-β and $\alpha + \beta$ hydrolases.

Knowing the structure of a domain, what can be inferred about its function? Many folds are compatible with very different activities. The five most 'versatile' folds are the TIM barrel, $\alpha + \beta$ hydrolase, the NAD-binding fold, the P-loop-containing NTP hydrolase fold and the ferredoxin fold. Conversely, the functions carried out by the most different types of structure are glycosidases and carboxylases. These two functions are carried out by seven different fold types, from three different fold classes.

What we are looking for, however, are cases where structure provides reliable clues to function. In their cross-table, Hegyi and Gerstein (1999) show several folds that appear in combination with only one function. These appear to have predictive significance for function. Of course one cannot tell whether this is just because they are rare folds, and whether the correlation will hold up as the databases grow.

Several authors have sought to extend motif searching to three dimensions. Given that motifs tend to correspond to regions of conserved structure linked to function, Wallace, Laskowski and Thornton (1996) searched known protein structures for the Ser–His–Asp catalytic triad of trypsin-like serine proteinases. They identified all known serine proteinases in their dataset, plus triglycerol lipases which share the catalytic triad. de Rinaldis *et al.* (1998) derived three dimensional profiles from a single protein structure or a set of aligned structures. They applied their results to identifying proteins with matching surface patches. Analysis of the three dimensional profiles of ATP- and GTP-binding P-loop proteins identified a positively charged phosphate-binding residue (Arg or Lys) in a position conserved in space but not in sequence. In a similar approach, Jackson and Russell (2000, 2001) have identified regions with conformations similar to those of PROSITE motifs, but not necessarily sharing sequence similarity with them. They were able to identify serine proteinase inhibitors that contain regions similar in conformation to the loops in known inhibitors that have a common structure that docks to the proteinase.

Methods making use of structural data

Shapiro and Harris (2000) and Teichman, Murzin and Chothia (2001) illustrate the power of structure, including but not limited to identifying distant relationships not derivable from sequence comparisons.

1. Identification of structural relationships unanticipated from sequence can suggest similarity of function. The crystal structure of AdipoQ, a protein secreted from adipocytes, showed a similarity of folding pattern to that of tumour necrosis factor. The inference that AdipoQ is a cell signalling protein was subsequently verified.

2. The histidine triad proteins are a broad family with no known function. Analysis of their structures indicated a catalytic centre and nucleotide binding site, identifying them as a nucleotide hydrolase. Note that this did *not* depend on detection of a distant homology.

3. Structural similarity of a gene product of unknown function from *Methanococcus jannischii* and other proteins containing nucleotide-binding domains led to experiments showing it to be a xanthine or inosine triphosphatase (Hwang *et al.*, 1999).

As with some sequence-based methods, these structure-based methods proceed by searching for homologues. Although distant relationship is frequently more easily detectable in structure than in sequence, the returns are diminishing because the more distant the relationship the less reliable the inference of common function.

Lichtarge, Bourne and Cohen (1996a) have developed an evolutionary trace method to define binding surfaces common to protein families. They extract functionally important residues from sequence conservation patterns and map them onto the protein surface to identify functional clusters.

Successful predictions by the Evolutionary Trace method include identification of the functional surface in families of G protein α subunits (Lichtarge, Bourne and Cohen, 1996b) and regulators of G protein signalling (Sowa *et al.*, 2000, 2001). Both cases were *blind* predictions subsequently verified by experiment. The success of the Evolutionary Trace method has led to its being taken up and developed by a number of groups (Aloy *et al.*, 2001; Madabushi *et al.*, 2002; Lichtarge and Sowa, 2002; Yao *et al.*, 2003).

10.5 Applications of Full Organism Information: Inferences from Genomic Context and Protein Interaction Patterns

For proteins encoded in complete genomes, approaches to function prediction making use of contextual information and intergenomic comparisons are useful (Marcotte *et al.*, 1999; Huynen and Snel, 2000; Kolesov, Mewes and Frishman, 2001, 2002).

1. *Gene fusion.* A composite multifunctional gene in one genome may correspond to separate genes in other genomes. The implication is that there is a relationship between the functions of these genes.

2. *Local gene context.* It makes sense to coregulate and cotranscribe components of a pathway. In bacteria, genes in a single operon are usually functionally linked.

3. *Interaction patterns.* As part of the development of full organism methods of investigation, data are becoming available on patterns of protein–protein interactions (Xenarios *et al.*, 2002). The network of interactions reveals the function of a protein.

4. *Phylogenetic profiles.* Pellegrini *et al.* (1999) have exploited the idea that proteins in a common structural complex or pathway are functionally linked and expected to coevolve. For each protein encoded in a known genome, they construct a phylogenetic profile that indicates which organisms contain a homologue of the protein in question. Clustering the profiles identifies sets of proteins that co-occur in the same group of organisms. Some relationship between their functions is expected.

There need be no sequence or structural similarity between the proteins that share a phylogenetic distribution pattern. One unusual and very welcome feature of this method is that it is one of the few that derives information about the function of a protein from its relationship to *nonhomologous* proteins (Pellegrini *et al.*, 1999; Marcotte *et al.*, 1999).

10.6 Conclusions

The problem of prediction of function from amino acid sequence and protein structure is far from being satisfactorily solved.

It appears that the most general and wide ranging cross-species classification of function is that produced by The Gene Ontology[TM] Consortium. Their results have the advantage of being appropriate to both biochemistry and biology, at the expense of greater logical complexity.

Many of the methods that have been applied to function prediction work part of the time but none is perfect. Morever, the more expert analysis of the results is applied, the better the predictions are. This makes it difficult to envisage a purely 'black-box' automatic annotation machine for new whole genome sequences. In most cases, predictions suggest, but do not determine, the general class of function. Their most useful effect is to guide investigations in the laboratory to confirm, or refute, the prediction, and, even if correct, to define the function in greater detail.

We conclude that predictions are useful but no substitute for work in the laboratory. Indications from theory may indict, but only experimental evidence can convict.

References

Aloy, P., Oliva, B., Querol, E., Aviles, F.X. and Russell, R.B. (2002). Structural similarity to link sequence space: new potential superfamilies and implications for structural genomics. *Protein Sci.* **11**, 1101–1116.

Aloy, P., Querol, E., Aviles, F.X. and Sternberg, M.J. (2001). Automated structure-based prediction of functional sites in proteins: applications to assessing the validity of inheriting protein function from homology in genome annotation and to protein docking. *J. Mol. Biol.* **311**, 395–408.

Andrade, M.A., Ouzounis, C., Sander, C., Tamames, J. and Valencia, A. (1999). Functional classes in the three domains of life. *J. Mol. Evol.* **49**, 551–557.

Ashburner, M. and Drysdale, R. (1994). Flybase: the *Drosophila* genetic database. *Development* **120**, 2077–2079.

Attwood, T.K. (2000). The quest to deduce protein function from sequence: the role of pattern databases. *Int. J. Biochem. Cell Biol.* **32**, 139–155.

Attwood, T.K. (2002). The PRINTS database: a resource for identification of protein families. *Brief Bioinform.* **3**, 252–263.

Attwood, T.K., Blythe, M., Flower, D.R., Gaulton, A., Mabey, J.E., Maudling, N., McGregor, L., Mitchell, A., Moulton, G., Paine, K. and Scordis, P. (2002). PRINTS and PRINTS-S shed light on protein ancestry. *Nucleic Acids Res.* **30**, 239–241.

Attwood, T.K., Bradley, P., Flower, D.R., Gaulton, A., Maudling, N. and Mitchell, A.L. (2003). PRINTS and its automatic supplement, prePRINTS. *Nucleic Acids Res.* **31**, 400–402.

Bateman, A., Birney, E., Cerruti, L., Durbin, R., Etwiller, L, Eddy, S.R., Griffiths-Jones, S., Howe, K.L., Marshall, M. and Sonnhammer, E.L.L. (2002). The Pfam protein families database. *Nucleic Acids Res.* **30**, 276–280.

Chen, R. and Jeong, S.S. (2000). Functional Prediction: identification of protein orthologs and paralogs. *Protein Sci.* **9**, 2344–2353.

de Rinaldis, M., Ausiello, M., Cesareni, G. and Helmer-Citterich, M. (1998). Three-dimensional Profiles: a new tool to identify protein surface similarities. *J. Mol. Biol.* **284**, 1211–1121.

Devos, D. and Valencia, A. (2000). Practical limits of function prediction. *Proteins: Structure, Funct., Genet.* **41**, 98–107.

Eddy, S.R. (1996). Hidden Markov models. *Curr. Opin. Struct. Biol.* **6**, 361–365.

Falquet, L., Pagni, M., Bucher, P., Hulo, N., Sigrist, C.J., Hofmann, K. and Bairoch, A. (2002). The PROSITE database, its status in 2002. *Nucleic Acids Res.* **30**, 235–238.

Ganfornina, M.D. and Sánchez, D. (1999). Generation of evolutionary novelty by functional shift. *Bioessays* **21**, 432–439.

Gene Ontology Consortium. (2000). Gene Ontology: tool for the unification of biology. *Nature Genet.* **25**, 25–28.

Gerlt, J.A. and Babbitt, P.C. (2000). Can sequence determine function? *Genome Biol.* **1**, REVIEWS0005.

Golding, G.B. and Dean, A.M. (1998). The structural basis of molecular adaptation. *Mol. Biol. Evol.* **15**, 355–369.

Gough, J., Karplus, K., Hughey, R. and Chothia, C. (2001). Assignment of homology to genome sequences using a library of hidden Markov models that represent all proteins of known structure. *J. Mol. Biol.* **313**, 903–919.

Grishin, N. (2001). Fold change in evolution of protein structures. *J. Structural Biol.* **134**, 167–185.

Gu, X. and Vander Velden, K. (2002). DIVERGE: phylogeny-based analysis for functional–structural divergence of a protein family. *Bioinformatics* **18**, 500–501.

Hannenhalli, S.S. and Russell, R.B. (2000). Analysis and prediction of functional sub-types from protein sequence alignments. *J. Mol. Biol.* **303**, 61–76.

Hegyi, H. and Gerstein, M. (1999). The Relationship between Protein Structure and Function: a comprehensive survey with application to the yeast genome. *J. Mol. Biol.* **288**, 147–164.

Henikoff, J.G., Greene, E.A., Pietrokovski, S. and Henikoff, S. (2000). Increased coverage of protein families with the Blocks database servers. *Nucleic Acids Res.* **28**, 228–230.

Holm, L. and Sander, C. (1999). Protein Folds and Families: sequence and structure alignments. *Nucleic Acids Res.* **27**, 244–247.

Huynen, M.A. and Snel, B. (2000). Gene and Context: integrative approaches to genome analysis. *Adv. Protein Chem.* **54**, 345–379.

Huynen, M., Snel, B., Lathe, W. III and Bork, P. (2000). Predicting Protein Function by Genomic Context: quantitative evaluation and qualitative inferences. *Genome Res.* **10**, 1204–1210.

Hwang, K.Y., Chung, J.H., Kim, S.-H., Han, Y.S. and Cho, Y. (1999). Structure-based identification of a novel NTPase from *Methanococcus jannaschii*. *Nature Struct. Biol.* **6**, 691–696.

Jackson, R.M. and Russell, R.B. (2000). The Serine Protease Inhibitor Canonical Loop Conformation: examples found in extracellular hydrolases, toxins, cytokines and viral proteins. *J. Mol. Biol.* **296**, 325–334.

Jackson, R.M. and Russell, R.B. (2001). Predicting Function from Structure: examples of the serine protease inhibitor canonical loop conformation found in extracellular proteins. *Comput. Chem.* **26**, 31–39.

Jeffery, C.J. (1999). Moonlighting proteins. *Trends Biochem. Sci.* **24**, 8–11.

Jeffery, C.J., Bahnson, B.J., Chien, W., Ringe, D. and Petsko, G.A (2000). Crystal structure of rabbit phosphoglucose isomerase, a glycolytic enzyme that moonlights as neuroleukin, autocrine motility factor and differentiation mediator. *Biochemistry.* **8**, 955–964.

Kinch, L.N., Wrabl, J.O., Krishna, S.S., Majumdar, I., Sadreyev, R.I., Qi, Y., Pei, J., Cheng, H. and Grishin, N.V. (2003). CASP5 assessment of fold recognition target predictions. *Proteins Struct. Funct. Genet.* **53**, (Suppl. 6), 395–409.

Kolesov, G., Mewes, H.W. and Frishman, D. (2001). SNAPping up Functionally Related Genes Based on Context Information: a co-linearity-free approach. *J. Mol. Biol.* **311**, 639–656.

Kolesov, G., Mewes, H.W. and Frishman, D. (2002). SNAPper: gene order predicts gene function. *Bioinformatics.* **18**, 1017–1019.

Lan, N., Jansen, R. and Gerstein, M. (2002). Towards a Systematic Definition of Protein Function that Scales to the Genome Level: defining function in terms of interactions. *Proc. IEEE* **90**, 1848–1858.

Lan, N., Montelione, G.T. and Gerstein, M. (2003). Ontologies for Proteomics: towards a systematic definition of structure and function that scales to the genome level. *Curr. Opin. Struct. Biol.* **7**, 44–54.

Lichtarge, O., Bourne, H.R. and Cohen, F.E. (1996a). An evolutionary trace method defines binding surfaces common to protein families. *J. Mol. Biol.* **257**, 342–358.

Lichtarge, O., Bourne, H.R. and Cohen, F.E. (1996b). Evolutionarily conserved $G_{\alpha\beta\gamma}$ binding surfaces support a model of the G protein–receptor complex. *Proc. Nat. Acad. Sci. USA* **93**, 7507–7511.

Lichtarge, O. and Sowa, M.E. (2002). Evolutionary predictions of binding surfaces and interactions. *Curr. Opin. Struct. Biol.* **12**, 21–27.

LoConte L., Brenner S. E., Hubbard T.J.P., Chothia C. and Murzin A. (2002). SCOP Database in 2002: refinements accommodate structural genomics. *Nucleic Acid Res.* **30**, 264–267.

Madabushi, S., Yao, H., Marsh, M., Kristensen, D.M., Philippi, A., Sowa, M.E. and Lichtarge, O. (2002). Structural clusters of evolutionary trace residues are statistically significant and common in proteins. *J. Mol. Biol.* **316**, 139–154.

Marcotte, E.M., Pellegrini, M., Thompson, M.J., Yeates, T.O. and Eisenberg, D. (1999). A combined algorithm for genome-wide prediction of protein function. *Nature* **402**, 83–86.

Murzin A.G. (1998). How far divergent evolution goes in proteins. *Curr. Opin. Struct. Biol.* **8**, 380–387.

Murzin A.G., Brenner S.E., Hubbard T. and Chothia C. (1995). SCOP: a structural classification of proteins database for the investigation of sequences and structures. *J. Mol. Biol.* **247**, 536–540.

Natale, D.A., Shankavaram, U.T., Galperin, M.Y., Wolf, Y.I, Aravind, L. and Koonin, E.V. (2000). Towards understanding the first genome sequence of a crenarchaeon by genome annotation using clusters of orthologous groups of proteins (COGs). *Genome Biol.* **1**, Research0009.1–0009.19.

Pellegrini, M., Marcotte, E.M., Thompson, M.J., Eisenberg, D. and Yeates, T.O.E (1999). Assigning Protein Functions by Comparative Genome Analysis: protein phylogenetic profiles. *Proc. Natl. Acad. Sci. USA* **96**, 4285–4288.

Perutz, M.F. (1983). Species adaptation in a protein molecule. *Mol. Biol. Evol.* **1**, 1–28.

Riley, M. (1997). Genes and proteins of *Escherichia coli* K-12 (GenProtEC). *Nucleic Acids Res.* **25**, 51–52.

Riley, M. (1998). Systems for categorizing functions of gene products. *Curr. Opin. Struct. Biol.* **8**, 388–392.

Quackenbush, J. (2002). Microarray data normalization and transformation. *Nat. Genet.* **32**, (Suppl.) 496–501.

Schonbrun, J., Wedemeyer, W.J. and Baker, D. (2002). Protein structure prediction in 2002. *Curr. Opin. Struct. Biol.* **12**, 348–354.

Serres, M.H., Gopal, S., Nahum, L.A., Liang, P., Gaasterland, T. and Riley, M. (2001). A functional update of the *Escherichia coli* K-12 genome. *Genome Biol.* **2**, research0035.1–0035.7.

Shapiro, L. and Harris, T. (2000). Finding function through structural genomics. *Curr. Opin. Biotech.* **11**, 31–35.

Shrager, J. (2003). The fiction of functions. *Bioinformatics* **19**, 1934–1936.

Sowa, M.E., He, W., Slep, K.C., Kercher, M.A., Lichtarge, O. and Wensel, T.G. (2001). Prediction and confirmation of a site critical for effector regulation of RGS domain activity. *Nat. Struct. Biol.* **8**, 234–237.

Sowa, M.E., He, W., Wensel, T.G. and Lichtarge, O. (2000). A regulator of G protein signaling interaction surface linked to effector specificity. *Proc. Natl. Acad. Sci. USA* **97**, 1483–1488.

Spiess, C., Beil, A. and Ehrmann, M. (1999). A temperature-dependent switch from chaperone to protease in a widely conserved heat shock protein. *Cell* **97**, 339–347.

Teichmann, S.A., Murzin, A.G. and Chothia, C. (2001). Determination of protein function, evolution and interactions by structural genomics. *Curr. Opin. Struct. Biol.* **11**, 354–363.

Teichmann, S.A., Rison, S.C., Thornton, J.M., Riley, M., Gough, J. and Chothia, C. (2001a). The evolution and structural anatomy of the small molecule metabolic pathways in *Escherichia coli*. *J. Mol. Biol.* **311**, 693–708.

Teichmann, S.A., Rison, S.C., Thornton, J.M., Riley, M., Gough, J. and Chothia, C. (2001b). Small-molecule Metabolism: an enzyme mosaic. *Trends Biotechnol.* **19**, 482–486.

Todd, A.E., Orengo, C.A. and Thornton, J.M. (2001). Evolution of function in protein superfamilies, from a structural prospective. *J. Mol. Biol.* **307**, 1113–1143.

Tramontano, A. (2003). Of men and machines. *Nat. Struct. Biol.* **10**, 87–90.

Wallace, A.C., Laskowski, R.A. and Thornton, J.M. (1996). Derivation of 3D coordinate templates for searching structural databases: application to Ser–His–Asp catalytic triads in the serine proteinases and lipases. *Protein Sci.* **5**, 1001–1013.

Wilson, C.A., Kreychman, J. and Gerstein, M. (2000). Assessing annotation transfer for genomics: quantifying the relations between protein sequence, structure and function through traditional and probabilistic scores. *J. Mol. Biol.* **297**, 233–249.

Wistow, G. and Piatigorsky, J. (1987). Recruitment of enzymes as lens structural proteins. *Science* **236**, 1554–1556.

Xenarios, I., Salwinski, L., Duan, X.J., Higney, P., Kim, S.M. and Eisenberg, D. (2002). DIP, the Database of Interacting Proteins: a research tool for studying cellular networks of protein interactions. *Nucleic Acids Res.* **30**, 303–305.

Yao, H., Kristensen, D.M., Mihalek, I., Sowa, M.E., Shaw, C., Kimmel, M., Kavraki, L. and Lichtarge, O. (2003). An accurate, sensitive and scalable method to identify functional sites in protein structures. *J. Mol. Biol.* **326**, 255–261.

III
Database Design and Integration

11 Information Flow and Data Integration of Databanks

C. H. Wu and W. C. Barker

Abstract

The large scale genome projects have resulted in a rapid accumulation of genome sequences and other high throughput data. Associated with the large volume and complexity of data is the growing number of molecular databases being maintained in heterogeneous and distributed sources. To fully exploit the value of the data, we need to address issues that hamper information flow and data integration. Major problems include non-standard representation of primary database objects (genes and proteins), disparate syntax and semantics of distribution formats, as well as genome annotation errors and error propagation among databanks. It requires wide adoption of common nomenclature and ontology for database annotation, common exchange formats and concise database definition for database distribution and evidence attribution for annotation error control. Furthermore, data integration facilitates knowledge discovery, allowing researchers to answer complex biological questions that may typically involve querying multiple sources, as illustrated by the iProClass database framework.

Keywords

data integration, database distribution format, error propagation, genome annotation, iProClass database, knowledge discovery, ontology, syntax and semantics

11.1 Introduction

The high throughput genome projects have resulted in a rapid accumulation of genome sequences for a large number of organisms. Meanwhile, scientists have

Database Annotation in Molecular Biology Edited by Arthur M. Lesk
© 2005 John Wiley & Sons, Ltd. ISBN: 0-470-85681-5

begun to systematically tackle gene functions and other complex regulatory processes by studying organisms at the global scale of genomes (genes, regulatory and noncoding sequences), transcriptomes (RNA and gene expression), proteomes (protein expression), metabolomes (metabolites and metabolic networks), interactomes (protein–protein interactions) and physiomes (physiological dynamics and functions of whole organisms). Associated with the enormous number and variety of data being produced is the growing number of molecular databases that are being generated and maintained. Meta-databases (databases of databases) have been compiled to catalogue and categorize these databases, such as the Molecular Biology Database Collection (Baxevanis, 2003). This online collection (http://nar.oupjournals.org/cgi/content/full/31/1/1/DC1) lists over 400 key biological databases that add new value to the underlying data by virtue of curation, provide new types of data connection, or implement other innovative approaches to facilitate biological discovery. Based on the type of information they provide, these databases can be conveniently classified into subcategories. Examples of major database categories include genomic sequence repositories (e.g. GenBank (Benson *et al.*, 2003)), gene expression (e.g. SMD (Gollub *et al.*, 2003)), model organism genomes (e.g. MGD (Blake *et al.*, 2003)), mutation databases (e.g. dbSNP (Sherry *et al.*, 2001)), RNA sequences (e.g. RDP (Cole *et al.*, 2003)), protein sequences (e.g. PIR-PSD (Wu *et al.*, 2003), Swiss-Prot (Boeckmann *et al.*, 2003)), protein family (e.g. InterPro (Mulder *et al.*, 2003)), protein structure (e.g. PDB (Westbrook *et al.*, 2003)), intermolecular interactions (e.g. BIND (Bader, Betel and Hogue, 2003)), metabolic pathways and cellular regulation (e.g. KEGG (Kanehisa *et al.*, 2002)) and taxonomy (e.g. NCBI taxonomy (Wheeler *et al.*, 2003)).

To fully explore these valuable data, advanced bioinformatics infrastructures must be developed for biological knowledge management. New approaches need to be devised for data collection, maintenance, dissemination, query and analysis. One major challenge lies in the volume, complexity and dynamic nature of the data, which are being collected and maintained in heterogeneous and distributed sources. To facilitate scientific discovery from these data sources, it is important to consider database information flow and issues concerning data integration. This paper describes information flows among databanks (Section 11.2), discusses issues of database distribution format (Section 11.3) and error propagation (Section 11.4) and illustrates our approach for data integration to facilitate knowledge discovery (Section 11.5).

11.2 Information Flow Among Databanks

While there are a large variety of databases, some databases constitute the primary data sources upon which secondary databases are derived. To analyse the information flow among databanks, it is useful to distinguish primary, underlying databases from secondary, derived databases. Major examples of the primary databases are DNA sequence databases such as GenBank, as well as protein sequence databases such as PIR-PSD and Swiss-Prot. Entries in these databases represent basic gene and protein objects that constitute the primary database objects of numerous secondary databases. With the genome sequencing projects, the vast majority of sequences in protein databases are now derived from conceptual translation of gene sequences rather than direct protein determination. The information, thus, flows from DNA sequence repositories to protein sequence databases to secondary databases that may provide value-added information or specialized properties for genes or proteins, such as protein family, function and pathway databases.

Representation of primary database object

In primary sequence databases, each object (gene or protein) is described by a varying degree of detail in different annotation fields, such as those listed by Barker and Wu (2004). However, only four fields, namely, database unique identifier, name, source organism and sequence, are commonly used to identify a gene or protein object in secondary databases. Still, the representation of gene or protein objects in these four fields is associated with several problems that may hinder information flow and data integration. Major problems for protein object representation are discussed below and summarized in Table 11.1.

Table 11.1 Format problems and annotation errors in the representation of protein object that hamper information flow and data integration

Field	Format problems or annotation errors
Unique identifier (UID)	No standard UID; ID or accession number no longer accessible
Protein name	No standard nomenclature; alternative names/synonyms not available; inconsistent usage of protein name fields; protein name too long or uninformative; wrong functional assignment for protein name or EC number
Source organism/ taxonomy	Contradictory taxonomy ID and organism name; missing ID or name; representation at different hierarchical level (genus, species, strain)
Protein sequence	Sequence variation due to alternate splice/initiator forms, allelic variants and post-translational modification; sequence discrepancy due to choices of reading frame initiation, splice boundary, genetic code or RNA editing

Database unique identifier

The database unique identifier (UID) is the ID and/or accession number assigned by individual databases to uniquely identify each sequence entry. Unlike the gene object where there is a widely acceptable UID (i.e. GenBank/EMBL/DDBJ ID), there is no standard UID as the central reference point for a protein object. Various secondary databases often use different UIDs to reference the same object from different protein sequence databases. For example, the human DNA-directed RNA polymerase II 14.4 kDa polypeptide can be identified using seven sets of UIDs from PIR-PSD (S38627), Swiss-Prot (RPB6_HUMAN or P41584), GenePept (AAH03582.1 or 13097771, CAB62981.1 or 18254493, CAA81629.1 or 415388), RefSeq (NP_068809 or 11527390) and PDB (1QKL:A) (see http://pir.georgetown.edu/cgi-bin/ nfEntry.pl?id = NF00104599). This is due to a high level of redundancy in GenePept (annotated GenBank translations), and the lack of one unified, central protein sequence database. PIR has recently joined forces with EBI (European Bioinformatics Institute) and SIB (Swiss Institute of Bioinformatics) to establish the Universal Protein Resource (UniProt), a central resource of protein sequence and function that merges PIR-PSD, Swiss-Prot and TrEMBL databases.

Protein name

Protein name is the form by which a protein object is referred to and communicated in the scientific literature and biological databases. There is, however, a long standing problem of nomenclature for proteins, where 'profligate and undisciplined labeling is hampering communication', as discussed in *Nature* (1997). Scientists may name a newly discovered or characterized protein based on its function, sequence features, gene name, cellular location, molecular weight or other properties, as well as their combinations or abbreviations. The same protein is often named differently in different databases, and occasionally different proteins may share the same name. For example, the human ATP-dependent RNA helicase is variably named based on function at different hierarchical levels ('ATP-dependent RNA helicase' versus 'RNA helicase'), molecular weight ('protein p68'), motif sequence similarity ('DEAD/H box-5'), combinations of properties ('RNA helicase p68') and even a misnomer ('RNA-dependent helicase') (see http://pir.georgetown.edu/cgi-bin/nfEntry.pl?id = NF00113874). Protein name standardization requires community effort – only a small fraction of all proteins has standard nomenclature, most notably, the Enzyme Nomenclature of the IUBMB (http://www.chem.qmul.ac.uk/iubmb/enzyme/). Alternative names or synonyms often are not available in databases.

Taxonomy

To unambiguously identify a protein object, one also needs to know the source organism of the protein, as different organisms may share the same protein sequence. While there is a widely adopted standard for taxonomy (i.e. NCBI taxonomy), several problems are associated with the taxonomy of source organisms and their mapping among primary sequence databases. The problem may stem from non-specific names provided by biologists during direct submission of DNA sequence entries to GenBank. Often such names cannot be mapped to the taxonomy even at the species level (such as *Mus* sp.). To be useful, the source organism information should be specific, including the strain (or cultivar for plant) if possible, but many early submissions do not contain this information. There may also be a mapping problem when two databases describe the same protein object at different taxonomy levels, such as species versus strain. The taxonomy in sequence databases is represented by both taxonomy ID and name, which sometimes may be discrepant due to update propagation problems (i.e. different update schedules between NCBI taxonomy and sequence databases).

Protein sequence

The primary source of protein sequences is conceptual translation of GenBank DNA sequences. The translations may be made with an incorrect genetic code, in the wrong reading frame, with incorrect splice boundaries, or without corrections for RNA editing and translational frame shifting. In some complete bacterial genome reports where peptide sequences were available, early initiators had been chosen 20 per cent of the time. Cases have been observed of late initiators having been chosen, revealed as carboxyl ends of incomplete homology domains at amino ends of translations. Other types of sequence variation may result from representations of alternative splice/initiator forms, precursor and mature forms, identical sequences from different loci, allelic variants, and post-translational modifications. For example, the seleno-cysteine TGA codon sometimes is translated as residue 'U' in GenBank, as found in GenPept entry AAA16579.2 (see http://pir.georgetown.edu/cgi-bin/nfEntry.-pl?id = NF00163996), while residue 'C' is used in PIR and Swiss-Prot (see http://pir.georgetown.edu/cgi-bin/nfEntry.pl?id = NF00160560).

Representation of protein object in PIR-NREF database

The PIR-NREF database (Wu *et al.*, 2003) has been developed to provide a timely and comprehensive collection of protein objects from all major sequence databases with source attribution (i.e. protein IDs, accession numbers, and protein names from each underlying database). It is a non-redundant reference database where identical protein sequences from the same source organism (species) reported in different databases are presented as a single entry, as illustrated in Figure 11.1. Also included in the entry report are amino acid sequence, taxonomy and composite bibliographic data, as well as related sequences identified by all-against-all BLAST (Altschul *et al.*, 1997) search, including identical sequences from different organisms, identical subsequences and highly similar sequences (≥95 per cent identity).

The collective protein names and bibliography of all published protein sequences in PIR-NREF can be utilized to develop a protein name thesaurus or ontology

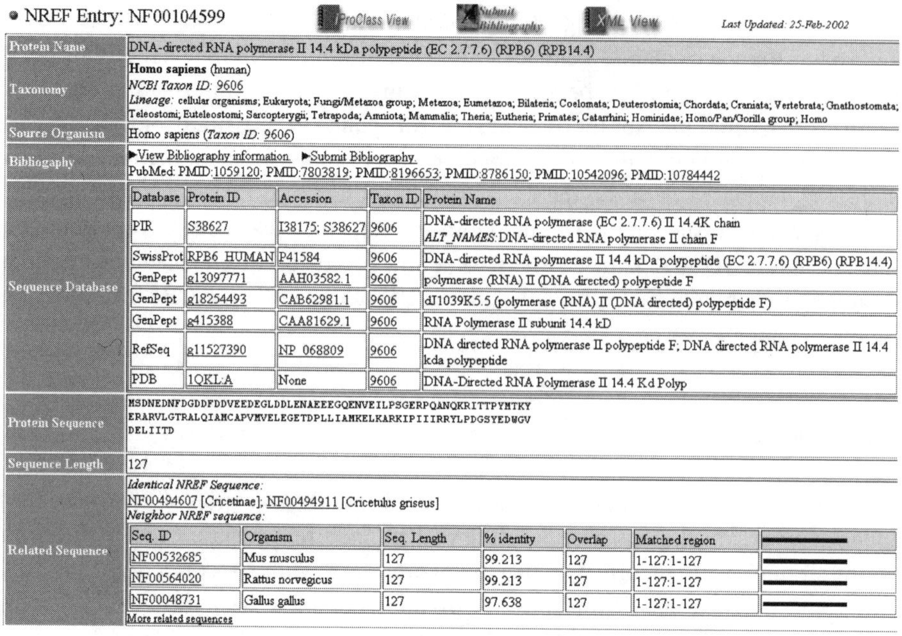

• NREF Entry: NF00104599 ProClass View Submit Bibliography XML View *Last Updated: 25-Feb-2002*

Protein Name	DNA-directed RNA polymerase II 14.4 kDa polypeptide (EC 2.7.7.6) (RPB6) (RPB14.4)
Taxonomy	**Homo sapiens** (human) *NCBI Taxon ID:* 9606 *Lineage:* cellular organisms; Eukaryota; Fungi/Metazoa group; Metazoa; Eumetazoa; Bilateria; Coelomata; Deuterostomia; Chordata; Craniata; Vertebrata; Gnathostomata; Teleostomi; Euteleostomi; Sarcopterygii; Tetrapoda; Amniota; Mammalia; Theria; Eutheria; Primates; Catarrhini; Hominidae; Homo/Pan/Gorilla group; Homo
Source Organism	Homo sapiens (*Taxon ID:* 9606)
Bibliography	▶View Bibliography information. ▶Submit Bibliography. PubMed: PMID:1059120; PMID:7803819; PMID:8196653; PMID:8786150; PMID:10542096; PMID:10784442

Sequence Database

Database	Protein ID	Accession	Taxon ID	Protein Name
PIR	S38627	I38175; S38627	9606	DNA-directed RNA polymerase (EC 2.7.7.6) II 14.4K chain *ALT_NAMES:* DNA-directed RNA polymerase II chain F
SwissProt	RPB6_HUMAN	P41584	9606	DNA-directed RNA polymerase II 14.4 kDa polypeptide (EC 2.7.7.6) (RPB6) (RPB14.4)
GenPept	g13097771	AAH03582.1	9606	polymerase (RNA) II (DNA directed) polypeptide F
GenPept	g18254493	CAB62981.1	9606	dJ1039K5.5 (polymerase (RNA) II (DNA directed) polypeptide F)
GenPept	g415388	CAA81629.1	9606	RNA Polymerase II subunit 14.4 kD
RefSeq	g11527390	NP_068809	9606	DNA directed RNA polymerase II polypeptide F; DNA directed RNA polymerase II 14.4 kda polypeptide
PDB	1QKL:A	None	9606	DNA-Directed RNA Polymerase II 14.4 Kd Polyp

Protein Sequence

```
MSDNEDNFDGDDFDDVEEDEGLDDLENAEEEGQENVEILPSGERPQANQKRITTPYMTKY
ERARVLGTRALQIAMCAPVMVELEGETDPLLIAMKELKARKIPIIIRRYLPDGSYEDWGV
DELIITD
```

Sequence Length: 127

Related Sequence

Identical NREF Sequence:
NF00494607 [Cricetinae]; NF00494911 [Cricetulus griseus]
Neighbor NREF sequence:

Seq. ID	Organism	Seq. Length	% identity	Overlap	Matched region
NF00532685	Mus musculus	127	99.213	127	1-127:1-127
NF00564020	Rattus norvegicus	127	99.213	127	1-127:1-127
NF00048731	Gallus gallus	127	97.638	127	1-127:1-127

More related sequences

Figure 11.1 Representation of protein object in PIR-NREF (http://pir.georgetown.edu/cgi-bin/nfEntry.pl?id = NF00104599)

(Hirschman *et al.*, 2002). The collective protein names, including synonyms, alternative names and even misspellings, constitute an initial dictionary of terms. The bibliography is hypertext linked to PubMed for direct online abstract retrieval to create annotated corpora. The different protein names assigned by different databases may also reflect annotation discrepancies and provide clues to incorrectly annotated proteins.

11.3 Database Distribution Format

In addition to the representation of gene or protein objects as discussed above, there are other problems associated with the database distribution format that may impact information flow among databanks.

Distribution format problems

The format issues may relate to syntax of the databases, which provides specifications for the data record and each annotation field (including constraints such as required or optional, repeating or non-repeating, and single valued or multi-valued) that are derived from the database schema, as well as specifications such as data types, punctuation and delimiters, and field lengths. The format problems may also relate to semantic issues that involve the use of standard nomenclature, controlled vocabulary or ontology to communicate the same database concept or object, as well as the proper usage of annotation fields. The distribution format problems are illustrated using examples from GenBank/GenPept, where annotations are provided via third party submissions from genome centres and individual researchers who may not adhere to strict database specifications.

The first example shows that protein names assigned to GenBank/EMBL/DDBJ protein coding regions are often uninformative concatenations of computational predictions from programs such as GENSCAN (Burge and Karlin, 1997) and BLAST. In the GenPept entry CAB72284.1, the protein name appears in two fields, the 'Protein' lines of the 'FEATURES' field, which is over 4000 characters long, and the 'DEFINITION' field, where the name is truncated to about 500 characters, as '/ prediction=(method:"genefinder", version:"084", score:"105.71")~/prediction= (method:"genscan", version:"1.0")~/match = (desc: "BASEMENT MEMBRANE-SPECIFIC HEPARAN SULFATE PROTEOGLYCAN CORE PROTEIN PRECURSOR (HSPG) (PERLECAN) (PLC)", species:"Homo sapiens (Human)", ranges:(query: 24292..24549, target:SWISS-PROT::P98160: 3713..3628, score: "201.00"),...' (see http://www.ncbi.nlm.nih.gov:80/entrez/query. fcgi?cmd = Retrieve&db = protein&list_ uids = 6946669&dopt = GenPept).

The second example shows the undisciplined usage of the GenBank annotation fields, where proteins names of the 'CDS' region may appear in either 'Product' or 'Note' lines for sequences from different genomes. For GenBank entry AE007317 that contains the complete genome of *Streptococcus pneumoniae* R6, the protein names are indicated in the 'Product' line, as in *product='DNA biosynthesis, initiation, binding protein'* for CDS (1..1362) (see http://www.ncbi.nlm.nih.gov/ entrez/viewer.fcgi?val = AE008385.1). On the other hand, in the GenBank entry AE007870 of the complete genome of *Agrobacterium tumefaciens* strain C58 linear chromosome, the protein names are displayed in the 'Note' line as in */note='(AP000731) alanine acetyl transferase-like protein'* for CDS (606..1208), while the 'Product' lines are used to indicate gene origins as in */product="AGR_L_4p"* (see http://www.ncbi.nlm.nih.gov/entrez/viewer.fcgi?val = AE008197.1).

Common distribution formats

Even with a concise database definition and a distribution format conforming to database schema, it is still a non-trivial task for database developers to parse and extract annotations from molecular databases of interest. Different database parsers need to be written and tailored for parsing databases distributed using different formats. There are numerous flat file formats just for the primary sequence databases alone, including GenBank format, EMBL format, Swiss-Prot format (for Swiss-Prot/

TrEMBL) and CODATA and NBRF formats (for PIR-PSD). To alleviate data exchange problems associated with format incompatibility, major database providers have started to adopt common, exchangeable distribution formats. Gaining wide acceptance is the adoption of XML (eXtensible Markup Language) as the data exchange format and the formulation of standardized models and interfaces by the Object Management Group (OMG).

XML (eXtensible Markup Language)

Ratified by the World Wide Web Consortium (W3C), XML (http://www.w3.org/TR/REC-xml) is quickly becoming a universal standard for data exchange. Like HTML, XML is a subset of SGML (Structured Generalized Markup Language). A key advantage of XML is that its structure and content, defined by the XML data, is separate from its presentation, defined by a stylesheet using the XSL (eXtensible Stylesheet Language). Another key advantage of XML is that users create their own tags to represent the meaning and structure of their data. Tags may be defined directly in an XML document or formally defined in a document type definition (DTD). Common XML definitions are being developed, including Genome Annotation Markup Elements (GAME), Bioinformatic Sequence Markup Language (BSML) (http://www.bsml.org/), BIOpolymer Markup Language (BIOML) and BioPerl XML (http://bio.perl.org/Projects/XML/).

Standard models and interfaces

To standardize models and interfaces for software tools, services, frameworks and components in life sciences research, the Life Sciences Research (LSR) Domain Task Force (http://www.omg.org/lsr/) of the OMG is coordinating with other standards organizations and information providers to ensure common standards. Specifications that have already been developed by the OMG-LSR include Biomolecular Sequence Analysis, Genome Maps, Bibliographical Query Service, Macromolecular Structure and Gene Expression.

PIR XML and MySQL distribution

Besides CODATA and NBRF flat file formats and FASTA sequence format, PIR-PSD is also distributed in XML and MySQL formats from the PIR anonymous FTP site (ftp://ftp.pir.georgetown.edu/pir_databases/). The XML distribution has an associated DTD file (http://pir.georgetown.edu/pirwww/xml/psdml.dtd). The MySQL open source relational database distribution file contains data files (in relational tables), SQL scripts for creating the database and a user's guide with the database schema.

11.4 Genome Annotation Errors and Error Propagation

Another factor that impacts information flow among databanks is the annotation quality of the primary databases. A general approach for genome annotation is to infer protein functions based on sequence similarity to annotated proteins in sequence databases. However, numerous genome annotation errors have been detected (Devos and Valencia, 2001), often due to transitive identification. Also termed 'transitive catastrophe', such identification errors frequently result from functional annotation of proteins based on the most similar sequence, which is itself incorrectly identified, or on local similarity without regard to end-to-end similarity and domain architecture. The functional annotation errors, in particular those reflected in protein names or EC (Enzyme Commission) numbers, are prone to propagate from one sequence to another or from primary to secondary databases, as in the IMP dehydrogenase example below.

Misannotation of IMP dehydrogenase

During the PIR curation process, at least 18 proteins were found to be misannotated as inosine-5′-monophosphate dehydrogenase (IMPDH) or related in various complete genomes. These 'misnomers', all of which have been corrected in the PIR-PSD and some corrected in Swiss-Prot/TrEMBL, still exist in GenPept and RefSeq. The misannotation apparently resulted from local sequence similarity to the CBS domain, named for the protein in which it was first described, cystathionine beta synthase (Shan *et al.*, 2001). As illustrated in Figure 11.2, most IMPDH sequences (e.g., PIR-NREF: NF00078343) have two kinds of annotated Pfam domain, the catalytic IMP dehydrogenase/GMP reductase (IMPDH/GMPR) domain (PF00478), associated with the PROSITE signature pattern (PS00487), and two adjacent CBS domains (PF00571), which actually interrupt the IMPDH/GMPR domain. Structurally, the N- and C-terminal parts of the IMPDH/GMPR domain form the core catalytic domain

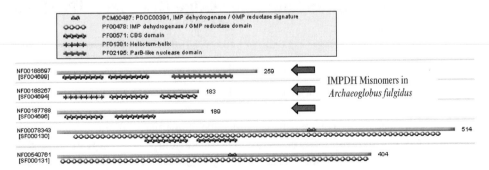

Figure 11.2 IMP dehydrogenase (IMPDH) and sequences misannotated based on CBS domains

and the two CBS regions form a flanking globular domain (Zhang *et al.*, 1999). There is also a well characterized IMPDH (PIR-NREF: NF00540761) (Zhou *et al.*, 1997) that contains the catalytic domain but lacks the CBS domains, showing that CBS domains are not necessary for enzymatic activity. The three misnomers from *Archaeoglobus fulgidus* shown in Figure 11.2 all lack the catalytic domain of IMPDH but contain adjacent CBS domains. Two of them also contain other domains.

Many of the genome annotation errors still remain in sequence databases and have been propagated to secondary, curated databases. IMPDH occurs in most species, as the enzyme (EC 1.1.1.205) is the rate-limiting step in the *de novo* synthesis of guanine nucleotides. It is depicted in the purine metabolism pathway for *Archaeoglobus fulgidus* (afu00230) in the KEGG pathway database based on the three misannotated IMPDH protein shown above. However, there is no evidence that a homologous IMPDH protein actually exists in the *Archaeoglobus fulgidus* genome to substantiate its placement on the pathway. Indeed, the only three proteins annotated by the genome centre as IMPDH are all misnomers. No IMPDH can be detected after genome-wide search using sequence similarity searches (BLASTP and TBLASTN) against known IMPDH proteins, or hidden Markov model search (HMMER (Eddy, Mitchison and Durbin, 1995)) against the IMPDH/GMPR domain.

Control of error propagation

We use several approaches at the PIR to partially control the propagation of genomic annotation errors: (i) systematic detection of annotation errors based on database integrity checks, such as identification of discrepant protein names in the PIR-NREF Database; (ii) systematic correction of annotation errors based on dynamic annotation, such as the PIR superfamily classification and rule-based annotation method, and (iii) prevention of error propagation based on evidence attribution to distinguish experimentally verified from computationally predicted annotations (Barker and Wu, 2004; Wu *et al.*, 2004).

11.5 Data integration and Knowledge Discovery: iProClass Case Study

The iProClass database system (Huang *et al.*, 2003) is designed to address the database integration issue arising from the voluminous, heterogeneous and distributed data. There are several general approaches for developing an integrated platform for heterogeneous databases (Davidson, Overton and Nuneman, 1995). These include hypertext navigation using links between related data sources, a data warehouse that provides a materialized solution and unmediated multi-database queries that provide view solution and database federation. Most data warehouses adopt a 'tightly coupled' approach that physically integrates a number of databases by converting the data into a unified database schema. While it allows local control of data, keeping data from the multiple databases up to date is not trivial. Hypertext navigation is a 'loosely coupled' approach that employs the browsing model wherein hypertext-linked web pages are followed for more information and are always one mouse click away.

iProClass uses database links as a foundation for interoperability (Karp, 1995) and combines both data warehouse and hypertext navigation methods. In our approach, we restrict the database content to the immediate needs of protein analysis and annotation and store a rich collection of links with related summary information. The latter will alleviate potential problems associated with timely collection of information from distributed sources over the Internet. The idea is similar to that of the Virgil database (Achard et al., 1998), which was developed to model the concept of rich links (the link itself and the related summary information) between database objects. Following the notation in LinkDB (Fujibuchi et al., 1998), the iProClass links may be roughly categorized into three types: (a) factual links for simple cross-references, such as literature data or reported sequence data; (b) similarity links compiled based on sequence similarity, such as members of a protein family, and (c) biological links associating biological meanings, such as interacting proteins or proteins in the same metabolic pathway. Another iProClass design principle that promotes database interoperation is the adoption of a modular and open architecture. The modular structure makes the system scalable, customizable and extendable for adding new components.

The database contains value-added descriptions of all proteins with up-to-date information from many sources, thereby providing much richer annotation than can be found in any single database. The annotation has source attribution and hypertext links to the underlying databases. The link mechanism is also attributed. For example, EC number is used to cross-reference functional databases such as EC-IUBMB, KEGG, BRENDA (http://www.brenda.uni-koeln.de/), WIT (Overbeek et al., 2000) and MetaCyc (Karp et al., 2002); PDB ID is used to link structure and structural classification databases, including PDB, SCOP (Lo Conte et al., 2002), CATH (Pearl et al., 2003), MMDB (Chen et al., 2003) and PDBsum (Laskowski, 2001); and PubMed ID links to NCBI's PubMed. The source attribution and hypertext links facilitate exploration of additional information and examination of discrepant annotations from different sources. Standard nomenclatures or accepted ontologies are adopted wherever applicable, such as IUBMB Enzyme Nomenclature, NCBI taxonomy and Gene Ontology (Gene Ontology Consortium, 2001).

The protein information in iProClass includes family relationships at both global (superfamily/family) and local (domain, motif, site) levels, as well as structural and functional classifications and features of proteins. Consisting of about 1.5 million non-redundant protein sequences from the PIR-PSD, Swiss-Prot and TrEMBL, iProClass is organized with more than 36 000 superfamilies, 7500 domains and 1300 motifs. It provides rich links to over 80 databases of protein sequences, families, functions and pathways, protein–protein interactions, post-translational modifications, protein expressions, structures and structural classifications, genes and

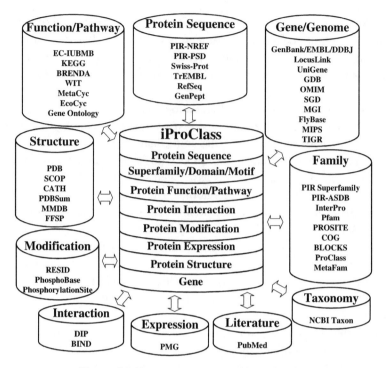

Figure 11.3 iProClass database integration

genomes, ontologies, literature and taxonomy (Figure 11.3). Protein and superfamily summary reports present extensive annotation information and include membership statistics and graphical display of domains and motifs.

11.6 Conclusions

The large volume and complexity of biological data being generated represents both a challenge and an opportunity for bioinformatics research and development. To maximize the utlization of these valuable data for scientific discovery, we need to address issues that hamper information flow and data integration. Major problems are raised in this chapter with illustrative examples in the areas of representation of primary database objects (genes and proteins) and the syntax and semantics issues of distribution formats, as well as genome annotation errors and error propagation among databanks. There are no simple solutions to these issues. They require that the bioinformatics community and database providers collectively adopt common nomenclature, controlled vocabulary and ontology for database annotation, adopt common data exchange formats and provide concise database definition for database distribution and control error propagation by systematic error detection, error correction and evidence attribution.

Data integration facilitates exploration of proteins, allowing users to answer complex biological questions that may typically involve querying multiple sources. In particular, interesting relationships between database objects, such as relationships among protein sequences, families, structures and functions, can be revealed readily. Functional annotation of proteins requires association of proteins based on properties beyond sequence homology – proteins sharing common domains connected via related multi-domain proteins (grouped by superfamilies); proteins in the same pathways, networks or complexes; proteins correlated in their expression patterns and proteins correlated in their phylogenetic profiles (with similar evolutionary patterns) (Marcotte *et al.*, 1999). Data integration as in iProClass is important in revealing protein functional associations beyond sequence homology (Wu *et al.*, 2004).

Acknowledgements

The PIR is supported by grant U01 HG02712 from the National Institutes of Health. The iProClass database and the protein name ontology projects are supported by DBI-0138188 and ITR-0205470 from the National Science Foundation.

References

Achard, F., Cussat-Blanc, C., Viara, E. and Barillot, E. (1998). The new Virgil Database: a service of rich links. *Bioinformatics* **14**, 342–348.

Altschul, S.F., Madden, T.L., Schaffer, A.A., Zhang, J., Zhang, Z., Miller, W. and Lipman, D.J. (1997). Gapped BLAST and PSI-BLAST: a new generation of protein database search programs. *Nucleic Acids Res.* **25**, 3389–3402.

Bader, G.D., Betel, D. and Hogue, C.W. (2003). BIND: the biomolecular interaction network database. *Nucleic Acids Res.* **31**, 248–250.

Barker, W.C. and Wu, C.H. (2004). Annotation of protein sequences (in this book).

Baxevanis, A.D. (2003). The Molecular Biology Database Collection: 2003 update. *Nucleic Acids Res.* **31**, 1–12.

Benson, D.A., Karsch-Mizrachi, I., Lipman, D.J., Ostell, J. and Wheeler, D.L. (2003). GenBank. *Nucleic Acids Res.* **31**, 23–27.

Blake, J.A., Richardson, J.E., Bult, C.J., Kadin, J.A. and Eppig, J. T. (2003). MGD: the mouse genome database. *Nucleic Acids Res.* **31**, 193–195.

Boeckmann, B., Bairoch, A., Apweiler, R., Blatter, M.C., Estreicher, A., Gasteiger, E., Martin, M.J., Michoud, K., O'Donovan, C., Phan, I., Pilbout, S. and Schneider, M. (2003). The SWISS-PROT protein knowledgebase and its supplement TrEMBL in 2003. *Nucleic Acids Res.* **31**, 365–370.

Burge, C. and Karlin, S. (1997). Prediction of complete gene structures in human genomic DNA. *J. Mol. Biol.* **268**, 78–94.

Chen, J., Anderson, J.B., DeWeese-Scott, C., Fedorova, N.D., Geer, L.Y., He, S., Hurwitz, D.I., Jackson, J.D., Jacobs, A.R., Lanczycki, C.J., Liebert, C.A., Liu, C., Madej, T., Marchler-Bauer, A., Marchler, G.H., Mazumder, R., Nikolskaya, A.N., Rao, B.S., Panchenko, A.R., Shoemaker, B.A.,

Simonyan, V., Song, J.S., Thiessen, P.A., Vasudevan, S., Wang, Y., Yamashita, R.A., Yin, J.J. and Bryant, S.H. (2003). MMDB: entrez's 3D-structure database. *Nucleic Acids Res.* **31**, 474–477.

Cole, J.R., Chai, B., Marsh, T.L., Farris, R.J., Wang, Q., Kulam, S.A., Chandra, S., McGarrell, D.M., Schmidt, T.M., Garrity, G.M. and Tiedje, J.M. (2003). The Ribosomal Database Project (RDP-II): previewing a new autoaligner that allows regular updates and the new prokaryotic taxonomy. *Nucleic Acids Res.* **31**, 442–443.

Davidson, S.B., Overton, C. and Nuneman, P. (1995). Challenges in integrating biological data sources. *J. Comput. Biol.* **2**, 557–572.

Devos, D. and Valencia, A. (2001). Intrinsic errors in genome annotation. *Trends Genet.* **17**, 429–431.

Eddy, S.R., Mitchison, G. and Durbin, R. (1995). Maximum discrimination hidden Markov models of sequence consensus. *J. Comput. Biol.* **2**, 9–23.

Fujibuchi, W., Goto, S., Migimatsu, H., Uchiyama, I., Ogiwara, A., Akiyama, Y. and Kanehisa, M. (1998). DBGET/LinkDB: an integrated database retrieval system. *Pac. Symp. Biocomput.* 683–694.

Gene Ontology Consortium. (2001). Creating the Gene Ontology Resource: design and implementation. *Genome Res.* **11**, 1425–1433.

Gollub, J., Ball, C.A., Binkley, G., Demeter, J., Finkelstein, D.B., Hebert, J.M., Hernandez-Boussard, T., Jin, H., Kaloper, M., Matese, J.C., Schroeder, M., Brown, P.O., Botstein, D. and Sherlock, G. (2003). The Stanford Microarray Database: data access and quality assessment tools. *Nucleic Acids Res.* **31**, 94–96.

Hirschman, L., Park, J.C., Tsujii, J., Wong, L. and Wu, C.H. (2002). Accomplishments and challenges in literature data mining for biology. *Bioinformatics* **18**, 1553–1561.

Huang, H., Barker, W.C., Chen, Y. and Wu, C.H. (2003). iProClass: an integrated database of protein family, function, and structure information. *Nucleic Acids Res.* **31**, 390–392.

Kanehisa M., Goto, S., Kawashima, S. and Nakaya, A. (2002). The KEGG databases at GenomeNet. *Nucleic Acids Res.* **30**, 42–46.

Karp, P.D. (1995). A strategy for database interoperation. *J. Comput. Biol.* **2**, 573–586.

Karp, P.D., Riley, M., Paley, S.M. and Pellegrini-Toole, A. (2002). The MetaCyc database. *Nucleic Acids Res.* **30**, 59–61.

Laskowski, R.A. (2001). PDBsum: summaries and analyses of PDB structures. *Nucleic Acids Res.* **29**, 221–222.

Lo Conte, L., Brenner, S.E., Hubbard, T.J.P., Chothia, C. and Murzin, A.G. (2002). SCOP Database in 2002: refinements accommodate structural genomics. *Nucleic Acids Res.* **30**, 264–267.

Marcotte, E.M, Pellegrini, M., Thompson, M.J., Yeates, T.O. and Eisenberg, D. (1999). A combined algorithm for genome-wide prediction of protein function. *Nature* **402**, 83–86.

Mulder, N.J., Apweiler, R., Attwood, T.K., Bairoch, A., Barrell, D., Bateman, A., Binns, D., Biswas, M., Bradley, P., Bork, P., Bucher, P., Copley, R.R., Courcelle, E., Das, U., Durbin, R., Falquet, L., Fleischmann, W., Griffiths-Jones, S., Haft, D., Harte, N., Hulo, N., Kahn, D., Kanapin, A., Krestyaninova, M., Lopez, R., Letunic, I., Lonsdale, D., Silventoinen, V., Orchard, S.E., Pagni, M., Peyruc, D., Ponting, C.P., Selengut, J.D., Servant, F., Sigrist, C.J., Vaughan, R. and Zdobnov, E.M. (2003). The InterPro database, 2003 brings increased coverage and new features. *Nucleic Acids Res.* **31**, 315–318.

Nature. (1997). Obstacles of nomenclature. *Nature* **389**, 1.

Overbeek, R., Larsen, N., Pusch, G.D., D'Souza, M., Selkov, E. Jr., Kyrpides, N., Fonstein, M., Maltsev, N. and Selkov, E. (2000). WIT: integrated system for high-throughput genome sequence analysis and metabolic reconstruction. *Nucleic Acids Res.* **28**, 123–125.

Pearl, F.M., Bennett, C.F., Bray, J.E., Harrison, A.P., Martin, N., Shepherd, A., Sillitoe, I., Thornton, J. and Orengo, C.A. (2003). The CATH Database: an extended protein family resource for structural and functional genomics. *Nucleic Acids Res.* **31**, 452–455.

Shan, X., Dunbrack, R.L. Jr., Christopher, S.A. and Kruger, W.D. (2001). Mutations in the regulatory domain of cystathionine beta synthase can functionally suppress patient-derived mutations in cis. *Hum. Mol. Genet.* **10**, 635–643.

Sherry, S.T., Ward, M.H., Kholodov, M., Baker, J., Phan, L., Smigielski, E.M. and Sirotkin, K. (2001). dbSNP: the NCBI database of genetic variation. *Nucleic Acids Res.* **29**, 308–311.

Westbrook, J., Feng, Z., Chen, L., Yang, H. and Berman, H.M. (2003). The protein data bank and structural genomics. *Nucleic Acids Res.* **31**, 489–491.

Wheeler, D.L., Church, D.M., Federhen, S., Lash, A.E., Madden, T.L., Pontius, J.U., Schuler, G.D., Schriml, L.M., Sequeira, E., Tatusova, T.A. and Wagner, L. (2003). Database resources of the national center for biotechnology. *Nucleic Acids Res.* **31**, 28–33.

Wu, C.H., Yeh, L.-S., Huang, H., Arminski, L., Castro-Alvear, J., Chen, Y., Hu, Z., Kourtesis, P., Ledley, R.S., Suzek, B.E., Vinayaka, C.R., Zhang, J. and Barker, W.C. (2003). The protein information resource. *Nucleic Acids Res.* **31**, 345–347.

Wu, C.H., Huang, H., Nikolskaya, A., Hu, Z. and Barker, W.C. (2004). The iProClass integrated database for protein functional analysis. *Comput. Biol. Chem.* **28**, 87–96.

Zhang, R., Evans, G., Rotella, F. J., Westbrook, E.M., Beno, D., Huberman, E., Joachimiak, A. and Collart, F.R. (1999). Characteristics and crystal structure of bacterial inosine-5′-monophosphate dehydrogenase. *Biochemistry* **38**, 4691–4700.

Zhou, X., Cahoon, M., Rosa, P., Hedstrom, L. (1997). Expression, purification, and characterization of inosine 5′-monophosphate dehydrogenase from *Borrelia burgdorferi*. *J. Biol. Chem.* **272**, 21 977–21 981.

12 Models of Database Interconnectivity

G. J. L. Kemp

Abstract

Our aim is to integrate and analyse biological data held in existing distributed, heterogeneous data resources. We highlight some of the different kinds of data management systems in use with bioinformatics data collections, and the problems and benefits that this heterogeneity brings. We look at features of the relational and functional data models, and their ability to represent the semantics of biological data. We describe the P/FDM database management system and illustrate its use with examples of queries against a database of antibody structures. Some limitations of web-based data collections are mentioned, and the data replication and database federation approaches to data integration are discussed. We describe the implementation of a bioinformatics database federation based on the P/FDM mediator, leading to an architecture that can take advantage of the different data management solutions used by each of the data resources in the federation.

Keywords

antibody structure, data models, database schema, federated database, functional data model, heterogeneous databases, list comprehension, mediator, query processing

12.1 Introduction

In recent years there has been a rapid expansion in the quantity and variety of biological data available to researchers. These include data on protein and genome

Database Annotation in Molecular Biology   Edited by Arthur M. Lesk
© 2005 John Wiley & Sons, Ltd.   ISBN: 0-470-85681-5

sequences and structure, gene and protein expression, molecular interactions and biological pathways. Scientists' ability to use these data resources effectively to explore hypotheses *in silico* is enhanced if it is easy to ask precise and complex questions that span across several different kinds of data resource in order to find the answer. Developments in our ability to integrate and analyse data held in existing heterogeneous data resources can lead to an increase in our understanding of biological function at all levels. However, supporting *ad hoc* queries across multiple data resources and correlating data retrieved from these is still difficult.

In this chapter we consider some of the different kinds of data management in use with bioinformatics data collections, and look at the features of two different data models. Different approaches to data integration are outlined in Section 12.4, and this is followed by a description of a prototype implementation of a bioinformatics database federation.

12.2 Heterogeneity in Bioinformatics Data Management

Many different file and database management systems are currently in use with biological data sets. Some examples are given in Figure 12.1. Many widely used

	Management	Examples
Flat files	UNIX ("grep", Perl, etc.) SRS Text editor	PDB, SWISS-PROT
Relational	Sybase, Oracle, MySQL	Ensembl, ArrayExpress
Object-based	P/FDM, AceDB, OPM, VODAK, POET	C.elegans genomic data, antibody database (P/FDM)

Figure 12.1   Heterogeneous bioinformatics data resources

databanks consist of readable flat files of data – each databank containing different kinds of data, and each having its own format for its entries. Some biological data are held in relational databases, e.g. Ensembl (Hubbard *et al.*, 2002) and ArrayExpress (Brazma *et al.*, 2003) projects both use relational database management systems. Object models are gaining in popularity in the genome community – the Genome Database (GDB) uses the Object-Protocol Model (OPM) (Chen and Markowitz, 1995), and the ACEDB model (Durbin and Thierry-Mieg, 1992) is widely used with various specialized collections of genetic data.

Many Internet resources are intended for interactive inspection and interpretation by users observing a screen. Images, such as a metabolic pathway diagram or a graphical representation of an enzyme with its active site highlighted, or free text descriptions, such as journal abstracts or descriptions within PROSITE entries, contain information which is readily digested by scientists viewing these. However, the information contained within these is not easily available to programs. Image processing and natural language processing technologies still have a long way to advance before they can be used by remote programs to interpret the content of such data resources, let alone relate these observations to data from other sources and form scientific hypotheses. Many web-based data resources only provide this kind of access. The World-Wide Web has evolved to suit human users, who tend to search for particular pages of interest, controlling navigation interactively. The search techniques used are generally those developed by the information retrieval community for free-format text. Since the search programs do not understand the text, they uses probabilistic matching, for example by scoring keywords, and expect to retrieve some *false matches*. Database queries, by contrast, are expected to return sets which *exactly* fit the given criteria, and may involve numerical comparisons. The data model they use effectively describes the meaning of data in the form of carefully checked formatted records, and does not have to deal with free-format natural language sentence structures. This is what allows queries to be more precise.

Formatted data files, such as SWISS-PROT entries and Protein Data Bank entries, can be used more easily by programs. Many such collections are now accessible via the World-Wide Web. It is possible for programs (e.g. UNIX and Perl scripts or application programs written in C or Java) to fetch a web page automatically and then process it like any other external file. However, this requires the user to have programming skills, knowledge of the data file formats and time to write a new program whenever they wish to access different data values or different data banks or to use these for a different purpose. The SRS system (Etzold and Argos, 1993) goes some way towards providing indexes and a query interface for flat file data banks on the same server, but the querying capabilities are not as expressive or flexible as database query languages.

Database management systems (DBMSs) provide *ad hoc* querying capabilities, enabling complex data retrieval requests to be expressed in a high level query language. These requests can include sophisticated data selection criteria and may traverse the data in ways not envisaged by those who created the database. The DBMS will provide optimization capabilities that can use all of the information in the query in designing an efficient execution strategy.

There are several reasons for heterogeneity across bioinformatics data resources. The custodians of these data collections are likely to use whatever tools are known and available to them. They may choose a simple physical representation to make porting and exchanging data easy. A more significant reason is that certain physical representations are more appropriate than others for particular kinds of data, and are better suited to the kinds of search performed against those data. Frequently a great deal of effort goes into developing customized programs to search through the data and answer particular kinds of query efficiently. We should like to take advantage of this earlier investment by making use of such existing search capabilities whenever possible.

12.3 Data Models

A *data model* specifies the rules according to which data are structured and also the associated operations that are permitted. The three classical data models are the *relational* model, the *hierarchical* model and the *network* model (Date, 1977). These data models have relatively limited expressive power and it is often difficult to map the user's conceptual view of the application onto these models. Consequently, a lot of effort is often needed to coerce the data into a suitable form for storage.

To address this difference, or 'semantic gap', *semantic data models* (Hull and King, 1987; Peckham and Maryanski, 1988) were developed in which the logical organization of data more closely resembles the conceptual model. Semantic data models represent entities and the relationships between these directly, and match closely our conceptual view of data. Examples of semantic data models include the entity-relationship model (Chen, 1976), which is often used when designing conceptual schemas, and the functional data model (Shipman, 1981).

In this section we shall give a brief introduction to two different data models: the relational data model and the functional data model (FDM). We then illustrate some of the features of P/FDM, which is a database management system based on the FDM, by looking at its use with antibody structure and sequence data.

The relational data model

In the relational data model (Codd, 1970) data are organized in rectangular tables (called *relations*). Each row in a relation consists of a data record (or *tuple*). Each column in a relation can be thought of as representing an attribute, and contains data values of the same type. An example of a relation is shown in Figure 12.2.

pdb_code	compound	resolution
7FAB	IMMUNOGLOBULIN FAB' NEW (LAMBDA LIGHT CHAIN)	2.0
1TLD	BETA-TRYPSIN (ORTHORHOMBIC) AT $P*H 5.3	1.5
1CRN	CRAMBIN	1.5

Figure 12.2   A relation with three tuples

In answering queries in a relational database it is often necessary to *join* two or more relations together by finding tuples in these relations that have matching values in specified columns.

The relational data model has enjoyed considerable commercial success, and many database management systems based on this data model are available today. The relational data model's simplicity and the existence of robust and efficient implementations have made relational database management systems a popular choice for bioinformatics projects. However, the relational model has some limitations; for example, the data model does not directly support all of the relationships that we see when designing a conceptual model of some domain. An earlier paper compares relational databases and a database based on a semantic data model for storing and accessing protein structure data (Gray *et al.*, 1990).

Ideally, we would like to use a data model that is sufficiently expressive to enable us to capture the semantics of the data we want to model. One example of the relational model's limited expressive power is seen with subtype–supertype relationships. For example, we can consider *enzyme* to be a subtype of *protein* that has additional attributes that are relevant for enzymes (e.g. enzyme classification (EC) number indicating the kind of reaction that an enzyme catalyses), but which are not relevant to proteins in general (non-enzymes do not have EC numbers). While we can invent tables to store the information of interest, the relational model does not allow us to represent the subtype–supertype relationship between enzymes and proteins in a direct, intuitive way.

Another example of the relational model's limited expressive power is many-to-many relationships. For example, there is a many-to-many relationship between enzymes and the metabolic pathways in which they play a role: each pathway can require many enzymes, and a particular enzyme may be involved in several pathways. To model this relationship using the relational data model we need to introduce an additional binary table that serves to map between enzyme identifiers in one column and pathway identifiers in the other. Again, the relational data model does not allow us to represent these relationships in a direct, intuitive way.

The functional data model

The basic concepts in the functional data model (FDM) (Shipman, 1981) are entities and functions. Entities are used to represent conceptual objects, while functions represent the properties of an object. Functions are used to model both scalar attributes, such as a protein structure's resolution and the number of amino acid residues in a protein chain, and relationships, such as the relationship between chains and the residues that these contain. Functions may be single-valued or multi-valued, and their values can either be stored or computed on demand. Entity classes can be arranged in subtype hierarchies, with subtypes inheriting the properties of their supertype, as well as having their own specialized properties.

The FDM has its roots in the Multibase project (Landers and Rosenberg, 1982). Although it is an old data model it has adapted well to developments in computing because it was based on very good principles. Firstly, it was based on the use of values denoting persistent identifiers for instances of entity classes, as noted by

Kulkarni and Atkinson (1986). This later became central to the object database manifesto (Atkinson *et al.*, 1989). Also, it had the notion of a subtype hierarchy, and it was not difficult to adapt this to include methods with overriding. Secondly, the notions of an entity, a property and a relationship (as represented by a function and its inverse) corresponded closely to the entity-relationship model and E-R diagrams, which have stood the test of time. Thirdly, it used a query language based on applicative expressions, which combined data extraction with computation. Thus it was a mathematically well formed language, based on the functional languages (Buneman and Frankel, 1979; Turner, 1985).

P/FDM database and antibody data

P/FDM is a database management system that is based on the functional data model (Gray, Kulkarni and Paton, 1992). The query language associated with the functional data model is called Daplex, and this section contains some example queries that illustrate this language's syntax.

P/FDM has been used in several projects with protein structure data, and we describe some of P/FDM's features here through our use of the system with antibody structure and sequence data (Kemp *et al.*, 1994b). Figure 12.3 shows the schema diagram for this database, and Figure 12.4 shows a pictorial representation of some instances in this database.

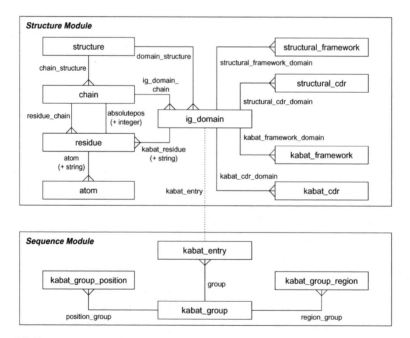

Figure 12.3 Antibody database schema diagram. Object classes are represented by rectangular boxes. Labelled lines between object classes represent relationships

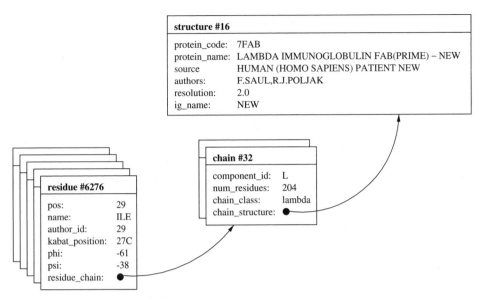

Figure 12.4 Some instances in the antibody database

Several different numbering conventions are used by scientists to identify particular residues in an immunoglobulin domain. The most widely used numbering convention is that used in the multiple alignments produced by Kabat *et al.* (1992). These codes are assigned so that residues at equivalent positions in different structures have the same position code. However, crystallographers will be familiar with the residue codes assigned by the authors in the PDB files. These are sometimes the same as those used by Kabat, but not always. A third way to number residues is to start at one end of the chain, and to assign consecutive numbers to the residues starting at one. Therefore, three code numbers are recorded with each residue from an antibody chain – the residue identifier used in the PDB entry; the Kabat position code; the ordinal position within the chain. Our schema includes a two argument function called *absolutepos* that takes a chain and an integer representing an ordinal position as its arguments and returns the residue object found at that position in the given chain. This function provides an index for accessing particular residues within a chain quickly, enabling navigation from a chain to particular residues of interest directly, compared with join operations that would be necessary if we were using relational storage. An important requirement for structure searches is that residues at topologically equivalent positions in different structures can be identified easily and quickly. Therefore, another index function, *kabat_residue*, takes an *ig_domain* object and a Kabat position code as its arguments and gives direct access to the residue at that position in the given domain.

We are interested in the orientation of the CDRs because these regions are important for specificity in binding antigens. Groups of variable domains whose CDRs have similar conformations have been identified (Chothia and Lesk, 1987;

Chothia *et al.*, 1989). It was observed in those studies that in Vλ domains, a particular class of VL domain, the first five residues of the L1 region have a similar conformation, and that the side-chain of the isoleucine residue at the fifth position in the L1 region points inwards towards the centre of the domain. We can query the database to investigate this observation.

First we must devise a way to express 'side-chain pointing inwards'. The first bond in the side-chain connects the alpha-carbon (Cα) atom to the beta-carbon (Cβ), and the direction of this bond can be used as the direction of the side-chain. Now, VL domains have a disulfide bond connecting the cysteine residues at Kabat positions 23 and 88. Visual inspection of any one of the known VL domain structures shows this disulfide bridge to be located in the middle of the VL domain, between the two beta-sheets. Therefore, the angle defined by the Cβ of the fifth residue in the L1 loop, the Cα of that residue and the Cα of residue 23 will be acute if the fifth residue in the L1 loop is directed towards the centre of the VL domain. A function called *angle* takes three atoms as its arguments and returns the angle (in degrees) defined by their centres. This function calls out to a routine written in C to calculate this value. The following query finds all L1 regions from Vλ domains and prints their PDB code, the names of the residues at the relevant positions and the calculated angle:

```
for each c in structural_cdr such that name(c) = 'L1'
   for the d in structural_cdr_domain(c) such that
       chain_class(d) = 'lambda'
     for the r1 in residue(c,5)
       for the r2 in kabat_residue(d,'23')
print(protein_code(d), name(r1), name(r2),
   angle(atom(r1,'CB'), atom(r1,'CA'),
     atom (r2,'CA')));
```

The results for this query are as follows:

```
1FB4 ILE CYS 19.3
2FB4 ILE CYS 19.3
2RHE ILE CYS 18.8
3FAB ILE CYS 16.6
7FAB ILE CYS 15.8
8FAB ASN CYS 116.2
```

The first five results support the observations made by Chothia and Lesk (1987). The structure 8FAB has been determined since that earlier study. It has a very different L1 conformation and its fifth residue is an outward pointing asparagine rather than an inward pointing isoleucine.

An alternative way to compare the conformations of the L1 regions is to superpose a pair of L1 regions and measure how well they fit. Fitting is done using a FORTRAN implementation of an algorithm for fitting two sets of points (McLachlan, 1979). This routine calculates the transformation that best fits the first set of points onto the second and measures the root mean square (RMS) distance between the two sets. The following query finds each pair of Vλ domains in turn and for each pair prints their codes and the RMS distance calculated when main chain atoms of five residues starting at Kabat position 26 (the start of the L1 loop) in the first domain are fitted to the corresponding atoms in the second domain.

```
for each d1 in ig_domain such that
    chain_class(d1) = 'lambda'
  for each d2 in ig_domain such that
      chain_class(d2) = 'lambda' and d1 ⟨⟩ d2
  print(protein_code(d1), protein_code(d2),
    main_chain_similarity(d1, d2, '26', 5));
```

We find that, apart from 8FAB, these have a similar conformation, giving an RMS distance less than 0.6 Å when compared. When 8FAB L1 region is compared with any of the others, the RMS distance is greater than 1.7 Å.

Rather than superposing L1 regions on each other, a variation on this query is to superpose the two strands flanking this loop from two different domains to find the three dimensional transformation that achieves the best fit. Applying this transformation to L1 loop atoms and comparing their transformed positions with the corresponding atoms in the target L1 loop shows this conformational difference more strongly.

The queries described in this section demonstrate the usefulness of augmenting the data from the Protein Data Bank (Berman *et al.*, 2000) with codes for residues that indicate a residue's position with reference to a structural template for a family of proteins. Annotating residues in this way facilitates inter-structure comparisons, and makes it possible to use the database to explore hypotheses about protein structure.

These queries also demonstrate the value of being able to combine arbitrary computations with data retrieval. In addition to calling code that derives a value by performing an arithmetic calculation, it is also possible to call out to code that retrieves a value from a remote data resource. This ability to encapsulate a remote data retrieval operation within an FDM function helps make the FDM a good data model for multi-database work.

12.4 Architectures for Data Integration

We are aiming to develop a system that will provide uniform access to heterogeneous databases via a single high level query language or graphical interface and will enable multi-database queries. This objective is illustrated in Figure 12.5. Data replication and multi-databases are two alternative approaches that could help us to meet this objective. This section contains an overview of these two approaches, but we start by

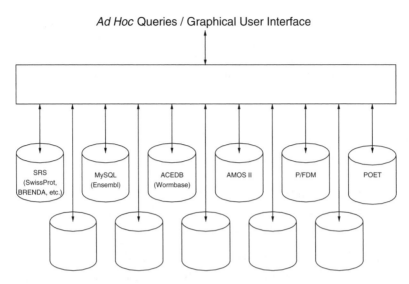

Figure 12.5 Users should be able to access heterogeneous distributed bioinformatics resources via a single query language or graphical user interface

describing some of the limitations of treating a collection of linked web pages as an integrated data resource.

Web-based data collections

Some may argue that a collection of indexed web pages constitutes a primitive database. However, the search capabilities provided are far below what one would expect from a database management system. When web pages are indexed for searching, this usually takes the form of a keyword index which enables searches for links to pages containing a specified word or phrase. Hypertext links between web pages do provide a kind of index for interactive browsing, but these links cannot be queried easily by automatic programs. If one does implement an automatic searching program which can follow links to retrieve related pages, then it is still necessary for the related pages to be retrieved one at a time and for these to be processed on the client machine; each would have to be scanned sequentially to see if it matches the search criteria. It is more efficient to send selection conditions across to a remote part of a distributed database and to send back just the items required than it is to transport the data as whole web pages including images, only to reject much of it on arrival.

Data replication

In a 'data replication' architecture, all data from the various databases and databanks of interest would be copied to a single local data repository, under a single database

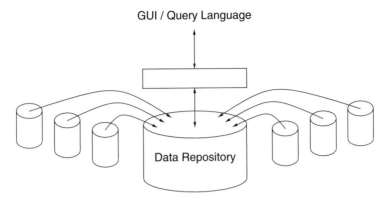

Figure 12.6   In a data replication approach, data are copied from various data resources into a single centralized system

management system, as illustrated in Figure 12.6. This approach is taken by Rieche and Dittrich (1994) who propose an architecture in which the contents of biological databanks including the EMBL nucleotide sequence databank and SWISS-PROT are imported into a central repository.

However, we believe that a data replication approach is not appropriate for this application domain for several reasons. Significantly, by adopting a data repository approach the advantages of the individual heterogeneous systems are lost. For example, many biological data resources have their own customized search capabilities that have been tailored to the particular physical representation that best suits that data set. Rieche and Dittrich (1994) acknowledge the need to use existing software and propose implementing 'exporters' to export and convert data from the data repository into files that can be used as input to software tools.

Another disadvantage of a data replication approach is the time and effort required to maintain an up-to-date repository. Scientists want access to the most recent data as soon as these have been deposited in a databank. Therefore, whenever one of the contributing databases is updated the same update should be made to the data repository.

Federated system

We favour a multi-database approach which makes use of existing remote data sources, with data described in terms of entities, attributes and relationships described in a high level schema. The schema is designed without regard to the physical storage format(s). Queries are expressed in terms of the conceptual schema and it is the role of a complex software component called a *mediator* (Wiederhold, 1992) to decide what component data sources need to be accessed to answer a particular query, to organize the computation and to combine the results. Robbins (1996) and Karp (1995) have also advocated a federated multi-database approach.

In contrast to a data replication approach, with a multi-database approach we can take advantage of the customized search capabilities of the component data sources in the federation, by sending requests to these from the mediator. The component resources keep their autonomy, and users can continue to use these exactly as before. There is no local mirroring, and updates to the remote component databases are available immediately. A multi-database approach does not require that large data sets be imported from a variety of sources, and it is not necessary to convert all data for use with a single physical storage schema. However, extra effort is needed to achieve a mapping from the component databases onto the conceptual model.

12.5 Implementing a Database Federation

The prototype P/FDM Mediator (Kemp, Angelopoulos and Gray, 2000, 2002) is based on the P/FDM object database system (Gray, Kulkarni and Paton, 1992). Tasks performed by the P/FDM Mediator include determining which external databases are relevant in answering users' queries, dividing queries into parts that will be sent to different external databases, translating these subqueries into the language(s) of the external databases and combining the results for presentation. This approach is particularly well suited to situations where the subqueries sent to the external databases are highly selective and return relatively small result sets.

Schema levels in a database federation

It is useful to think of the federation having a clear separation between schemas at the five distinct levels shown in Figure 12.7 since this makes it easier to build the database federation in a modular fashion (Kemp, Angelopoulos and Gray, 2000).

First, let us consider an external data resource. Each external resource has two pre-existing schema levels, shown below the dashed line in Figure 12.7. The resource's *conceptual schema* (which we call C_R) describes the logical structure of the data contained in that resource. If the resource is a relational database then this will include information about table names and column names, and type information about stored values. With ACEDB (Durbin and Thierry-Mieg, 1992), this is the classes and tags defined in the model description. With SRS (Etzold and Argos, 1993), it is the databank names and field names. These systems also provide a mechanism for querying the data resource in terms of the table/class/databank names and column/tag/attribute/field names that are presented in the conceptual schema.

The *internal schema* (or *storage schema*, which we call I_R) contains details of allocation of data records to storage areas, placement strategy, use of indexes, set ordering and internal data structures that impact on efficiency and implementation details (Gray, Kulkarni and Paton, 1992). We do not need to concern ourselves with the internal schemas of individual data resources. Others have already implemented

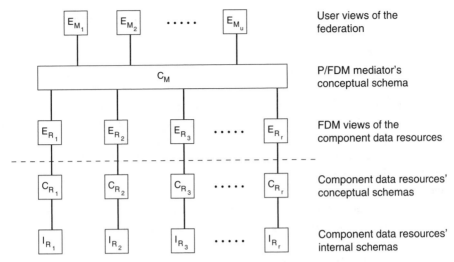

Figure 12.7   Schemas in a database federation

the mapping from the conceptual schema to the internal schema within each of the individual resources that we use, and we assume that this has been done to make best use of the resources' internal organization.

We implemented the three schema levels that are shown above the dashed line in Figure 12.7 within the P/FDM mediator. Our approach does not require that the participating sites use the same data model. Rather, it is sufficient for the mediator to hold descriptions of the participating sites that are expressed in a common data model – in our system the FDM. All of the schemas above the dashed line in Figure 12.7 are implemented using the FDM.

The first step in adding a new external resource to the federation is to describe the structure of that resource using the FDM. In doing this we choose entity names and functions that represent, as closely as possible, the contents and structure of the data in the external resource. The result of this step is an FDM view of the external resource, which we call E_R.

The mediator's conceptual schema, C_M, describes the content of the (virtual) data resources that are members of the federation, including the semantic relationships that hold between data items in these resources. We also refer to this as the federation's integration schema. We have chosen to express this schema using the functional data model because it makes computed data in a virtual resource, both the derived results of arithmetic expressions and derived relationships, look no different from stored data. Both are the result of functions – one calculates, the other extracts from storage. It is at this level that mappings between data items in different data resources are made explicit. Through functional mappings, different attributes of the same conceptual entity can be spread across different external data resources, and subclass–superclass relationships between entities in the conceptual model of the domain might not be present explicitly in the external resources (Grufman *et al.*, 1997).

We cannot expect scientists to agree on a single schema. Different scientists are interested in different aspects of the data, and will want to see data structured in a way that matches the concepts, attributes and relationships in their own personal model. The principle of logical data independence means that the system can provide different users with different views onto the integration schema. We use E_M to refer to an external schema presented to a user of the mediator.

The role of the mediator is to process queries expressed against the federation's integration schema (C_M). The mediator holds metadata describing the integration schema and also the external schemas of each of the federation's data resources (E_R). In P/FDM, these metadata are held, for convenience of pattern matching, as Prolog clauses that are compiled from high level schema descriptions.

P/FDM mediator architecture

The main components of the P/FDM mediator are shown inside the dashed box in Figure 12.8, and are described below.

The *parser* reads a Daplex query (Daplex is the query language for the FDM), checks it for consistency and produces a *list comprehension* containing the essential elements of the query in a form that is easier to process than Daplex text (we call this internal form '*ICode*').

The *simplifier*'s role is to produce shorter, more elegant and more consistent ICode, mainly through removing redundant variables and expressions, and flattening out nested expressions where this does not change the meaning of the query. Simplifying the ICode form of a query makes the subsequent query processing steps more efficient because this reduces the number of equivalent ICode combinations that need to be considered.

The *rule-based rewriter* can be used to perform semantic query optimization by replacing parts of a query with equivalent expressions that can be evaluated more efficiently. This capability is important since graphical interfaces make it easy for users to express inefficient queries which cannot always be optimized using general purpose query optimization strategies. This is because transforming the original query to a more efficient one may require domain knowledge e.g. two or more alternative navigation paths may exist between distantly related object classes but domain knowledge is needed to recognize that these are indeed equivalent. A recent enhancement to the mediator is an extension to the Daplex compiler that enables generic rewrite rules to be expressed using a declarative high level syntax (Kemp, Gray and Sjöstedt, 2001). This will make it easier to add new query optimization strategies to the mediator in the future.

The *optimizer* performs generic query optimization.

The *reordering module* reorders expressions in the ICode to ensure that all variable dependencies are observed, thus ensuring that each variable is assigned a value before that variable is used.

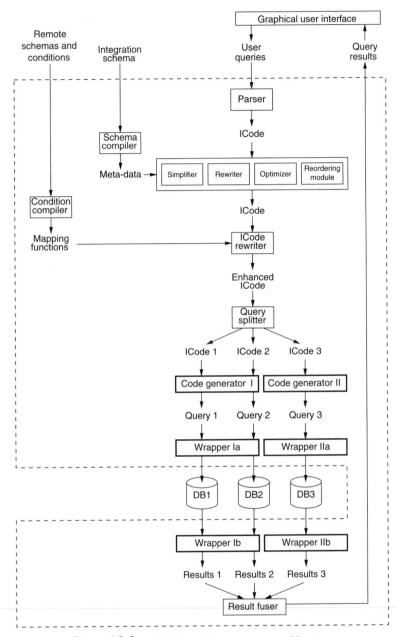

Figure 12.8 P/FDM mediator system architecture

The *condition compiler* reads declarative statements about conditions that must hold between data items in different external data resources in order that these values can be mapped on to the integration schema. These declarative statements will usually identify corresponding key attributes in different data resources.

The *ICode rewriter* expands the original ICode by applying mapping functions that transform references to the integration schema into references to the federation's component databases. Essentially the same rewriter that was mentioned above is used here, but with a different set of rewrite rules. These rewrite rules enhance the ICode by adding tags to indicate the actual data sources that contain particular entity classes and attribute values. Thus, the ICode rewriter transforms the query expressed against the C_M schema into a query expressed against the E_R schemas of one or more external databases.

The *query splitter* identifies which external databases hold data referred to by parts of an integrated query, and those parts that refer to the same database are grouped together into 'chunks'. Query 'chunks' are shuffled and variable dependencies are checked to produce alternative execution plans. A generic description of costs is used to select a good sequence of instructions for accessing the remote databases. The crucial idea is to move selective filter operations in the query down into the appropriate chunks so that they can be applied early and efficiently using local search facilities as registered with the mediator (Kemp, Iriarte and Gray, 1994a).

Each ICode chunk is sent to one of several *code generators*. These translate ICode into queries that are executable by the remote databases, transforming query fragments from E_R to C_R. New code generators can be linked into the mediator at runtime. We have implemented code generators that translate ICode into SQL, OQL, AMOSQL, SRS code, ACEPERL and Prolog. Our modular design should make it easy to add further code generators for other database management systems.

Wrappers deal with communication with the external data resources. They consist of two parts: code responsible for sending queries to remote resources, and code that receives and parses the results returned from the remote resources. Wrappers for new resources can be linked into the mediator at runtime. Note that a wrapper can only make use of whatever querying facilities are provided by the federation's component databases. Thus, the mediator's conceptual model (C_M) will only be able to map onto those data values that are identified in the remote resource's conceptual model (C_R). Thus, queries involving concepts such as 'gene' and 'chromosome' in C_M can only be transformed into queries that run against a remote resource if that resource exports these concepts. We have implemented wrappers for ACEDB, SRS and the P/FDM object database system, and we have used our system to integrate protein data from remote P/FDM systems with data accessed through the SRS system at the European Bioinformatics Institute, and Wormbase (ACEDB) at Cold Spring Harbor Laboratory.

The *result fuser* provides a synchronization layer, combining results retrieved from external databases so that the rest of the query can proceed smoothly. It interacts tightly with the wrappers.

12.6 Conclusions

Different bioinformatics data resource provide different kinds of access to their data. Often they depend on the user observing the screen and working interactively. This prevents one from using automatic programs to assist end users to work with a variety of resources simultaneously. Other resources present data in well defined text formats that can also be used by automatic programs. Other data resources go further and provide access through database management software, thus enabling remote programs to query the data efficiently and providing the structured framework of a schema which is necessary for integration with data from other resources.

Storing annotations in a database in a form that can be used by automatic programs enables us to use the database to explore scientific questions in a way that otherwise might not be convenient, or even possible. The use of Kabat position codes described above is an example of this.

In order to relate data values from different data resources it is necessary that the criteria for establishing an association between related data items are explicit. Here the choice and use of key attributes is vital.

Autonomy and heterogeneity across different bioinformatics data resources is inevitable and desirable, since individual groups compiling and curating data should adopt the data management systems that are best suited to the characteristics and search requirements of their data. A federated architecture is compatible with this heterogeneous environment and can take advantage of the different customized data management solutions employed by each of the component data resources in the federation.

References

Atkinson, M., Bancilhon, F., DeWitt, D., Dittrich, K., Maier, D. and Zdonik, S. (1989). The object-oriented database system manifesto. In Kim, W., Nicolas, J.-M. and Nishio, S., eds, *Proceedings of 1st International Conference on Deductive and Object-Oriented Databases*, Kyoto, Japan. North-Holland-Elsevier, Amsterdam, pp. 223–240.

Berman, H., Westbrook, J., Feng, Z., Gilliland, G., Bhat, T. Weissig, H., Shindyalov, I. and Bourne, P. (2000). The protein data bank. *Nucleic Acids Res.* **28**, 235–242.

Brazma, A., Parkinson, H., Sarkans, U., Shojatalab, M., Vilo, J., Abeygunawardena, N., Holloway, E., Kapushesky, M., Kemmeren, P., Lara, G., Oezcimen, A., Rocca-Serra, P. and Sansone, S. (2003). ArrayExpress – a public repository for microarray gene expression data at the EBI. *Nucleic Acids Res.* **31**, 68–71.

Buneman, P. and Franek, R. (1979). FQL – a functional query language. In Bernstein, P., ed., *SIGMOD 79 Conference*, Boston. ACM Press, pp. 52–58.

Chen, I.-M.A. and Markowitz, V.M. (1995). An overview of the Object-Protocol Model (OPM) and the OPM data management tools. *Information Systems* **20** (5), 393–418.

Chen, P. (1976). The Entity-Relationship Model – toward a unified view of data. *ACM Trans. Database Syst.* **1** (1), 9–36.

Chothia, C. and Lesk, A. (1987). Canonical structures for the hypervariable regions of immunoglobulins. *J. Mol. Biol.* **196**, 901–917.

Chothia, C., Lesk, A., Tramontano, A., Levitt, M., Smith-Gill, S., Air, G., Sheriff, S., Padlan, E., Davies, D., Tulip, W., Colman, P., Spinelli, S., Alzari, P. and Poljak, R. (1989). Conformations of immunoglobulin hypervariable regions. *Nature* **342**, 877–883.

Codd, E. (1970). A relational model of data for large shared data banks. *Commun. ACM* **13**, 377–387.

Date, C. (1977). *An Introduction to Database Systems*, 2nd edn, Addison-Wesley, Reading, MA.

Durbin, R. and Thierry-Mieg, J. (1992). *Syntactic Definitions for the ACEDB Data Base Manager*, included as part of the ACEDB distribution.

Etzold, T. and Argos, P. (1993). SRS – an indexing and retrieval tool for flat file data libraries. *CABIOS*, **9**, 49–57.

Gray, P., Kulkarni, K. and Paton, N. (1992). *Object-Oriented Databases: a Semantic Data Model Approach*, Prentice-Hall Series in Computer Science, Prentice-Hall, Hemel Hempstead.

Gray, P., Paton, N., Kemp, G. and Fothergill, J. (1990). An object-oriented database for protein structure analysis. *Protein Eng.* **3**, 235–243.

Grufman, S., Samson, F., Embury, S. and Gray, P. (1997). Distributing semantic constraints between heterogeneous databases. In Gray, A. and Larson, P.-Å., eds, *Proceedings: 13th International Conference on Data Engineering*, IEEE computer society press, Los Alamitos, CA, pp. 33–42.

Hubbard, T., Barker, D., Birney, E., Cameron, G., Chen, Y., Clark, L., Cox, T., Cuff, J., Curwen, V., Down, T., Durbin, R., Eyras, E., Gilbert, J., Hammond, M., Huminiecki, L., Kasprzyk, A., Lehvaslaiho, H., Lijnzaad, P., Melsopp, C., Mongin, E., Pettett, R., Pocock, M., Potter, S., Rust, A., Schmidt, E., Searle, S., Slater, G., Smith, J., Spooner, W., Stabenau, A., Stalker, J., Stupka, E., Ureta-Vidal, A., Vastrik, I. and Clamp, M. (2002). The Ensembl genome database project. *Nucleic Acids Res.* **30**, 38–41.

Hull, R. and King, R. (1987). Semantic Database Modeling: survey, applications and research issues. *ACM Comput. Surveys* **19**, 201–260.

Kabat, E., Wu, T., Perry, H., Gottesman, K. and Foeller, C. (1992). *Sequences of Proteins of Immunological Interest*, 5th edn, Public Health Service, NIH, Washington, DC.

Karp, P. (1995). *A Vision of DB Interoperation*. Meeting on the interconnection of molecular biology databases, Cambridge.

Kemp, G., Angelopoulos, N. and Gray, P. (2000). A schema-based approach to building a bioinformatics database federation. In *Proceedings IEEE International Symposium on Bio-Informatics and Biomedical Engineering*, IEEE Computer Society Press, Los Alamitos, CA, pp. 13–20.

Kemp, G.J.L., Angelopoulos, N. and Gray, P.M.D. (2002). Architecture of a mediator for a bioinformatics database federation. *IEEE Trans. Information Technol. Biomed.* **6**, 116–122.

Kemp, G.J.L., Gray, P.M.D. and Sjöstedt, A. R. (2001). Improving federated database queries using declarative rewrite rules for quantified subqueries. *J. Intell. Information Syst.* **17**, 281–299.

Kemp, G., Iriarte, J. and Gray, P. (1994a). Efficient access to FDM objects stored in a relational database. In Bowers, D., ed., *Directions in Databases: Proceedings of the Twelfth British National Conference on Databases*, lecture notes in computer science, Vol. 826, Springer, Heidelberg, pp. 170–186.

Kemp, G., Jiao, Z., Gray, P. and Fothergill, J. (1994b). Combining computation with database access in biomolecular computing. In Litwin, W. and Risch, T., eds, *Applications of Databases: Proceedings of the First International Conference*, lecture notes in computer science, Vol. 819, Springer, Heidelberg, pp. 317–335.

Kulkarni, K. and Atkinson, M. (1986). EFDM: extended functional data model. *Comput. J.* **29** (1), 38–46.

Landers, T.A. and Rosenberg, R.L. (1982). An overview of MULTIBASE. In Schneider, H.-J., ed., *Distributed Data Bases, Proceedings of the Second International Symposium on Distributed Data Bases, Berlin, 1982,* North-Holland, Amsterdam, pp. 153–184.

McLachlan, A. (1979). Gene duplication in the structural evolution of chymotrypsin. *J. Mol. Biol.* **128**, 49–79.

Peckham, J. and Maryanski, F. (1988). Semantic data models. *ACM Comput. Surveys* **20**, 153–189.

Rieche, B. and Dittrich, K. (1994). A federated DBMS-based integrated environment for molecular biology. In French, J.C. and Hinterberger, H., eds, *Proceedings of the Seventh International Working Conference on Scientific and Statistical Database Management, Charlottesville, VA, 1994,* IEEE computer society.

Robbins, R.J. (1996). Bioinformatics: essential infrastructure for global biology. *J. Comput. Biol.* **3**, 465–478.

Shipman, D. (1981). The functional data model and the data language DAPLEX. *ACM Trans. Database Syst.* **6** (1), 140–173.

Turner, D.A. (1985). Miranda: a non-strict functional language with polymorphic types. In Jouannaud, J.-P., ed., *Proceedings of the IFIP Int. Conf. on Functional Programming Languages and Computer Architecture*, lecture notes in computer science, Vol. 201, Springer, Heidelberg, pp. 1–16.

Wiederhold, G. (1992). Mediators in the architecture of future information systems. *IEEE Comput.* **25** (3), 38–49.

13 The European Bioinformatics Institute Macromolecular Structure Relational Database Technology

H. Boutselakis, D. Dimitropoulos, K. Henrick, J. Ionides, M. John, P.A. Keller, P. McNeil, J. Pineda and A. Suarez-Uruena

Abstract

The MSD database is derived from Protein Data Bank (PDB) entries, which are loaded into the deposition database. Relational database technologies, in Oracle, are used in a comprehensive cleaning procedure to ensure data uniformity across the whole archive. The deposition database is highly normalized to facilitate this procedure. This database is then transformed into the denormalized search database, which is specifically designed to facilitate complex queries. The search database contains an extensive set of derived properties, goodness-of-fit indicators and links to other EBI databases including InterPro, GO and SWISS-PROT, together with links to SCOP, CATH, PFAM and PROSITE. The search database is updated using an incremental transformation and is replicated and distributed to other sites. It makes use of Oracle cartridge technology; e.g., a chemical database cartridge (for small molecules, drugs and amino acids) has been implemented in java. These are aspects of our continuous process of enhancing the quality and consistency of macromolecular structure data working towards the integration of various bioinformatics data resources.

Keywords

Protein Data Bank, macromolecular, structure, relational, database, Oracle, normalized, data integrity, metamodel, transformation, denormalized, data warehouse, replication, cartridge

Database Annotation in Molecular Biology   Edited by Arthur M. Lesk
© 2005 John Wiley & Sons, Ltd.   ISBN: 0-470-85681-5

The challenge for the next decade will be to harness the wealth of protein sequence, structural and functional information being generated by the international genome initiatives (Service, 2000), in order to reveal the molecular mechanisms of protein evolution, and the regulatory processes which control the observed phenotypes. Exploiting this genomic data will depend on integrating key sequence and structural data for protein families and providing common views onto this data and standardized nomenclature. It will also depend on building robust interfaces between the plethora of sequence and structure databases, which have been set up by experts in complementary areas of genome analysis.

The E-MSD, EBI Macromolecular Structure Database, for the Protein Data Bank (PDB) (Berman *et al.*, 2000), http://www.ebi.ac.uk/msd, was set up in 1996 to give Europe an autonomous and trusted facility to collect, organize and make available data about biological macromolecular structures and to integrate structure with the other biological databases at the EBI. Since then, the E-MSD group has been working in the following areas:

- Accepting and processing depositions to the (PDB)

- Transforming the PDB flat file archive to a relational database system

- Developing services to search the PDB

- Developing standards for 3D database information design and models that describe the conceptual framework, in which all data are collected, stored and disseminated

- In partnership with projects to address an urgent need to develop an end user environment to take advantage of the rapid development of high throughput facilities associated with protein crystallography.

The EMSD relational database project brings together diverse ideas and approaches for the searching and use of a new relational database for macromolecular structure. The database stores PDB information enriched with procedures designed to derive important taxonomical, structural and functional properties. The MSD relational database system is made up of two main components: the deposition database, and the search database. Both use Oracle (Awai *et al.*, 2000) as the database engine and are designed and managed using the CASE tool Oracle Designer.

The PDB is a collection of formatted flat files with the disadvantages of (a) uncontrolled redundancy, (b) inconsistent data, (c) inflexibility, (d) limited data sharing, (e) poor enforcement of standards, (f) low programmer productivity, (g) excessive program maintenance and (h) excessive data maintenance. The MSD relational database takes advantage of all the power of a relational database management system of (a) controlled redundancy, (b) consistency of data and integrity constraints, (c) integration of data, (d) data and operation sharing, (e) multiple interfaces, (f) security and privacy controls, (g) backup and recovery, (h) enforcement of standards, (i) flexibility, (j) data independence, (k) data accessibility, (l) reduced program maintenance and (m) ease of application development. In addition, a relational database is more adaptable to new hardware, new functions, new users, new storage, new techniques and linkage to other databases.

A database is a representation of the real world and changes in the real world need to be reflected in the database. To achieve this aim the database design is maintained in the form of a logical (entity-relationship) model, in which entity subtyping is permitted. This model is validated using both Oracle Designer tools and programs developed by the MSD database group, and all relationships are verified and semantically characterized. The logical model is transformed into a description of the physical implementation of the database (the server model), in which each root entity is implemented by one table. Each table has a primary key which is a single integer column populated by values generated internally by Oracle sequence objects. In the Oracle Designer tools, these are referred to as 'surrogate primary keys'. Natural unique identifiers (i.e. those defined using values contained in external data) are implemented as unique key constraints. Additional validation operations are performed after the generation of the server model. These operations include the hierarchical structuring of all relationships to determine the proper load order. Additionally, all leaf entities (entities representing subtypes that have no subtypes themselves) of the logical model are transformed into views on the root tables that are implementing the root entities. Finally, additional code is automatically generated for unique key selection and for insertion triggers of the views that implement the leaf entities. Oracle Designer is used to store, manipulate, validate and maintain the entity-relationship model and the server model in a separate Oracle database (currently Oracle 9i Enterprise Edition).

The design of the core of the relational database in which deposition information is loaded, curated and validated has evolved to expand its knowledge to related areas, to improve its data precision and to host data originating in the application of new technologies. Changes are incorporated in the logical model. The revised model is used to generate a new server model, from which existing implementations of the model can be updated in a controlled fashion.

The server model described above is used to generate the Data Definition Language scripts to create an Oracle database schema. This schema is enriched with a set of Designer-generated PL/SQL packages and table triggers called the table API, which standardizes the operations of insertion, deletion, modification and selection, and provides public structures to access the database tables and views in a common way. Code developed using the table API is less affected by database modifications among versions, simplifying its maintenance.

13.1 Database Design Process

The MSD database uses Oracle Designer/Repository for the entity-relationship (ER) design and the Oracle Designer built-in utility Database Design Transformer (DDT) to generate server models. The entity-relationship model, ERM (Chen, 1976), is the most commonly applied modelling technique. With a small model, the normal path would be to use the DDT to generate a first cut server (physical) model from the ER (logical) model, and then edit the server model by hand as required. The MSD contains ca. 400 tables, and therefore this approach is not practical. We have opted to extend the repository to hold extra information in the logical model. This is then used by code written against the repository API to carry out the edits on the server model that would otherwise have to be done by hand. These edits include

- Changing the names of foreign key columns, foreign key constraints and foreign key indexes where the names generated by the DDT are not suitable.

- Setting server-side delete rules for individual foreign keys to cascade, restrict or nullify.

- Setting unique and foreign key constraints to defer validation until the end of transaction.

Often we also have to use the repository API to work around Designer limitations and bugs.

As mentioned above, all primary keys in the deposition database are surrogate primary keys (i.e. the primary key is an abstract identifier with no meaning outside the database). All foreign keys refer to these surrogate primary keys. The data model has some deep hierarchies. If natural unique identifiers were used as primary keys, the primary keys of tables at the bottom of the hierarchies would contain a large number of columns. Also, updating values of primary key columns would require cascading them down the hierarchy. Using foreign keys that join to abstract primary keys avoids this potentially expensive operation. The downside of this is that creating a meaningful representation of data at the bottom of the hierarchy requires joining all the tables in the hierarchy, which is why we transform into a flatter structure and de-normalize heavily for the search database. This design also requires frequent querying using natural unique keys (which are present in external data) to find the corresponding surrogate primary key values. We auto-generate code that encapsulates the select statements on natural unique keys and caters correctly for SQL tri-valued logic to treat null values in external data correctly.

13.2 Loading and Exporting Data in mmCIF

The loading of a new PDB deposition (and the load of all the legacy PDB files) is a process which involves not only the database schema but also an mmCIF parser, a database meta-model that maps the different mmCIF (macromolecular Crystallographic Information File; Bourne *et al.*, 1997) items and categories onto database views, and a binary dictionary which stores the semantics of all the structured mmCIF files. These views (and triggers defined on them) perform the task of maintaining high level thematic data integrity and perform some additional calculations.

Before using this schema for the loading of depositions, it is necessary to provide it with some core reference data which are used to look up controlled vocabulary terms during the database load. Internally we convert PDB files to mmCIF formatted files for database loading. The mmCIF format was designed for expressing complex information about a macromolecular structural determination experiment. There are strong similarities between mmCIF on the one hand, and a relational data model and its implementation on the other. In particular, mmCIF categories correspond to entities and tables, and mmCIF data names to attributes/relationships and columns. Data within mmCIF categories can be 'looped', and each row within a loop corresponds to a row in a relational table. Categories can also have 'keys', i.e. combinations of data items whose values uniquely identify a row within a loop. Pairs of items can be related by defining child–parent links, and this can be used to express relationships between categories.

Mapping between the two types of data representation is not always straightforward. Basically, the mmCIF standard does not enforce the rules that are required by relational theory. This means that, whereas an mmCIF dictionary can be used to express the essential features of a relational model, the reverse is not true, namely constructions that are allowed in mmCIF cannot be easily encapsulated in a fully relational description. In practice, the publicly distributed COMCIFS-approved mmCIF dictionary, as well as a number of others that are in use, exploits this freedom, and so cannot be mapped to a relational model in a straightforward way. Moreover, mmCIFs that are deposited under the data harvesting system (Henrick and Dodson, 1999; Winn, 1999) will have many mandatory relationships unspecified, and these will need to be constructed before the data can be loaded. In order to load data from mmCIFs into the deposition database, we have taken the following approach. On the server side (i.e. at the Oracle DBMS), views are written that correspond closely to mmCIF categories. Almost all of these views are join views. They have 'instead of' triggers (an Oracle-specific SQL feature) defined on them, such that an insert operation will invoke server-side code (which can be written in the Oracle specific language PL/SQL or in Java) rather than attempting the insert operation. This code then handles the actual insertion into database tables. The code is generated semi-automatically and maintained manually thereafter. Any heuristics or informal interpretations of mmCIF specifications that are necessary to loading the data are coded manually in these triggers or in other server-side code that they invoke.

The correspondence between mmCIF items and categories on the one hand, and Oracle views and columns on the other, is handled in the 'metadatabase'; this is a small database that is separate from the deposition database. Apart from the correspondences, the metadatabase contains information that allows the splitting and joining of mmCIF categories. Splitting occurs where one mmCIF category corresponds to several tables in the database and joining, where corresponding rows from two mmCIF categories have to be loaded into the same row of a database table (e.g. cell and space group are in different mmCIF categories, but the same database table). Other information maintained in the metadata includes

- Server-side callback functions to be invoked when all rows of a category have been loaded
- Discriminator information that allows different rows within a category to be handled differently depending on the data that they contain
- Grouping of the loading views, to allow loading of a single entry in several passes
- For any mmCIF item, special values that must be mapped to SQL null values for loading.

This information is manually maintained in a source file for the Oracle SqlLoader utility, to allow easy re-generation of the metadatabase as required.

The order in which data from mmCIF categories is loaded is also extremely important, since mmCIF data are unordered within the file. All foreign keys join via surrogate primary keys whose values are only generated at the time of data insertion. This means that populating mandatory foreign key columns in the database from mmCIF data requires that, for virtually all the foreign keys, the table from which the foreign key is migrated must be loaded before the table that contains the foreign key column. Even if this were not the case, it would be necessary to load the data such that mandatory foreign key constraints were satisfied at all times (inserting 10^5 rows with constraints deferred can hit database resource limits, and disabling and re-enabling foreign keys is expensive for large tables.) Accordingly, the metadata contain information that specifies the order in which mmCIF categories are read and inserted into the corresponding views. We use a modified breadth-first graph traversal of logical and server models to automatically derive a load order that will not leave any (mandatory) foreign keys unsatisfied at any intermediate stage of the load. This load order is stored in the repository in the server model (in fact in the table entity associations). Where cycles exist, one of the relationships is annotated in the logical model as not expecting its parent to be present at load time (i.e. a relationship that would normally be populated by an update rather than an insert, and is not mandatory). The logical model is partitioned into deposition data and reference data (complex controlled vocabulary data). Load order derivation operates independently within each partition.

Once an entry is loaded, it is available for the derivation of scientific information not only from its own self-contained information but also from aggregating data across multiple entries. Some of the results of the calculation are incorporated in the deposition database and the most important of them are used to populate the search database.

13.3 Exporting mmCIFs or XML Files from the Deposition Database

The metamodel stores additional mappings of the database, for example a mapping to an mmCIF dictionary defined for information exchange with the parent PDB in the United States. A local package has been developed in PL/SQL as a dynamic generator of other server-side PL/SQL procedures that handle each mmCIF category independently. The generated procedures extract the information from one or more different databases and output mmCIF or XML files. In addition, the package permits the use of mmCIF terminology to specify the set of depositions for export, produces UTL files in the server and loads the mmCIF dictionary. The package automatically handles all the hierarchy, relationships and table order and manages the correct export of standardized database entries.

The use of server-side trigger code to handle the less structured aspects of mapping mmCIFs to the deposition database structure allows programs that load and export data to be fairly simple. Any such program requires two simultaneous database connections: one to the deposition database, and the other to the metadatabase. The loading application is written in Pro*Fortran: this was dictated by the availability of a suitable library to parse mmCIFs and access their contents in the manner required for this purpose. We expect to port it to Pro*C or Java in the near future.

13.4 Subtypes and 'Leaf Views'

A separate but related issue is how the many supertype–subtype relationships in the logical model are implemented in the server model. Currently, they are always implemented as 'supertype tables'. Code has been written to generate views that correspond to the lowest level entities in this kind of relationship. These views look exactly like the tables that would be generated in implementations where tables representing the subtypes are defined. The practical upshot of this is that instead of writing SQL that requires knowledge of the subtype discriminator column

SELECT...FROM SUP_CHEM_COMP WHERE SCC_TYPE = 'DCC'...

The following will do the same:

SELECT...FROM DEP_CHEM_COMP...

This simplifies both writing the 'instead of' views in the trigger code, and the writing of the select statements that are used to construct the search database. It also provides robustness with respect to changes in implementation of supertype–subtype relationships. Like the code that works out the order of loading, this code is written against the Oracle Repository API.

13.5 Maintenance Aspects

Maintaining mmCIF dictionaries has always been a challenge. While there are various tools available to check a dictionary for problems, the actual maintenance has to be done by the use of standard text editors. The COMCIFs dictionary is about 1.5 Mb in size, and contains over 2300 data names, category names and aliases. A lot of effort has been expended over the years by various people involved with the mmCIF project in tracking down various typographical errors and inconsistencies, and extending dictionaries is a major effort. We have expanded the metadatabase to hold much of the mmCIF dictionary information. Modifications to the dictionary can be carried out inside the metadatabase, and the text form of the dictionary exported from the metadatabase as required. The mmCIF DDL (a dictionary-like definition of the mmCIF dictionary structure) contains all the information necessary to do this.

The triggers can also be problematic to maintain, although much of the trigger code is pretty straightforward to write. The main problems arise from inadequacies in the mmCIF dictionaries, problems in the PDB data and difficulties in representing certain types of datum in the PDB files in a manner that conforms to mmCIF dictionaries. PDB knowledge about the real world has to be encoded somewhere, and the trigger code carries out much of this task. A large number of the PDB problems are dealt with by a complex suite of Fortran90 software that converts a PDB entry into an in-house form of mmCIFs that are passed to the loader. This software also determines the most important classification of the coordinate data into database 'assemblies' (Henrick and Thornton, 1998; Boutselakis *et al.*, 2003).

Maintaining the metadata itself is not a major problem. The SQL Loader source file that contains this information is simple and concise.

Maintenance of the deposition database requires some additional code to customize the Oracle database design methodology to standard practice within the MSD group. This code is mainly related to the following.

Creation of new database objects. As mentioned above, the Oracle Designer server model is augmented with some objects that participate actively in the database implementation. These objects, mainly views and packages, are derived from the logical model and transformed into the server model and provide the implementation of various features, such as sub-entities.

Reporting of impact information. PL/SQL code has been developed for impact analysis when preparing to upgrade an existing schema to a newer version of the server model. These impact reports are particularly useful before a new release of the MSD database is issued, because they enable the database programmers to preview and estimate the effort required to implement any database structural change before this change is effectively made.

Entry replication. This enables the MSD Database to make a copy of a particular database entry (known as a 'deposition') respecting all the primary and foreign keys. This is a generic algorithm that uses the semantic information contained in the logical model and generates the particular calls to the table API to duplicate rows in the hierarchically associated tables.

Determination of topographical variants. Amino acid residues and nucleic acid bases are represented differently in the database according to whether they are at one or other of the termini or at an intermediate position in the protein or nucleic acid chain. PL/SQL code has been developed that uses both entry replication and graph isomorphism to identify and create these variants, and to maintain information that is common to the variants (such as atomic information).

Determination of chemical entities. This PL/SQL code identifies and organizes chemical information, based on supplied and calculated connectivity information.

13.6 Data Clean-up

The design of the deposition database has followed an important policy of modelling the real world and not the PDB-format files, as far as possible. This means going beyond the PDB file specification and think about the real world entities that they represent – the ultimate goal of relational design.

Data quality has a direct effect on the value of the database and the validity of conclusions or decisions based on it. The data clean-up operation of the legacy data is a laborious and important phase of the project, since over the years the PDB collection has included a lot of inaccurate data, and also there has been some variation in terminology. Clean-up of this type of data is a difficult, error-prone task requiring considerable thought and discussion to resolve contentious issues. It is important to keep a record of clean-up operations together with a mechanism to make the original values available. It is necessary to justify the validity of clean-up operations and indicate the scale of the effort involved.

An important question is how to deal with incomplete and incorrect information. Of course, the effort of a comprehensive data clean-up cannot be ultimately avoided, but the arrangement of the clean-up may have serious effects in timing of the project tasks. At one extreme, one could try to correct all data errors prior to loading in a trial and error fashion, by manually fixing the data in the files that fail to load and attempting the load once more. The problem with this approach is that many other tasks would have to wait until the clean-up is complete, and the delay would be prohibitive.

At the other extreme, one could initially load data as is, and follow a straightforward design approach, planning to improve its quality later, by direct database manipulation. This approach allows for the development of applications that use the intermediate quality data, risking the possibility that the clean-up is postponed indefinitely.

The MSD has adopted a somewhat middle road, in developing sophisticated fuzzy methods that attempt automatic clean-up operations that can be checked manually at a later stage. In this way, the effort of manual checking is reduced, applications can immediately use the final form of the model and the quality of loaded data is reasonably high in the first place. In order to facilitate the automatic correction process and perform fuzzy matches with controlled vocabulary data, we have developed a similarity score algorithm for strings. This works by finding the largest common regions of two strings together with regions that do not match and calculating a similarity score, counting positively the matched regions (taking their size into account) and negatively the unmatched regions (also taking their size into account). The score is normalized using the sizes of the input strings, and the result is a real number in the range of zero to unity, where a value close to zero means low similarity while a value close to unity means high similarity.

By following this semi-automatic clean-up procedure we have the flexibility to postpone manual checking for a long period (other than for entries that fail to load completely) and still around 95 per cent of the data is available for use and more than 97 per cent of it is immediately correct. Finally, a record of the clean-up process is generated in the database that can be used to support the validity of the clean-up operations.

13.7 The Search Database

The MSD uses data warehouse technologies (Inmon, 2002) to integrate biochemical information data with PDB structure data. A data warehouse is a subject-oriented, integrated, time-variant and non-volatile collection of data in support of decision-making processes. Data warehouses are not just large databases. They are large, complex environments that integrate many different technologies, including extracting, cleansing and transformation tools. Cleansing the data in data warehousing, i.e. to ensure the integrity of data, is a major problem in commercial systems. However, in the MSD search database the data-cleansing process is carried out in the deposition database. The MSD search database (data warehouse) has different principles and guidelines that are followed during the design phase in order to cope with the different set of needs and objectives. In the Deposition database normalization is always the golden rule to ensure consistency and data integrity. Query performance can be met by clever design at the application level. The Deposition database design is rigid and simplicity is not important; application statements are predefined and will be carefully written and tuned.

On the other hand, the search database should be considered as a long-term asset and the ways that it will be used cannot be foreseen. Since modifications are performed in batches and come from already consistent sources, normalization is disregarded in favour of performance and simplicity while database constraints are not enabled. The search database is easy to understand and a new user will be able to rapidly formulate efficient ad hoc queries. Simplicity is important and strict normalization that would result in a highly hierarchical complex schema is very unlikely to facilitate the development of efficient queries.

Denormalization and hierarchy collapse is a common practice in a data warehouse. Frequently used attributes of parent and reference entities are propagated in child entities so that users do not have to join many tables to collect all the attributes that they are interested in. Often, entire levels of parent–child relation hierarchies may collapse and their attributes are merged in a single entity. The focus of this process is deciding on the entities and attributes to denormalize. Obviously, denormalization has to be planned carefully and to be applied only up to an extent, since it may result in administrative and maintenance problems as well as waste of storage space. Natural keys and naming attributes are obvious candidates for denormalization while any further attributes should be considered conservatively on an individual basis. Additional denormalization is one of the main reasons for the non-static character of a data warehouse, since often further changes in the database schema are required in order to improve performance in particular queries.

In a typical data warehouse the dimensions (generic reference information) and fact tables (detailed information) are organized in a star-shaped schema and fact data are typically analysed over one or several dimensions. While in the MSD search database there is no strict distinction between fact and dimension entities, the same pattern of star-shaped design applies. This does not mean that there is a single star schema that involves each one of the hundreds of entities in the database. Instead, there is a star schema around every entity that has been considered as a possible target of data analysis. The hierarchical network of stars resembles what is often called starflake or snowflake design in the data warehouse world (Anahory and Murray, 1997). For example, in a query that requires the number of heavy atoms in a protein, the protein atom table has the role of the fact table, but when the query is in the number of residues that contain a molecule fragment, then the protein residue table is the fact table. The design of the warehouse is built on the hierarchical nature of the data and follows the Deposition, Assembly, Chain, Residue, and Atom hierarchy. A similar pattern can be seen in the secondary structure module where residues make strands, and strands make sheets.

The MSD search database is modular. Each module contains a different type of information. Each module can be loaded, updated and distributed separately from the rest. Modules can contain derived information in which case programs and procedures are run to populate them. These events can be collectively called post-transformation events.

Currently the modules contain information on the following areas:

- Entry-specific data

- Keywords

- Authors

- Experimental details

- Bibliography

- Coordinate- and sequence-related data

- Taxonomy references

- Derived data as active site information and secondary structure

- Mapping to other databases (CATH, Orengo *et al.*, 1997; SCOP, Murzin *et al.*, 1995; SWISS-PROT, Bairoch and Apweiler, 2000; MEDLINE, National Library of Medicine, 1989).

The modules are equivalent to data marts as subsets of the search database that support the requirements of a particular aspect of macromolecular structure. The data marts focus on only the requirements of one function to give selected users access to the data they need to analyse most often.

13.8 Transformation

Data transformation operations are very common in databases when information stored in different tables is combined and reshaped to present a different view. Data warehouse transformation is different in that it is not performed on the fly for each individual query. Instead, it is applied in advance and the results become the basis of defining a new table. In that way, user queries can directly access a single pre-transformed table and do not have to join, filter or aggregate data themselves, benefiting from a substantial performance improvement. Denormalization is introduced during the transformation for performance reasons since the data analysis operations expected on a data warehouse use the whole set of available data (full table scan queries). Simplicity is an additional reason for data transformation. The MSD database is to be distributed and used directly by end users who are familiar neither with complex queries nor with MSD's normalized design. Therefore tuning for speedy query retrieval is paramount in a warehouse and traditionally warehouses are hardware resource hungry. Denormalization commands repetition of information and the storage prerequisites of a warehouse are immense. The MSD Search database requires in excess of 200 GB disk space, although a distribution that does not contain atomic coordinate data would require an order of magnitude less.

13.9 Incremental Transformation

Often the complexity of the join and the number of data is so large that the transformation query execution may take several hours or days. When the source data change rather slowly, such operations are not cost effective. Suppose, for example, that just a single row changes in a particular week in one of the source tables. This modification may affect a single record in the search database, but if we simply re-execute the query, we will re-join and store again every other row, even though it remained constant in the last week.

What is needed is an incremental transformation: a mechanism that identifies which of the source data rows have been modified and which rows in the transformed results they affect. Then we will refresh only the rows that have really changed. Unfortunately, there are several limitations on the types of query that can use the Oracle mechanism based on fast refreshable materialized views. We have developed an incremental transformation process that is equivalent to Oracle materialized views. Conventional materialized views could not handle the increased complexity of protein structure information. The MSD system uses an SQL parser using javaCC to analyse the transformation queries. The search database metadata were extended to include a dictionary for queries that is able to store analysed information about the transformation queries. The next step was to develop generators based on the metadata in order to create the query statement from its analysed form, as well as to generate triggers for the source tables. These triggers follow up the defining queries to find the records of the result tables that are affected by each single modification (insert, update, delete) in the source tables and keep an appropriate log. At a later stage when the actual transform takes place another generated PLSQL procedure re-evaluates all marked records of the transformed tables, to examine whether they need updating.

13.10 Replication

An important function for the MSD search database is to be distributed and replicated to enable utilization of the systems required in order to cope with the massive computational needs of data analysis and complex ad hoc queries. Even the most powerful in-house database servers will eventually not manage to support user demand. Users will become more information and resource hungry as they gain familiarity with the search database and start to utilize its data mining potential. The MSD has to impose some limits for on-line web operations in order to ensure operability of its public search database. It will allow users to carry out database replication on their own equipment, so that they may use its full potential without conflicting with other users.

Inter-vendor master–slave database replication over the web is not a straightforward task. Despite the adoption of relational standards such as ANSI SQL and standard database APIs such as ODBC (Sanders, 2000) and JDBC (White *et al.*, 1999), it is hard to find off-the-shelf utilities for data exchange between different databases. The MSD database development includes a replication system based on java serialized objects. We have produced a generic, platform and database vendor independent replication mechanism that allows for schema export in SQL variants for other databases and ANSI SQL, trigger generation for keeping track of changes in master source tables (similar to materialized view logs), export of the changes in the data in files in the form of java serialized objects through JDBC, download of the files by the import mechanism on the slave sites through HTTP or FTP and finally an import mechanism for changes through JDBC in Oracle or other databases such as MySQL (DuBois, 1999).

A further issue with relational database replication is the difficulty in maintaining a replicated database up to date. The granularity of flat files is manageable and there are straightforward methods of mirroring a data collection based on their last modification date in order to identify the ones to be refreshed. Even if just a single byte changes, the file has to be refreshed, but at least this will not happen to files that have not been modified at all. In relational databases data are usually kept in a relatively small number of binary files that change very frequently, with no efficient way of identifying the changed sections within the file, making synchronizing a replicated relational database a demanding task.

The Oracle materialized views that address the issue of incremental replication are limited in scope. Oracle does not allow remote materialized views to be built on top of existing ones, while with the current versions of the Oracle server the incremental back-up mechanism based on archive logs would mean replication of the whole database. Still, the concept of incremental replication is simple. All that is needed is a mechanism of keeping track of every single modification that has taken place in the master database since the last incremental update. The modifications will be then extracted and applied to the slave database. We decided to implement this mechanism in java, using JDBC technology, and managed to provide an inter-vendor incremental replication solution that overcomes the limitations set by the Oracle materialized views.

This solution has the form of an incremental export and an incremental import script, while the incremental update files contain data in the form of java-serialized objects. A third script translates the replicated schema to DDL statements that are compatible with several commercial and freeware databases such as Oracle and MySQL. Additionally, the replication mechanism is configurable and flexible, allowing for the master and slave schemas to be different. The user may choose to replicate some of the tables or to map them to different tables and columns.

13.11 Oracle Cartridge Applications

Ligand chemistry

The MSD curators ensure that the basic structure of every ligand is correct. This means that the atoms and their names and elements as well as the bonds between atoms and the bond orders are defined and checked manually during deposition processing. In-house developed software as well as the CACTVS (Ihlenfeldt *et al.*, 1994) and CORINA (Sadowski, Gasteiger and Klebe, 1994) packages are used to populate ligand tables with

- GIF image

- Smiles (Weininger, Weininger and Weininger, 1989; James, Weininger and Delany, 2004)

- Stereo hash

- Fingerprints (Fredenslund, Jones and Prausnitz, 1975). (see http://www2.che-mie.uni-erlangen.de/services/fragment/index.html for the software used)

- Rings, ring atoms and flags

- Idealized coordinates

- Atom stereochemistry (R/S)

- Bond stereochemistry (E/Z)

- Planes and plane atoms.

Using the complete information of the particular stereoisomer, curators use ACD-Labs software (Williams and Shear, 2002) to derive the systematic name for the molecule. Finally, VEGA (Pedretti, Villa and Vistoli, 2002) is used to obtain atomic energy types.

For advanced search operations on the ligand chemistry data, a chemical database cartridge (for small molecules, drugs and amino acids) implemented in java (in java packages wrapped by java stored procedures) has been developed. The cartridge includes an implementation of graph algorithms for sub-graph isomorphism (Ullman, 1976; Krissenel and Henrick, 2004) and a mechanism for indexing the chemical graph operations based on bit strings for the detection of segments (fingerprints). The cartridge integrates the chemical graph operations in normal SQL statements together with other SQL operators. Generators have been written to automatically generate a stored procedure layer that exposes the interface of a java class using the java type information (java.lang and java.lang.reflect). Additionally the dictionary contains a classification of the atoms by energy type, and associates them with the energy type reference dictionary for different library sets (AMBER, Cornell *et al.*, 1995; CHARMM, MacKerell *et al.*, 1998; CNS, Brunger *et al.*, 1998, and CCP4, Collaborative Computational Project, Number 4, 1994). Since every residue and every atom in the MSD database references a molecule and an atom in this dictionary, this is the repository that defines the link between proteins and chemistry.

The chempdb Service (MSD chempdb Service, 2004) provides a wide range of possibilities for exploring the ligand data collection. For example, one may start by using the classes in 'Molecule Classification' that their name match some criteria i.e. '*SACCHARIDES*', look at one of them, select one molecule in the class, have a look at their atoms and then their energy types; then find other atoms with the same energy types and their molecules. The underlying mechanism allows combination of questions with AND and OR operators, to follow relations in an arbitrary way and retrieve results in several formats. There are advanced search methods such as drawing the search fragment using the JME Molecular editor (Ertl and Jacob, 1997) and searching for molecules whose graph contains as a subgraph the query molecule. There is also a fuzzy similarity search operation where the result is the list of molecules that contain at least 99 per cent of the same segment composition as the search object, from a predefined set of 500 segments.

For all instances of the ligands contained in the PDB, additional tables are generated for all contacts between different residues. Covalent, ionic, van der Waals and hydrogen bonds are recorded together with inter-planar contacts (using a 6 Å cut-off between plane centres). This information is stored in the search database at the assembly/model levels.

13.12 Related Data Warehouse

DataFoundry (Critchlow *et al.*, 2000) is a data warehouse that integrates scientific data from several distributed, autonomous, heterogeneous information sources, including PDB information.

Acknowledgements

E-MSD gratefully acknowledges the support from the Wellcome Trust (GR062025MA), the EU (TEMBLOR, NMRQUAL, SPINE, AUTOSTRUCT and IIMS), CCP4, the BBSRC, the MRC and EMBL.

References

Anahory, S. and Murray, D. (1997). *Data Warehousing in the Real World*, Addison Wesley Longman.
Awai, M. (ed.), Bortniker, M., Carnell, J., Cox, K., O'Connor, D., Zucca, M., Dillon, S., Kyte, T., Horton, A., Hubeny, F., Mitchell, G.E. II, Mukhar, K., Nicol, G. and Ruth, G. (2000). *Professional Oracle 8i Application Programming with Java, PL/SQL and XML*, Wrox New York.
Bairoch, A. and Apweiler, R. (2000). The SWISS-PROT protein sequence database and its supplement TrEMBL. *Nucleic Acid Res.* **28**, 45–48.
Berman, H.M., Westbrook, J., Feng, Z., Gilliland, G., Bhat, T.N., Weissig, H., Shindyalov, I.N. and Bourne, P.E. (2000). The protein data bank. *Nucleic Acids Res.* **28**, 235–242.
Bourne, P., Berman, H. M., Watenpaugh, K., Westbrook, J. D. and Fitzgerald, P. M. D. (1997). The macromolecular crystallographic information file (mmCIF). *Meth. Enzymol.* **277**, 571–590.

Boutselakis, H., Dimitropoulos, D., Fillon, J., Golovin, A., Henrick, K., Hussain, A., Ionides, J., John, M., Keller, P.A., Krissinel, E., McNeil, P., Naim, A., Newman, R., Oldfield, T., Pineda, J., Rachedi, A., Copeland, J., Sitnov, A., Sobhany, S., Suarez-Uruena, A., Swaminathan, J., Tagari, M., Tate, J., Tromm, S., Velankar, S. and Vranken, W. (2003). E-MSD: the European bioinformatics institute macromolecular structure database. *Nucleic Acids Res.* **31**, 458–462.

Brunger, A.T., Adams, P.D., Clore, G.M., Delano, W.L., Gros, P., Grosse-Kunstleve, R.W., Jiang, J.-S., Kuszewski, J., Nilges, M., Pannu, N.S., Read, R.J., Rice, L.M., Simonson, T. and Warren, G.L. (1998). Crystallography & NMR system. *Acta Crystallogr.* **D54**, 905–921.

Chen, P. P.-S. (1976). The entity-relationship model – toward a unified view of data. *ACM Trans. Database Syst.* **1**, 9–36.

Collaborative Computational Project, Number 4. (1994). The CCP4 suite programs for protein crystallography. *Acta Crystallogr.* **D50**, 760–763.

Cornell, W.D., Cieplak, P., Bayly, C.I., Gould, I.R., Merz, K.M., Jr., Ferguson, D.M., Spellmeyer, D.C., Fox, T., Caldwell, J.W. and Kollman, P.A. (1995). A second generation force field for the simulation of proteins, nucleic acids, and organic molecules. *J. Am. Chem. Soc.* **117**, 5179–5197.

Critchlow, T., Fidelis, K., Musick, R., Ganesh, M. and Slezak, T. (2000). DataFoundry: *Information Management for Scientific Data* **4**, 52–57. http://www.llnl.gov/CASC/datafoundr/

DuBois, P. (1999). *MySQL*. New Riders, Indianapolis, IN.

Ertl, P. and Jacob, O. (1997). WWW-based chemical information system. *Theochem.* **419**, 113–120.

Fredenslund A., Jones R.L. and Prausnitz J.M. (1975). Group-contribution estimation of activity coefficients in nonideal liquid mixtures. *AIChE J.* **21**, 1086–1099.

Henrick, K. and Dodson, E. (1999). *Report from the Joint CCP4/EBI Software Developers and Data Harvesting Workshop.* http://www.dl.ac.uk/CCP/CCP4/newsletter36/03_harvest.html

Henrick, K. and Thornton, J. M. (1998). PQS: a protein quarternary file server. *Trends Biochem. Sci.* **23**, 358–361.

Ihlenfeldt, W.D., Takahashi, Y., Abe, H. and Sasaki, S. (1994). Computation and Management of Chemical Properties in CACTVS: an extensible networked approach toward modularity and flexibility. *J. Chem. Inf. Comput. Sci.* **34**, 109–116.

Inmon, W.H. (2002). *Building the Data Warehouse*, 3rd edn, Wiley, New York.

James, C.A., Weininger, D. and Delany, J. (2004). *Daylight Theory Manual*, Daylight, Irvine, CA, chapter 3.

Krissinel, E. and Henrick, K. (2004). Common subgraph isomorphism detection by backtracking search. *Softw. Pract. Exp.* **34**, 591–607.

MacKerell, A. D. Jr., Brooks, B., Brooks, C.L. III, Nilsson, L., Roux, B., Won, Y. and Karplus, M. (1998). CHARMM: the energy function and its parameterization with an overview of the program. In Schleyer, P. v. R. *et al.*, eds, *The Encyclopedia of Computational Chemistry*, Wiley, Chichester, Vol. 1, 271–277.

MSD chempdb Service. (2004). http://www.ebi.ac.uk/msd-srv/chempdb

Murzin, A. G., Brenner, S. E., Hubbard, T. and Chothia, C. (1995). SCOP: a structural classification of proteins database for the investigation of sequences and structures. *J. Mol. Biol.* **247**, 536–540.

National Library of Medicine. (1989–). MEDLINE [database online], Bethesda, MD. Updated weekly.

Orengo, C. A., Michie, A. D., Jones, S., Jones, D. T., Swindells, M. B. and Thornton, J. M. (1997). CATH – a hierarchic classification of protein domain structures. *Structure* **5**, 1093–1108.

Pedretti, A., Villa, L. and Vistoli, G. (2002). VEGA: a versatile program to convert, handle and visualize molecular structure on windows-based PCs. *J. Mol. Graph.* **21**, 47–49.

Sadowski, J., Gasteiger, J. and Klebe, G. (1994). Comparison of automatic three-dimensional model builders using 639 X-ray structures. *J. Chem. Inf. Comput. Sci.* **34**, 1000–1008.

Sanders, R.E. (2000). *ODBC 3.5 Developer's Guide (McGraw-Hill Series on Data Warehousing and Data Management)*, Osborne McGraw-Hill, Berkeley, CA.

Service, R.F. (2000). Structural genomics offers high-speed look at proteins. *Science* **287**, 194–196.

Ullman, J.R. (1976). An algorithm for subgraph isomorphism. *J. Assoc. Comput. Mach.* **23**, 31–42.

Weininger, D., Weininger, A. and Weininger, J.L. (1989). SMILES2 algorithm for generation of unique smiles notation. *J. Chem. Inf. Comput. Sci.* **29**, 97–101.

White, S., Fisher, M., Cattell, R., Hamilton, G. and Hapner, M. (1999). *JDBC(TM) API Tutorial and Reference: Universal Data Access for the Java(TM) 2 Platform.* 2nd edn, Addison-Wesley Longman, Boston, MA.

Williams, A. and Shear, G. (2002). Completing the cycle of relating systematic names and chemical structures. *ACD Labs Users Meeting*, Fujitsu, Japan, http://www.acdlabs.com/download/publ/2002/jum2002/naming.pdf

Winn, M. (1999). *Implementation of Data Harvesting in the CCP4 Suite.* http://www.dl.ac.uk/CCP/CCP4/newsletter37/13_harvest.html

IV
Conclusions and Prospects

14 Looking Around, Looking Ahead

Arthur M. Lesk

Recognition of the importance of data and of data quality, as the underpinning of research and applications, has been a tenet of science for centuries. Recognition of the importance of the organization of data, into structured databanks interfaced with information-retrieval systems, is more recent but is universally accepted. Integral to the organization of data in contemporary molecular and cellular biology, raw data are supplemented with annotation. Some annotation is based on experiment, some on inference and some on combinations of the two. (Indeed, the distinction between raw data and annotation by no means as clear is it might superficially appear.)

The importance of high quality annotation has led to the emergence of annotators as professional specialists, having to draw on a specific combination of skills. At first, annotators were recruited from related fields, importing some of the required techniques and acquiring the others. As the field matures still further, one can envisage specific courses, degree programs and probably a learned society and a journal. This book is a step in that direction. The preceding chapters have described the current state of the art. What may change in the future?

One ongoing problem is that the development of high throughput experiments that generate data is not matched by correspondingly reliable high throughput methods of annotation. Automation of annotation is possible to only a limited extent. Getting annotation right remains labour intensive. However, the importance of proper annotation cannot be underestimated, and – for purposes of applications – errors in annotation degrade the quality of the data.

As progress in our field becomes ever more data driven, it is likely that there will be moves to expand the kinds of information conserved by archives. For example, at

Database Annotation in Molecular Biology Edited by Arthur M. Lesk
© 2005 John Wiley & Sons, Ltd.   ISBN: 0-470-85681-5

present the deposition of structure factors associated with atomic coordinates determined by X-ray crystallography is not mandatory. Deposition of structure factors would help resolve some of the problems in distinguishing real outliers from errors in structures. Moreover, as software for crystal-structure determination improves, it will be possible in some cases to redetermine the structure from the experimental data to produce more accurate results. In addition to mandating what data are required adequately to record an experimental result, the format of data storage will become more formally specified, in order to facilitate exchange of data among databanks and the support of query systems that interrogate multiple data archives.

Looking ahead, it is reasonable to expect development towards *distributed* and *dynamic* error-correction and annotation processes. Distributed, in that databank staff – even the professional corps of annotators to whose training this book will contribute – will have neither the hours nor the specialized expertise for the job; other practicing scientists, masters of particular topics, will have to act as curators. Dynamic, in that improvements in annotation and error identification/correction will permit updating database contents. We will have to sacrifice the reassuring idea of a stable databank composed of entries that are correct when first distributed in mature form and that stay fixed thereafter. Databanks will become a seething broth of information, not only growing in size, but maturing in quality.

Of course this will create problems in organizing applications. Many institutions maintain local copies of databanks: at present 'maintain' means 'top up'; this will no longer be the case. In the face of dynamically changing databanks, can we avoid proliferation of versions in different and uncharacterized states? How will it be possible to reproduce a scientific investigation based on a database search that was carried out at a particular time on a database that has since undergone many changes? It will be necessary to maintain adequate history records in the databanks to be able to reconstruct its form on any date. This is analogous to the information in the *Oxford English Dictionary* that permits construction of a English dictionary appropriate for 1616 or 1756.

More generally, the biomedical community as a whole will have to play an active role in making intelligent decisions about the contents, form and accessibility of the archives. In the end, we will get the resources that we deserve.

Index

absolutepos 209
accession number 31, 138
AceDB database 10–11, 13, 204
added value and knowledge 121–5
ADIT 69
ADIT deposition interface 150
Affymetrix system 83
Agrobacterium tumefaciens 193
alanine acetyl transferase-like protein 193
AMBER 237
annotation
   attribution to validated experimental
      sources 140
   automation 143, 243
   database distribution formats 193–4
   design and sources 113–30
   efficiency and quality 4
   errors 138–9
   errors and error propagation 189,
      195–6
   form of 2
   genomic data 3–5
   high quality 243
   levels 5
   miscellaneous issues 161–3
   position specific 141–2
   processes 3–4, 244
   protein sequence databases 131–47
   protein structures 149–65
   rule-based 142–4
   stages 4
   structure 133
   summarized 123
   use of term 132–3
annotation databases
   access 12–13

nature of information stored in 14
annotation tools 92
ANSI SQL 236
antibody database schema diagram 208–9
antibody structure 206
Apollo 16
Archaeoglobus fulgidus 196
archival databases 25–6, 68–73, 138–9
arginase, structure of 153
ARPANET-based internet 67
Array Definition Format (ADF) 92
array design 86
ArrayExpress 91–5
   submissions 95
Artemis 16
ascorbate oxidase, structure of 153
association between genes 7
asymmetric unit (ASU) 152
AT content 116
AutoDep 69, 151, 157
automated access facilities 16–19

Bacillus, growth of multiple strains 109
Bacillus coagulans 109
Bacillus stearothermophilus 109
BioAssayData 90
Biodas project 17
biodiversity 102
Bioinformatics Research and Development of
     Japan Science and Technology
     Corporation (BIRD-JST) 71
biological annotation 32
   nucleotide sequence databases 31
Biological Macromolecule Crystallization
     Database (BMCD) 70, 74
biological process 123, 173

Database Annotation in Molecular Biology   Edited by Arthur M. Lesk
© 2005 John Wiley & Sons, Ltd.   ISBN: 0-470-85681-5